PRINCIPLES AND PRACTICE OF PUBLIC HEALTH IN AFRICA

VOLUME 2

Second Edition

FSG MEDIMEDIA LTD

Reach, Cambridge, UK.

PRINCIPLES AND PRACTICE OF PUBLIC HEALTH IN AFRICA

VOLUME 2

Second Edition

Edited by
G.O. Sofoluwe
R. Schram
D.A. Ogunmekan

University Press Plc
Ibadan
1998

University Press PLC
IBADAN ABUJA AKURE BENIN ENUGU ILORIN JOS KANO LAGOS OWERRI UYO ZARIA

First Edition 1985
Second Edition 1997

ISBN 978 030 032 5 (General)
ISBN 978 030 490 8 (Volume II)

Printed by Intec Printers Limited, Ibadan
Published by University Press PLC
Three Crowns Building, Jericho, PMB 5095, Ibadan, Nigeria

Contents

PART THREE

Environmental Health – Principles

PART FOUR
Prevention and Abatement of Communicable Diseases in Africa

PART FIVE
Prevention and Abatement of Non-Communicable Diseases in Africa

PART SIX

Personal Health Services in Africa

PART SEVEN

Public Health Administration and Health Planning in Africa

PART EIGHT

Health Care Services in Economically Developed Countries: Lessons for Africa

PART NINE
Medical Sociology, Nutrition, Health Education and Training in Public Health in Africa

PART TEN

Health and Wealth in Africa – Ventures for Generating Wealth and Employment Opportunities through Active and Better Health Promotion

Preface

Many of our colleagues from other faculties have often asked why it has been necessary to change the name of our department so often – first from Public Health to Preventive and Social Medicine; then recently to Community Health. Even as recently as 1990 in the United Kingdom it was again changed to Public Health Medicine. Medical students get confused and many regard the subject as one to be learnt but not practised because legislations in most parts of Africa have not yet made practical achievements readily possible.

The first principle of public health practice is the identification of the root cause or causes of all health problems. Invariably, these causes do not lie with the diseased individual alone, but are the effects on the individual of family, social, community, national, global, environmental, and other factors. The second principle is the utilization of the resources of the community, the nation and the world to effect a lasting and, often, a cheaper solution to health problems.

Hence, in the era when such environmental factors as failings in the town and country planning, housing, water supply and refuse and sewage disposal, and contaminated food and the like were identified as the root causes of many scourges, especially communicable diseases, the practice of the speciality was appropriately called Public Health. Later, as the family and some social factors were identified as causes of many human problems, the practice of the speciality was renamed Preventive and Social Medicine. In the same way, as the root causes of paediatric, obstetric, gynaecological and some medical problems were first identified, their solutions resulted in a change in the names of the corresponding departments to Child Health, Maternal Health, Social Obstetrics, Community Paediatrics and the like. The assessment of the cost-effectiveness of the billions of dollars spent by the United Nations and national agencies in the attempt to control or eradicate malaria has provided one singular example to emphasize the importance of the way in which health services are administered.

The above and many other operational research studies have heralded the inculcation of scientific principles in public health planning and practice. Many countries have accordingly reorganized their health services in an attempt to remove the 'iron curtain' between curative and preventive health services and to emphasize that health practice should be based, centred and focused on well-defined communities.

To impress the importance of these points on all graduates in medicine, irrespective of the speciality they will eventually practise, our medical schools have renamed Community Health and are now gradually returning to Public Health. Both the developed and developing countries have for the same reason extended the length of time for which the subject is taught from the usual period of two terms in one year to the entire five years of a medical undergraduate course. In addition, medical schools in Africa have created special communities both in urban and rural areas to offer practical opportunities for training, research and service to all medical undergraduates.

This book, which is in two volumes, is specifically aimed at undergraduate medical students. They will find it a ready source for most of what they need to know on the principles and practice of public and community health in African countries. It provides more practical advice than the earlier book, which did not cover all the aspects of a comprehensive public health practice sufficiently. It is also useful to the other members of the health care team and the supporting professionals.

Young graduate doctors in African countries who tend to be called upon to serve as public health physicians for about 50,000 to 100,000 people living in areas of 50 to 120 square kilometres will find the book a useful manual which will assist them to construct baseline data; to conduct a census of the area accurately; to assess the health status of the community, and then gradually, to introduce measures (the effects of which can be measured) to improve the physical, mental, social, moral and spiritual health of the community.

The chapters of the book are written by specialists who have contributed considerably to the improvement and promotion of health in their own particular sub-specialities of public health. In addition, colleagues in the clinical fields contributed chapters to indicate their present level of co-operation in public health practice.

The emphasis throughout the book is on bringing out the principles involved in identifying the root causes of all types of health problems and discovering practical and innovatory solutions for them in the ways which are best suited to African countries.

Efforts are made to list a number of obvious gaps in our current knowledge which will need to be filled by budding specialists and consultants in the field of public health.

O.O. Humponu-Wusu has reminded us about the large number of public health specialists needed in Nigeria to meet the minimum needs of the people. It is gratifying that African consultants in public health now hold important positions outside Africa, especially in the United Kingdom and in the United States of America. It is hoped that before the year 2000 or soon after, many will return home to elevate the status of Public Health practice in Africa.

In addition to the above, this edition has further been enriched with the following:

> It provides guidelines aimed at making Africa able to tackle her specific health problems through methods which are totally achievable by all Africans.
>
> It defines an African as a human being with the same anatomy and physiology as any other human being anywhere in the world, irrespective of colour, creed, race and nationality who is prepared to live in and contribute to the total development of Africa.
>
> It demonstrates that, like economically developed countries, Africa could generate wealth by actively promoting public, especially environmental health as ably pioneered by Edwin Chadwick in the United Kingdom, Shattuck in the United States of America, Semmelweiss in Austria, Moshe Prywes in Israel and Isaac Ladipo Oluwole of the Yaba Garden City fame in Lagos, Nigeria.
>
> Some of the new chapters indicate that like the developed countries, Africans can generate wealth through the active promotion of environmental health. They also emphasize the interdisciplinary conception of the promotion and practise of public health by all Africans.

Lastly, this second edition gives guidelines to assist all African countries in actively generating wealth by the provision of chlorinated pipe-borne water, water closets, sewage disposal, healthy housing which all Africans can afford, of electricity for lighting, refrigerating, radio and television.

Hopefully, by the year 2,000, through ardent adherence to the essence of this edition, the majority of Africa will have achieved considerable basic standards of healthy houses, water closets, jacuzzis, electricity and other basic health facilities as in Europe, USA, Japan and Singapore. Such advancement will, thus, be the measure of the success of this edition.

G.O.S.
R.S.
D.A.O.

LIST OF CONTRIBUTORS

Professor Z.A. Ademuwagun, c/o University of Ibadan, **Nigeria.**

Professor A. Adeyokunnu, Dept. of Paediatrics, University of Ibadan, Ibadan, **Nigeria.**

Dr K. V. Bailey; Chief Medical Adviser on Nutrition, World Health Organization Regional Office for Africa B.P. 6; **Congo-Brazzaville.**

Professor T.D. Baker, Department of International Health, The John Hopkins University, School of Hygiene and Public Health, 615 North Wolfe Street, Baltimore, Maryland 21205; **United States of America.**

Dr V. Barell, Faculty of Health Sciences, Ben Gurion University of the Negev, Beer Sheva, **Israel.**

Emeritus Professor F.J. Bennett, 12 Cranmer Close Off Spences Lane, Lewes, Sussex, **United Kingdom.**

Dr W.R. Brieger, Co-ordinator of Studies, The Ibarapa Community Programme, Department of Social and Community Medicine, University of Ibadan, Ibadan, **Nigeria.**

Prof J.W.K. Duncan, World Health Organization, P.O.Box 529. Freetown, **Sierra Leone.**

Dr A.O. Erinoso, Director of Medical Services, Health Centre, The Polytechnic, Ibadan, **Nigeria.**

Professor G.O. Esuruoso, Professor of Veterinary Public Health and Preventive Medicine, University of Ibadan, Ibadan, **Nigeria.**

Professor O.F. Esuruoso; Former Provost, College of Agricultural Sciences, Ogun State University, Ago Iwoye, **Nigeria.** [or P. O. Box 9756, U.I. Post Office, **Ibadan**].

Dr L. Frenkiel, Faculty of Health Sciences, Ben Gurion University of the Negev, Beer Sheva, **Israel.**

Professor J.R. Goldsmith; Department of Epidemiology, Faculty of Health Sciences, Ben Gurion University of the Negev, Beer Sheva, **Israel.**

Professor G. Hatful, University of Pittsburgh, Biological Sciences, A234 Langley Hall, Pittsburgh, P.A; **United States of America.**

C.E. and C. Hoppmann, Organic Farms, 529E Farmer Street, Dumas, Arkansas 71639 **United States of America.**

Professor O.O. Humponu-Wusu, Department of Community Medicine, College of Medicine, University of Lagos. P.M.B. 12003, **Lagos.**

Professor W.L. Kilama, Director General, National Institute for Medical Research, P.O.Box 9653, **Dar-Es-Salaam, Tanzania.**

Engr. I.O.A. Lasode, Director, Even Ezra, P.O.Box 51385, 1, Lasode Crescent, Maroko, Victoria Island, Lagos, **Nigeria.**

Professor O. Lloyd, Formerly of Wolfson Institute of Occupational Health, University of Dundee, **Scotland** and now Professor of Occupational Health, University of Hong Kong, **Hong Kong.**

Professor E.B. Lucas, Faculty of Technology, University of Ibadan, Ibadan, **Nigeria.**

Dr S.K. Lwanga, Statistician, Epidemiological and Statistical Methodology Unit, World Health Organization (WHO) Headquarters, Geneva, **Switzerland.**

Dr M. Mokrane, International Labour Office (I.L.O.), 4 rue des Morrilous, CH-1211 Geneva 22, **Switzerland.**

Dr F.D.E. Mtango, Senior Research Fellow, Epidemiology and Statistics, Faculty of Medicine, University of Dar-Es-Salaam, **Tanzania.**

Dr J.O. Mume, N.D; D.O; Ph.D; J.P; Tradomedical Naturopathic Physician, JOM Tradomedical Naturopathic Hospital, P.O.Box 25, Agbarho, Warri, **Nigeria.**

Dr F. Munema, Department of Community Medicine, Faculty of Medicine, University of Dar-Es-Salaam, **Tanzania.**

Professor J.M. Namboze, formerly Dean, Institute of Public Health, Makerere University, Kampala, **Uganda** recently Public Health Adviser, World Health Organization, Geneva, **Switzerland.**

Professor O. Ogbeide, Department of Community Health, School of Medicine, College of Medical Sciences, University of Benin, Benin City, **Nigeria.**

Professor E.O. Ogunba, Department of Medical Microbiology, University of Ibadan, Ibadan, **Nigeria.**

Professor D.A. Ogunmekan, Head of the Department of Community Health, College of Medicine, University of Lagos, P.M.B. 12003, Lagos, **Nigeria.**

Dr S. Ogston, Department of Epidemiology and Public Health, University of Dundee Medical School, Ninewells, Dundee, Scotland, **United Kingdom.**

Professor G.U. Oleru, Occupational and Environmental Health Unit, Department of Community Health, College of Medicine, University of Lagos, P.M.B. 12003, Lagos, **Nigeria.**

Chief E.O. Olofin, Director, World Soul Winning Evangelical Ministry (WOSEM), P.O.Box 151, Akure, **Nigeria.**

Professor P.A. Oluwande, Head of Department of Civil Engineering, Institute of Education, University of Ibadan, **Nigeria.**

Dr J.C. Omoruan, Department of Physical and Health Education, Ahmadu Bello University, Zaria, **Nigeria.**

Professor A.O. Osoba, Department of Microbiology, University of Ibadan, Ibadan, **Nigeria.**

Professor P.C. Osuhor, now Consultant in Public Health Medicine, Burnley General Hospital, Casterton Avenue, Burnley BB10 2PQ, Lancashire, **United Kingdom.**

Professor M. Oyediran, Department of Community Health, College of Medicine, University of Lagos, P.M.B. 12003, Lagos, **Nigeria.**

Prof J. Patrick, Department of Paediatrics, Faculty of Medicine, University of Ottawa, Ontario K1n 6N5, **Canada.**

Dr G.T. Pollock, Hon Senior Clinical Visiting Lecturer, School of Postgraduate Medical Education, University of Warwick, Coventry CV4 7AL, **United Kingdom.**

Rev. S.A. Popoola, World Communications Ministries, 20 Kudeti Avenue, Onireke, P.O.Box 1571, Ibadan, **Nigeria.**

Dr J. Riha; Director, World Health Organization (WHO), Regional Training Centre for Medical Equipment Maintenance, Freetown, **Sierra Leone.**

Rev. Dr R. Schram; 'Kufena' 78 Outram Road, Croydon, CRO 6XF **United Kingdom.**

Mr M.J. Simpson, Senior Deputy Clerk and Deputy Chief Executive Officer, Staffordshire County Council, Stafford, **United Kingdom**; now World Bank Consultant.

Chief Dr E.A. Smith, formerly Director of Public Health, Federal Ministry of Health; now Ademola Smith Holdings (Nig) Ltd, P.O.Box 616, Ikeja, Lagos, **Nigeria.**

Professor G.O. Sofoluwe, 35 Danta Way, Baswich, Stafford, ST17 0BA, **United Kingdom.**

Late Mr O.O. Sosan, past Chief Health Superintendent, Western Nigeria Ministry of Health and Principal Health Superintendent of the Department of Preventive and Social Medicine, Ibarapa Project, University of Ibadan, **Nigeria.**

Professor O.O. Soyinka, Head of Department of Dermatology and Venerology, Faculty of Health Sciences, Obafemi Awolowo University, Ile Ife, **Nigeria.**

Miss R.M. Taylor, Social Anthropologist, Edinburgh Council for Single Homeless, Cowgate, Edingburgh, Scotland, **United Kingdom.**

Professor O. Tomori, Postgraduate Institute for Medical Research and Training, College of Medicine, University of Ibadan, **Nigeria.**

Emeritus Professor Chief E. Topley, 1 Wickens Place, High Street, West Malling, Maidstone, Kent, ME19 6NB, **United Kingdom.**

Professor Wai-On Phoon, Professor of Occupational Health, University of Sydney and Director, Professional Education Program, Worksafe, **Australia.**

Dr R. Weintrab, Faculty of Health Sciences, Ben Gurion University of the Negev, Beer Sheva, **Israel.**

Professor M.K. Were, UNICEF, Africa Hall, P.O.Box 1169, Addis Abbaba, **Ethiopia.**

Dr M. Woodward, Department of Applied Statistics, University of Reading, Reading, Berkshire, **United Kingdom.**

Dr F.K. Wurapa, Chief Regional Adviser, World Health Organization Regional Office for Africa, P.O.Box 6, **Congo Brazzaville.**

Dr P. Zadka, Faculty of Health Sciences, Ben Gurion University of the Negev, Beer Sheva, **Israel.**

PART SIX

Personal Health Services in Africa

39

Maternal Health Services

J.M. Namboze

The term 'maternal and child health' refers to promotive, preventive, curative, and rehabilitative health care for mothers and children (WHO 1976). Maternal and child health (MCH) services embrace these services for mothers throughout the child-bearing period, that is from 15 to 45 years of age, and health services for children from conception through to adolescence. Men, as fathers, are not directly discussed in this chapter, but the important role of the father as head of the family and as traditional breadwinner is well recognized; his physical, mental, and social well-being as well as his active participation and support makes a great contribution to the health of the family.

Priority should be given to the health care of mothers and children. They are the most valuable members of the population, largely because of the biological demands inherent in reproduction, growth, and development. Mothers and children form the majority of the population, particularly in developing countries. For instance in Uganda, according to the 1969 census, children under 5 years constituted 25 per cent of the population; and women in the child-bearing ages of 15-45 years constituted 23 per cent of the population. These people taken together made up about two-thirds of the entire population of Ugânda. In countries such as the UK, for comparison, children under the age of 15 constituted only 20 per cent of the population in 1960. MCH services, therefore, provide a channel through which medical and other health services can be organized to reach the majority of the population.

The general aims of MCH services are to promote and preserve the lives of mothers and children by ensuring that:

> Every expectant and nursing mother maintains good health, learns the art of child care, has a normal delivery and bears healthy children and that every child whenever possible lives and grows up in a family unit with love and security in healthy surroundings, receives adequate nourishment, health supervision, and efficient medical attention, and is taught the elements of healthy living (WHO 1955).

MCH services deal with problems that cover a broad spectrum, their solution requires a great deal of interdependence action on the part of various disciplines, such as obstetrics and gynaecology, paediatrics, nutrition, health education, mental health, and environmental sanitation, for the promotive, preventive, curative, and rehabilitative aspects of these disciplines.

Pre-conceptional Care

Pre-conceptional care denotes the care of a woman to ensure that she is in optimum health before conception. It includes care during infancy, childhood, school age, and adolescence generally, through attending to the nutrition of the individual so that she attains optimal growth and development, and also through providing specific protection against the common communicable diseases. Among such diseases are measles and whooping cough, which themselves can produce adverse effects on the nutritional state of the individual, often precipitating kwashiorkor.

Health education in schools also makes a great contribution to the pre-conceptional care of a woman, as does attending to the nutritional requirements during this period and adolescence. Pre-marital medical examination of would-be couples is part of pre-conceptional care and is a requirement in certain countries. Furthermore, it involves knowing the history of the problem, followed by a physical examination, a serological test for syphilis, and a treatment depending on the examination's findings. Marriage counselling is also given. Genetics counselling can also be given when it is found to be indicated–as may be the case when the sickle-cell trait is recognized in both individuals. Another example of pre-conceptional care consists of the study of parents who have had at least one unfavourable outcome of pregnancy, for example foetal or neonatal death or a disabled infant, in order to remedy the causes before the next conception.

Antenatal Care

Antenatal care comprises the complete health supervision of the pregnant mother in order to maintain, protect, and promote her health and well-being and that of the foetus, and the new-born infant. There is enough evidence to suggest that mothers who have received early and continuous antenatal care of good quality have a lower incidence of prematurely born infants, and a lower prenatal mortality. Thus the quality and quantity of antenatal care may to a large extent determine the outcome of pregnancy in relation to the health of both the mother and child (Royal College of Obstetricians and Gynaecologists 1948; Kohl 1959).

I shall now focus on many of the activities that antenatal clinics cover.

(1) Group Health Education

Group health education is best given by a well-trained midwife or public health nurse or her equivalent before examination of the mothers begins.

(2) History-taking and Examination

At the first attendance at the clinic, the patient is registered and a history is taken. The height, weight and blood pressure are measured and a urine sample is tested. In addition, blood is taken for haemoglobin, blood grouping and Rh determination. On every subsequent visit the weight and blood pressure are measured and urine samples are tested.

(3) Identification of the High-risk Patients

It is not the purpose of this chapter to go into the details of the examination and health-care management of mothers, as these are dealt with in obstetric textbooks, but identification of high-risk mothers deserves special attention.

At present it is impossible to give the most skilled hospital services to every member of the community, and such services have to be limited to the few mothers that need them most; those mothers should be placed in a high-priority group, and should be known to every level of the medical personnel. Most of the antenatal clinics are conducted by midwives; and it is therefore very important that they should be taught the criteria for identifying high-risk mothers. These criteria include:

(1) age: under 16 and over 35 at conception;
(2) grand multiparity: sixth or later pregnancy (excluding abortions under 20 weeks);
(3) too short or too long intervals between births: under 2 years and over 4 years;
(4) any previous surgical delivery, caesarian section, or forceps delivery;
(5) any pregnancy with prolonged labour (of 24 hours or more);
(6) any pregnancy with antepartum or postpartum haemorrhage: the woman should be asked about antepartum bleeding on every visit and any history of this merits immediate referral;
(7) repeated abortions, stillbirths, or premature births; and
(8) features which should be discovered by examination, such as short women under 150 cm; any woman with a limp e.g from polio; hypertension with blood pressure BP. 130/80 and over; rapid weight gain; anaemia; oedema; multiple pregnancies; abnormal lie of the foetus; and cephalo-pelvic disproportion.

If a midwife is running the antenatal clinic alone, she should refer the high-risk patients to a doctor's clinic. If the doctor normally attends the clinic then it is advisable to arrange for these patients to attend a special clinic held on a particular day; or else they can be seen in a special part of a general clinic. These mothers should have an easily recognizable card, perhaps with a special coloured star for easy identification, particularly if admitted while in labour. Several antenatal cards have been devised which record the high-risk factors; and the midwife completing such a card also has guidelines for what she must do.

(4) Treatment

Treatment for any disorders,whether associated with pregnancy or not, will be provided.

(5) Individual Health Education

Any mother in the high-risk group requires some explanation as to why she is being singled out for special care; and she should be brought to understand that she has to continue to attend that particular clinic, and that once she has been advised to deliver in a hospital she should not attempt to deliver at home or in a small unit. Other mothers with conditions such as anaemia, malnutrition, or overwork need individual counselling on their need for special diets or on reducing the amount of work they do. Sometimes the mother herself may not be in a position to buy the extra foods that have been recommended to her, and may not be able to afford domestic help. If she is unable to convince her husband of the need to follow the doctor's instructions then it may be necessary to write a note to the husband or to invite him for a talk with a suitable member of the medical staff. A mother in need of family planning counselling should be introduced to the idea of family planning at this stage.

Attendance should ideally be monthly until the 28th week of pregnancy, then fortnightly until the 36th, and from then on weekly until term. Mothers with special problems may be seen more regularly, as required. In a health care centre the follow-up of patients who do not keep their appointments can be performed by a public health nurse or an assistant health visitor.

(6) Immunization and Prophylaxis

It is advisable that mothers should be immunized with two doses of tetanus toxoid spaced one month apart from the 16th week of pregnancy. This produces immunity which lasts about 40 months, after which a booster is required (Schofield 1971). The maternal antibodies are passed on to the foetus, and this protects the new born.

In an endemic malaria area pregnant women should be protected against malaria with weekly chloroquine.

Women in Industry

With increasing industrialization, more women are seeking employment. It is important for the employer to realize that at any time some of the women employed may be pregnant. Such women should be encouraged to report to clinics when they become pregnant; they should be permitted to attend the antenatal clinic during working hours, and should be assigned work appropriate to their pregnancy. Pregnant women should be relieved of duties involving prolonged standing, as this increases the risk of getting varicose veins; they should not undertake overtime or travel too much on rough roads, neither should they lift heavy weights. If the employer does not recognize the special needs of pregnant women, they may tend to conceal their pregnancies for fear of losing their jobs, and may seek antenatal care irregularly and late in pregnancy.

Maternity Leave

Many countries recognize the need for maternity leave. In the USSR, for example, a pregnant mother is entitled to 112 days leave; 56 days before birth and 56 days after birth. Leave is extended by 14 days if she has an abnormal or a premature birth. During her maternity leave she continues to draw her full salary *(Maternal and Child Health in the USSR)*. In some developing countries, for example Uganda, a pregnant woman may take maternity leave at between the 36th and 38th weeks of pregnancy, as determined by a doctor. Women are entitled to 45 days of maternity leave with full pay. If an additional period of absence from duty is required, this is regarded as part of her annual leave entitlement, or else such a period is regarded as leave without pay (Makerere University General Circular 1979).

Maternal and Natal Care

During labour, delivery, and the immediate post-natal period, care is crucial for the survival of the mother and the infant. In many cases, childbirth is a physiological process which proceeds without serious complications. But if the mother's health and development has been impaired by illness or malnutrition, if her physical resources have been depleted by the burden of frequent child bearing, child caring, and physical work, and if there is inadequate or improper care, excessive loss of life may occur, or disabilities can result for the mother and the offspring (Schmidt 1973). This is particularly true in developing countries, where, for example, a previous history of protein-calorie malnutrition can cause complications during delivery in what might otherwise be regarded as a normal patient.

In Uganda about 32 per cent of deliveries take place in medical institutions, while 68 per cent are home deliveries (Grech, Galas and Trussell 1967). The maternal mortality rate in Uganda is 40-60 per 10, 000 live births (1969 census), which may be compared with that of Sweden, which in the same year was 1.1 per 10, 000 live births.

The maternal mortality rate is regarded as a good index of the effectiveness of the obstetrical services in a country; but it can only be obtained if there is a good registration system for births and deaths. Because of the high maternal mortality rate in developing countries, the number of women between thirty and fifty years of age is lower than the number of men of those ages, in contrast to the situation in many other countries *(International Children's Centre 1972)*. (This statement does not apply to Uganda, according to the 1969 census).

The death of the mother can have many tragic implications for the health and welfare of the family. The mother may be survived by an infant who has to be looked after by relatives; and in some cases this infant may be taken to a children's home where he can receive institutional care for the first two to three years of life, after which he can be returned to his family.

In a few cases it may not be possible to trace the baby's family. Such babies can be taken to foster homes where they can stay temporarily, or even sometimes permanently until childhood. Sometimes the rest of the offspring of the deceased mother may also have to be separated and taken to various relatives, perhaps living in different physical and social environments, as the father may not be able to look after them.

It is important to give the best type of care to the mother during the crucial period of delivering a baby, so that she does not develop any complications such as VVF which may lead to chronic morbidity and limit her ability to look after herself and her family.

Supervision during labour, delivery and the early puerperium should, besides caring for the maternal health, aim at ensuring that a potentially healthy baby does not get any physiological deformity during this period. For instance, an infant who gets birth trauma and develops cerebral palsy is a tragedy for the family: the parents are very disappointed, and such a child is very difficult to look after; and since he is helpless the mother, who may have several other children to look after, as well as the routine domestic duties, may find herself in a very difficult situation. In some communities the mother may even be blamed for having delivered such a helpless child, and may face other unpleasant consequences.

Care at the Place of Delivery

(1) While in hospital or in a maternity clinic, mothers should receive health education encouraging them to attend the post-natal clinic for the first six weeks after delivery.

(2) The baby should receive BCG vaccination before discharge.

(3) Mothers should receive health education about diet for the nursing mother, to ensure that they lactate successfully.

(4) Mothers with abnormal deliveries such as caesarian section, forceps delivery, vacuum extraction, etc., should receive some explanation as to why the operation was carried out and be told that they should attend a hospital for any subsequent delivery.

(5) Mothers in need of family planning counselling should be identified and given the relevant advice, and should be directed to a clinic where they can receive guidance on the spacing of pregnancies.

(6) Mother whose babies have abnormalities should be informed about subsequent care. This is to avoid any bad advice and any mismanagement of the abnormalities through the use of home remedies, which may sometimes be harmful to the child. A mother with a baby with cleft palate should receive special instructions about the feeding of the baby until surgery can be carried out.

(7) Mothers with premature births should stay at the hospital for a fairly long time, and during this time they should receive health education about their premature infants and about child care in general – for example, attendance at young children's clinics, immunization,etc. Such mothers should be discharged with the baby on the breast and at a point at which lactation is continuing successfully.

Causes of Maternal Mortality

The leading causes of maternal mortality in a developing country are: haemorrhage; abortion; ruptured uterus mainly due to cephalo-pelvic disproportion; septicaemia; and anaesthetic factors; (Makerere Medical School 1969–69). This list was compiled at Mulago Hospital in Uganda, which is also a national reference hospital and a teaching hospital.

Prevention of Maternal Mortality

1. Good antenatal care, proper identification of the high-risk mothers and referral to a hospital for more specialized services. Mobile antenatal clinics may be conducted as part of the integrated MCH clinic.
2. Early diagnosis and treatment of mothers with anaemia during the antenatal period.
3. Supervision of mothers during labour, delivery and the immediate postnatal period, made possible by the training of more personnel. In a country where there is a great pressure on maternity beds this would be achieved in the following way:
   (a) Having a delivery centre where patients are discharged 24 hours after delivery. Ideally they should be visited daily for a period of about five days to ensure that the mother and baby are in a good condition. The high-risk mothers are not ideal patients for delivery centres.
   (b) Training more midwives and preferably having more maternity hospitals in a health centre set up so that as many healthy women as possible with normal obstetrical histories delivering their second to fifth babies can be delivered by a midwife.

(c) Provision of maternity villages or maternity waiting shelters. These are recommended in areas where the population is sparse and the distances great. A village consisting of simple buildings or dormitories is set up near a hospital. Mothers are advised at their antenatal clinics to come to a maternity shelter a few weeks before term. They can come with an attendant to do their cooking. Some can cook for themselves. A midwife visits the shelter daily to check on the condition of the mothers and to give them health education. As soon as labour starts the mother is taken to the maternity ward to be delivered. Typical examples of maternity shelters are the one at Mbarara hospital in Western Uganda and the one run by the Methodist Hospital at Ituk Mbang in Eastern Nigeria (Trussell 1966).

(d) An invitation to retired midwives by the government to return to active practice and by giving them an honorarium or providing them with equipment for delivery and antenatal care and giving them access to a consultation service. These midwives can practise in their home villages, and can either deliver in the mother's home or in their own delivery homes, and conduct the care during the puerperium.

(e) *Domiciliary midwifery*. Patients for a home delivery are selected at the antenatal clinic, and when labour starts the midwife at the maternity or health centre is informed by phone or by a runner. She goes with a delivery bag, and expects to find everything ready as the patient has been instructed to make it ready during the antenatal period. She conducts the delivery and visits the home daily for five to ten days. If any difficulty arises a doctor is called from the hospital or the patient is taken to hospital for admission.

Domiciliary midwifery can be practised in some countries, but at present it can only be practised in Uganda in urban areas such as housing estates where houses are fairly close and communication is fairly easy. It can however be quite expensive, as a midwife can be attending to just one patient at any given time.

(f) *Traditional birth attendants* (untrained midwives). These are the people who conduct deliveries in the villages. Some countries have recognized the services rendered by these women and have given them basic training. These women could be trained in conducting antenatal care, with emphasis on cleanliness, hand washing, and on the fact that there is no real need to interfere so much in the vagina. They should be taught how to care for the cord, and to make some observations during the puerperium and antenatal period. At the end of the training, they could be given simple midwifery equipment, a badge and a licence to practise under the supervision of the public health nurse or of a midwife in the area. Such women could be used to identify the high-risk mother and child, and could compile as well as notify births and deaths which occur under their care. Later they can be replaced by scientifically trained midwives as these become available in adequate numbers (Trussell 1966). Some people, however, argue against training these women, giving the following reasons:

(1) Such women are unlikely to change their ways even if they are trained;

(2) By training them you are creating a substandard cadre which will never pass an examination; and

(3) There is likely to be an increase to the time of delay in the village before antenatal care is sought, particularly in the case of the high-risk mother.

Additional Factors in the Prevention of Maternal Mortality

(1) ensuring that a baby does not get birth injury; because to give birth well one must have been born well;

(2) improving nutrition throughout life – i.e. during pregnancy, infancy, childhood and adolescence – to ensure that optimal growth and development is achieved;

(3) provision of rapid systems of communication and transportation;

(4) provision of specialist obstetrical services;

(5) improving the skill of doctors and midwives;

(6) giving health education to mothers concerning how to care for themselves during pregnancy;

(7) health education in schools and for the general public regarding this importance of attending the antenatal clinic.

Postnatal Care

After delivery, mothers are advised to return six weeks later with their babies for a postnatal examination. Even the mothers who deliver at home should be encouraged to attend the same clinic where the condition of the mother and the baby is checked again. This clinic provides the opportunity for early diagnosis and treatment of any complications of delivery and the puerperium such as vaginal tears, VVF, and breast abscesses; attention can also be given to any congenital abnormalities or diseases of the baby. Any relevant health education can be given to the mother; for instance a mother who is having poor lactation can be given nutrition health education to enable her to improve her lactation.

Procedure at the postnatal clinic

History. This includes the mother's general health and the health of the baby including the state of lactation, and the feeding, sleeping, and bowel habits of the baby. The mother should be asked if she has any worries or problems and if she is sleeping well. An early depression is often missed unless this sort of question is asked.

Examination. While conducting a general examination on the mother one should specifically examine for anaemia, condition of the breasts, size of the uterus and condition of the abdominal scar if the mother had a caesarian section; and then one should look for any peripheral tears, the condition of the cervix, and the type of lochia; and finally a *per vaginam* examination should be performed.

Treatment and health education. The mother should be treated for any abnormal conditions that may have been discovered, and should receive any relevant individual health education. She should be invited to bring the baby regularly to the children's clinic for health education, immunization, and checking on the growth progress.

Examination of the baby. This includes weighing, followed by a general physical examination of all the systems to make sure there are no congenital abnormalities. The condition of the umbilical stump should also be checked. Finally the mother should receive some health education depending on the examination's findings; for instance, if the baby has not gained weight, and the general examination has not revealed anything abnormal to which this could be attributed, then this may be accounted for by poor lactation, and the mother should receive individual health education to enable her to have her lactation well established. She should be advised to take a diet containing plenty of protein foods, fruits, and vegetables, and plenty of fluids such as milk, in addition to the staple food and fruit juice. She should also be advised to have some rest; this is particularly important for overworked African mothers.

Immunization. On the first postnatal visit, when the baby is six weeks old, he should receive the following immunization:

(1) BCG if not given at birth;
(2) first DPT and polio

Family planning. Mothers in need of family planning counselling should be identified and given appropriate advice, and should receive the first supply of contraceptives at this clinic. Subsequent supplies and checks may be given at the same clinic when the baby is brought for the children's clinic. In countries where family planning is not integrated with other MCH activities mothers in need of family planning should be directed to the place nearest to their homes where they can receive family planning advice (such a service might be rendered by a voluntary organization).

Organization of MCH Services as Part of Basic Health Services

MCH services can be organized at three main levels:

1. the peripheral level;
2. the intermediate level;
3. the central level.

The functions at the various three levels are represented diagrammatically in the figure 39.1.

Training

Training should be at all levels, i.e., specialists, general practitioners, nurses and other paramedical personnel. Training should include basic training and refresher courses.

Co-ordinating with other Units

In MCH co-ordination and co-operation with other sectors of government such as Community Development Associations and voluntary agencies is essential for the success of the programme.

Fig. 39.1

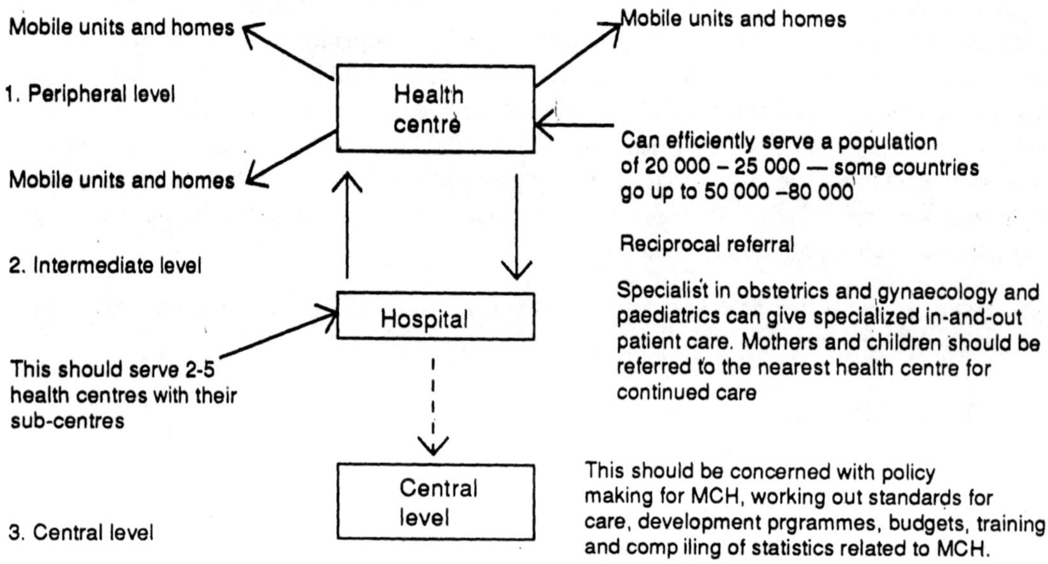

Planning of the MCH Programme and Evaluation

Basic steps in programme planning:

1. Identification of the problems: study available statistical data from all medical institutions – i.e. hospital, maternity unit, dispensaries, etc – to identify the causes of morbidity and mortality among mothers and children; and also scrutinize other causes of pathology – e.g. nutrition, immunization levels, and programmes of communicable disease control.
2. Setting objectives: i.e. defining what you want the programme to achieve.
3. Establishment of criteria: i.e. expected levels of achievement in numerical terms. These should be manageable and feasible.
4. Activities: procedures to be used to achieve the desired goal.
5. Timetable of activities: i.e. the duration of the programme's schedule and its phases, including what should be carried out first – e.g. staff training, awareness propaganda.
6. Resources: personnel (professional, administrative and technical), materials and equipment, and facilities – i.e, a hospital, clinic, etc., and the kind, size and location of these institutions.

7. Alternatives which can be tried: e.g. primary health care workers or else the training of traditional midwives.
8. Evaluation; this should be based on objective, and should include:
   (a) periodic evaluation to decide whether the programme should be revised, or re-directed; and
   (b) yearly evaluation which can be based on statistical reports, or on official surveys, and might also include useful but unreliable yardsticks such as personal judgement and public opinion.

Reference

International Children's Centre (1972). Children in The Tropics No. 84, p.3. International Children's Centre, Paris.

Grech. E.A., Galas. J. and Trussell, R.R. (1968). Maternal Mortality in Uganda 1967. *Uganda Atlas of Disease Distribution* p. 144. Department of Preventive Medicine and Department of Geography, Occasional Paper No. 12., Makerere University College, Kampala.

Kohl, S.G. (1959). *Community Obstetrical Study Progress Report,* April 1959, Hartford, Connecticut.

Makerere University (1979). General Circular No. 556.

Maternal and Child Health in the USSR. Public Health Papers 11. Geneva: WHO.

Royal College of Obstetricians and Gynaecologists and the Population Investigation Committee (1948). *Maternity in Great Britain,* Oxford University Press, New York.

Schofield, F.D. (1967). Maternal Immunization Against Neonatal Tetanus. *Proceedings of the Seminar on Immunization in Africa, Kampala,* Uganda, Dec. 1971. Children's International Centre, Paris.

Trusell, R. (1966). *Maternity Care. Medical Care in Developing Countries* (ed. Maurice King) Chapter 19. Oxford University Press.

WHO (1955). Second Report of the Expert Committee on Maternal and Child Health Services *Technical Report Series, World Health Organization 115.*

Further Reading

Lawson, J.B. & Stewart, D.B. *Obstetrics and Gynaecology in the Tropics and Developing Countries.* The English Language Book Society and Edward Arnold Publisher Ltd., London.

Schmidt, William (1973). A UNICEF Field Manual on Health Care of Mothers and Children. Monograph No. 26. *J. Trop. Paediatr. Envon. Chld. Hlth.*

Williams, D. Cicely & Jelliffe, B. Derrick (1972). *Mother and Child Health, Delivering the Services.* Oxford University Press.

Wallace, M. Helen. Gold M. Edwin & Lis F. Edward. *Maternal and Child Health Practices, Problems, Resources and Methods of Delivering.* Charles, C. Thomas, Springfield, Illinois.

WHO (1969). The Organization and Administration of Mother and Child Health Services: 5th Report, WHO Expert Committee on MCH. *Technical Report Series World Health Organization.* **428.**

— (1976). New Trends and Approaches in Delivering of Maternal and Child Care in Health Services. 6th Report of the WHO Expert Committee, *Technical Report SeriesWorld Health Organization,* **600.**

40

Infant and Under-five Child Health Services

J.M. Namboze

Introduction

Child health services aim at attaining optimal health, growth and development throughout infancy and childhood by means of good nutrition, health supervision and health protection.

Child health begins at the time of conception, and therefore good maternal supervision during the antenatal period, throughout labour and during the time of delivery makes a good contribution to child health. Diagnosis and treatment of maternal infections such as syphilis is a way of ensuring that the infant will be healthy. Similarly, health supervision of every woman, particularly during the period of growth and development, and attending to her nutrition can greatly minimize some obstetrical problems such as obstructed labour due to a generally contracted pelvis, which can lead to birth trauma, cerebral palsy, and a permanently incapacitated individual.

In child health one has to consider the following categories of individuals:

(1) the infant –0-11months;
(2) the pre-school child – 1 year-4 years;
(3) the school child – 5-14 years;
(4) the adolescent – 14-18 years.

The infant at birth may be either full-term or premature.

Prematurity

The definition of a premature infant is a neonate of 2, 500g (5 $^1/_2$ *lb*) or less at birth (WHO 1950, 1961). But it has been observed in some parts of the world that many babies under 2, 500g are physiologically mature; and for this reason the term low-birth-weight baby is used to refer to these babies. Some babies may be of low birth weight due to a short *gestational* period, and others may be *underweight at full term.* The truly premature babies are physiologically immature, and often cannot survive without special care. For instance, the level of the special care in Uganda is taken as 4 *lb*. 6 oz. (2 000*g*) (Williams and Jelliffe 1972).

The need for special care for premature infants is because of certain physiological peculiarities, such as unstable temperature control, irregular breathing in rate and volume, inability to suck, especially in very small infants, and lack of resistance to infections. Such premature infants should be looked after in a special care unit with special facilities to meet their particular requirements– viz. a warm environment, protection from infection, and special feeding techniques such as intragastric feeding as well as special nursing care. It is advisable to transfer a mother with premature labour to a hospital with a special care unit; if the mother arrives at a normal hospital too far advanced in labour, she should be delivered, but arrangements should be made for her immediate transfer together with the baby to a hospital with a special care unit. The long stay of the mother in such a hospital provides a good opportunity for health education.

The following are some of the causes of low birth weight: chronic malnutrition, malaria and other antenatal pyrexial infections, pre-eclamptic toxaemia, antepartum haemorrhage, multiple pregnancy, gross foetal abnormality and excessively short intervals between pregnancies. Other causes can lie in maternal behaviour, such as smoking and excessive consumption of alcohol. Good antenatal care and health education during pregnancy can make a great contribution to the prevention of prematurity.

The Neonate

The neonatal period lasts from birth to the end of the first month of life. This is especially important because during this period the infant begins his independent existence by gradually adapting himself to his new environment. The mortality during this period is quite high, and depends on prenatal, natal and postnatal causes. There is no concrete information regarding these factors in developing countries, mainly because of the incomplete reporting of births and deaths. A study conducted at Kasangati Health Centre between 1964 and 1971 (Namboze 1974) revealed that out of the 75 infant deaths, 44 (or 58 per cent) died during the first month of life, and 13 of these deaths were due to unknown causes because of the lack of a proper diagnosis before death and inadequate postmortem examinations after death. Of the deaths due to known causes prematurity was the leading cause, followed by birth trauma.

The following practices are likely to contribute to a high infant and neonatal morbidity and mortality, particularly as they apply to deliveries conducted outside the medical institutions:

(i) instructions to the mother to push as soon as labour starts (in some cultures) may result in early rupture of the membranes, and infection may ascend along the maternal birth canal to the unborn foetus, causing septicaemia; and

(ii) the unsuitability of the place of delivery, of the instruments used for cutting the cord, and of some of the rituals observed while cutting the cord are likely to expose the infants to infection. In some ethnic groups the mother who is about to deliver kneels on dry grass, dried cow dung, or dried banana leaves or a mat. Traditional midwives usually put on working clothes lest their clean ones become soiled. Washing of hands is not a routine practice. The mucus in the infant's nostrils is blown away, while that in the mouth is removed with an index finger; and these may be ways of introducing infection.

In some African communities, the umbilical cord is cut with a razor blade or a blade made from a reed or from elephant grass. In Uganda the cord may be held between the hands while it is being cut, or it may be cut over a hoe handle in the case of a girl and over a spear handle in the case of a boy, symbolizing the traditional roles of the two sexes (Namboze 1964). The severed end of the umbilical cord is then gently rolled between the thumb and the index finger of the attendant to prevent bleeding, and this may be accompanied by the application of umbilical dressings. Some individuals do not use any cord ligatures; while others may use a string torn from an old piece of cloth or from a strip of banana fibre.

The following conditions are likely to affect the new born as a result of the above practices: omphalitis, septicaemia, *tetanus neonatorum*, excessive umbilical bleeding, and birth trauma. The mother is also at risk of developing puerperal sepsis. The only way these problems can be overcome is by delivering a mother in a medical institution or by delivering her at home under the supervision of a skilled person, preferably a midwife.

The Infant

Infancy lasts from birth to the first birthday, but for statistical purposes it is defined as a period from 0-11 months. (This period includes the time between eleven and twelve months of age.) The infant is usually healthy, especially during the first six months of life when he is receiving an adequate amount of breast milk to meet his nutritional requirements; but if for some reasons the infant has to be artificially fed by the average village mother, without proper guidance, under unhygienic conditions then the problem of nutritional marasmus and gastroenteritis are liable to arise.

Respiratory tract infections and malaria, especially in endemic areas, are some of the principal problems during this period. After six months, when breast milk becomes inadequate by itself and when supplemental feeding is not properly practised, signs of early protein-calorie malnutrition start appearing, and increase as the child enters the pre-school period.

Infant Mortality Rate

Infant mortality rate is the number of live births dying in the first year of life divided by the number of live births that year x 1000. The infant mortality rate is the most widely used index of the state of child health, and is considered as one of the most sensitive indicators of the health of the community, as it also reflects the effects of environmental and social conditions. This rate is not available in many developing countries, and if it exists may not be completely reliable owing to an incomplete registration of births and deaths. Suggested ratings of the infant mortality rate given by the United Nations are as follows:

Low: under 50 per 1000 live births (many developed countries)
Medium: 50-100 per 1000 live births; and
High: over 100 per 1000 live births (many developing countries), (Jelliffe 1970)

In developed countries such as Sweden, the UK, and the USA the infant mortality rate is under 25 per 1000 live births. The infant mortality rate has two components, the *neonatal mortality rate*, defined as the number of live births that die in the first 28 days of life divided by the number of live births that year x 1000. The *post-neonatal mortality rate* is defined as infant deaths from 1 to 11 months in a year divided by the number of live births in that year x 1000. Table 40.1 gives an example of neonatal mortality, post neonatal mortality, and infant mortality rates in selected countries.

Table 40.1

Country	*Neonatal mortality rate per 1000 live births*	*Postneonatal mortality rate per 1000 live births*	*Infant Mortality rate per 1000 live births*
Uganda 1959 census	22.2	137.8	160
Sweden 1973*	7.8	2.0	9.9
UK (Eng. & Wales 1973)*	11.1	5.7	16.9
Madagascar 1972*	12.1	41.0	53.2
Kasangati health centre, Uganda 1971+	14.6	18.9	35.5

* WHO Statistics Annual 1973–1976
\+ Namboze, (1974)

In many developed countries one half to two thirds of infant deaths occur in the first seven days of life, and are mainly due to low birth weight, congenital malformation, and intrauterine anoxia due to toxaemia or APH (antepartum haemorrhage). In developing countries, where the mortality rate is high, about two thirds or more of the deaths occur during the post-neonatal period, and these are mainly due to infections, infestations, malnutrition, lack of adequate health services, other environmental factors, and low socio-economic levels. The infant mortality rate in developing countries is about three to ten times as high as in developed countries.

The infant mortality rate can be reduced by providing antenatal supervision to the mothers, through skilled supervision during the time of delivery, health education, nutrition, environmental sanitation, and a general increased availability of health services of the child. For example, attempts to meet these requirements are being made in the defined area of Kasangati Health Centre, which is the teaching health centre for the Institute of Public Health, Makerere University Medical School. The area is situated nine miles north of Kampala and has a population of approximately 12, 000 people. By 1971, 97% of mothers had received antenatal care, and 85% were delivered in medical institutions. The neonatal mortality rate was 14.6 per 1000 live births, while the post-neonatal mortality rate was 18.9 per 1000 live births.

Table 40.2 gives examples of the IMR in developing countries of Africa.

Table 40.2

Country	*Year*	*Infant mortality rate per 1000 live births*
Ghana	1970*	122
Kenya	1970*	126
Nigeria	1970*	157
Tanzania	1970*	165
Uganda	1970*	124

* Population Programme Assistance 1971.

The Pre-school child

The pre-school period is from 1 to 4 years. The pre-school child represents a major public health problem in developing countries. The leading causes of morbidity and mortality during this period are: diarrhoeal diseases; respiratory tract infections and protein-calorie malnutrition (kwashiorkor and nutritional marasmus). These are referred to as the 'Big Three'. The rest include tuberculosis, childhood infections (measles and whooping cough), intestinal helminths, which may be hookworm, roundworm, or tapeworm, depending on local circumstances, malaria, anaemia, and accidents. Almost all these diseases are preventable.

Table 40.3

Age-specific mortality rate 1-4 years in selected countries

Country	*Year*	*Deaths 1-4 years per 1000 population*
Uganda	1969+	30-40
Sweden	1968*	0.5
UK (Eng. & Wales)	1968*	0.8
USA	1968*	0.9
UAR	1968*	35.0

+ 1969 Census
* Wallace (1971)

Age-specific mortality rate 1-4 years

Definition: $\dfrac{\text{No of children 1-4 years dying in a year} \times 1000}{\text{Total population 1-4 years in that year.}}$

The age specific mortality rate 1-4 years is used as an index of the nutritional status of a community (WHO 1963). Deaths during this period in developing countries are mainly due to malnutrition and infections, while in developed countries they are mainly due to accidents. The age specific mortality rate 1-4 years is about 30-40 times as high as in developed countries (see Table 40.3).

Morbidity and mortality within this age group could be greatly reduced by the organization of Young Children's Clinics for regular supervision of the child's health, for early diagnosis and treatment, and for immunization and health education. This has been demonstrated in Western Nigeria by D. Morley (1963), where the under-five clinics reduced the IMR and the 1-4 years mortality (see Table 40.4).

Table 40.4

Reduction of IMR and 1-4 mortaility in Western Nigeria

	Before 1957	*After 1962*
IMR	295	72
1-4 Mortality	70	31

Young Children's (Under - fives) Clinics

In the Western countries in the past there has been a tendency to separate clinics for the sick and clinics for the 'well' children; clinics for well children were called child welfare clinics. These clinics started as stations for providing milk to healthy babies; later attention turned to instructions on the preparation and cleanliness of milk; and finally immunization was introduced. The present concept of a children's clinic is much broader; it is a place where a child is weighed and immunized, advice is given on general health care, and minor illnesses are treated; and it is more practicable thus to combine preventive, promotive, and curative services. The functions of these clinics are as follows:

(1) promotion of the health of the child by means of health education for the parents and the early finding of children with correctable abnormalities – this includes nutritional surveillance;
(2) prevention of diseases by immunization;
(3) treatment of sick children;
(4) malaria prophylaxis in endemic areas; and
(5) parasitic 'deworming' in some areas.

Organization of Young Children's Clinics

The clinic may be either static or mobile. It should be situated where it is most accessible to the people in the particular area it serves, and ample waiting space should be available. Static clinics can be organized at a hospital, health centre, or dispensary; while mobile clinics can be organized at a school, a village hall, or a private home. Most of these clinics are run by a public health nurse or an assistant public health nurse or her equivalent, who is assisted by other auxiliary staff. All these clinics should refer difficult cases to a central place which is visited by a doctor, preferably a health centre; if not, such cases can be referred to a hospital.

The young children's clinic, whether static or mobile, should be organized in such a way that patients move from one station to the next in the following order:

1. Arrival of mothers and children – ample waiting space and shelter from sun and rain is essential.
2. Group health education – suggestions of suitable subjects are listed in the chapter on maternal and child health.
3. Registration.
4. Weighing and charting of weights – the scales should be checked at the beginning of each clinic.

5. Consultation with a public health nurse or her equivalent to see if the child is gaining weight satisfactorily: she should remark on this to the mother, and then check the immunization record. If the child is not well, the public health nurse should either treat the child, or refer the case to the doctor at the same clinic (if one is available) or the nearest medical unit. Individual counselling should be given as required, and arrangements made for home visiting.
6. Immunization.
7. Issue of food supplements and/or medicine required.
8. Malaria prophylaxis if necessary.
9. Consultation with a doctor. Ideally a doctor should carry out a full physical examination of all the children attending the clinic for the first time, but this is seldom possible. Children with any correctable or treatable defects should be referred to the appropriate specialist. Severely malnourished children may be referred to the nearest nutrition rehabilitation centre. Besides prescribing treatment and referral to another medical unit, the doctor may send a child for immunization or refer it back to the health visitor for individual health education and/or home visiting.

Mobile Clinics

These clinics function only at specific times in certain places. They can be in any place which is convenient for the people whom the clinic services. This may be a private home, a court house, or a school. The aim of the mobile clinics is to reduce the distance walked by the mothers and children to the possible minimum. Usually a team for a mobile clinic requires a particular room at the base for the storage of their own equipment and for preparation.

Equipment

Transport (landrover or pick-up van), records, drugs, vaccines carried in a portable cooling apparatus with ice cubes, sterile needles, syringes and a Dermojet if possible, a Heaf gun, and a stove plus a large saucepan for sterilizing needles and syringes. A large number of needles and syringes can be sterilized in a pressure cooker operated at 15 lb. per square inch or its maximum setting for 15 minutes, and such cookers can easily be carried to a mobile clinic (Stanfield 1966). In addition scales, plus a weight standard for checking the scales, and folding tables and chairs, if none are available at the clinic, will be required. Milk and other food supplements, water (if necessary), soap, towels, and specimen containers will also be necessary. A portable microscope is ideal, provided somebody on the staff can do the laboratory work; otherwise request forms for investigations should be filled in at the clinic and mothers should be instructed to take the specimens such as stools and urine or the child itself for finger prick and blood investigations as, for example, tests for Hb, malaria parasites, sickling, etc., to the nearest medical institution. Prepacked drugs are also required.

Personnel

1. A doctor, if possible
2. A public health nurse. Being in charge of the clinic, she gives health education interviews and counsels parents, examines, treats, decides on children who should be immunized, refers children to the doctor, arranges for home visiting, and decides on the

need for investigations, such as, for example, a sickling test or stool and urine examination. She identifies mothers in need of family planning counselling.

3. An assistant public health nurse, whose concerns are the weighing and charting of weights and, later, the dispensing of drugs.
4. A second assistant public health nurse or nurse, who performs immunization.
5. A records clerk, whose role is registration and the keeping of immunization records.
6. A driver, whose functions are driving and helping with records and with the distribution of milk and other food supplements.

Some clinics may not have the suggested number of personnel, and in such cases the available personnel should be well utilized to cover the *required* clinic activities.

Weighing and the Weight Chart

Baby weight is widely used as an indicator of growth, and is very sensitive to changes in the nutritional status. The weight can be taken using various types of scales, for example:

(1) *A beam balance scale.* This scale has two movable weights, of which one moves in kilograms and the other in 10 gram steps up to one kilogram.

(2) *A simple hanging scale.* This is a scale on which the child can be suspended in a pair of strong locally made fabric trousers. A number of pairs of trousers should be made available; each child is then dressed into one pair and suspended on the hook of the hanging scale.

(3) *A bathroom scale.* This can be used for bigger children who do not fit in the fabric trousers, and who are able to stand up on the scale. It is essential that the child should be undressed before he is weighed; the weight record is then charted on the growth chart.

The Growth Chart

Fig. 40.1(b) illustrates a type of chart that is used in Uganda. At the bottom of the chart are rectangular spaces, each representing a month. The month of birth is heavily marked and the name of this month is written in all the heavily marked spaces, e.g. if the child was born in February and February has to be written in all the heavily marked spaces; after this all the other months are filled in. The child's weight is marked on the chart at a point corresponding to the child's age at the time. Other significant information and illness can also be written on the chart e.g. initiation of supplemental feeding,diarrhoea and vomiting, separation from the mother, etc. If the month of birth is not known it is not possible to construct a growth chart for the particular child.

On the reverse side of this chart is the immunization record of the child. The weight chart can be put in a polythene bag and taken away by the mother who brings it to subsequent clinics; this has the advantage that the mother can present the child's record in case of illness to any medical institution. She can also study it and take greater interest in her child's progress. The other alternative is for the growth charts to be kept at the clinic, where they can be used for teaching and research purposes; under such circumstances the mother should be given a form which bears the serial number of her child's card, and she should be given a separate immunization record to ensure that the child returns on the correct days for subsequent immunizations, so that he does not get superfluous immunizations.

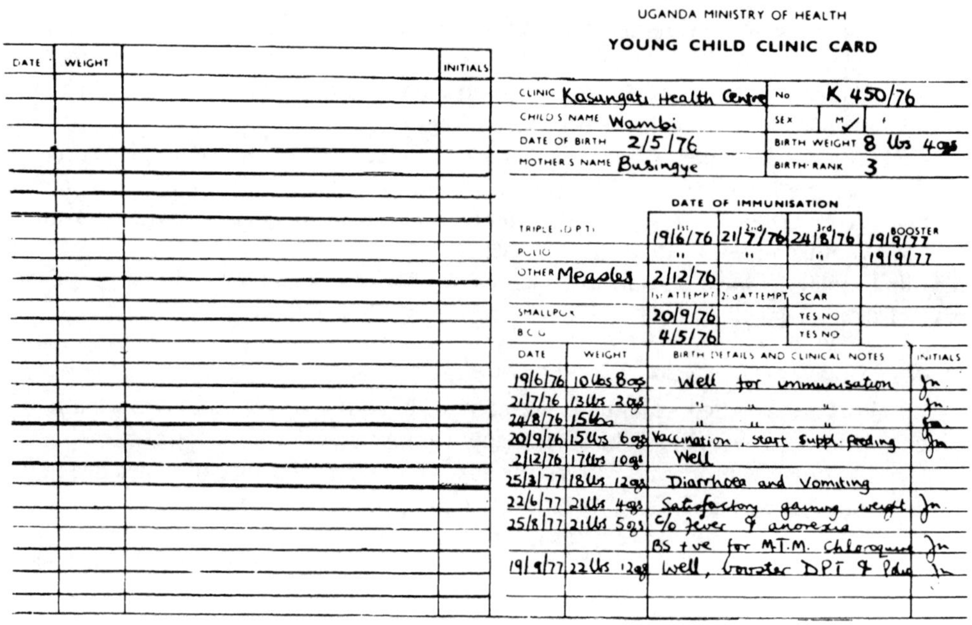

Fig. 40.1: (a) The weight chart

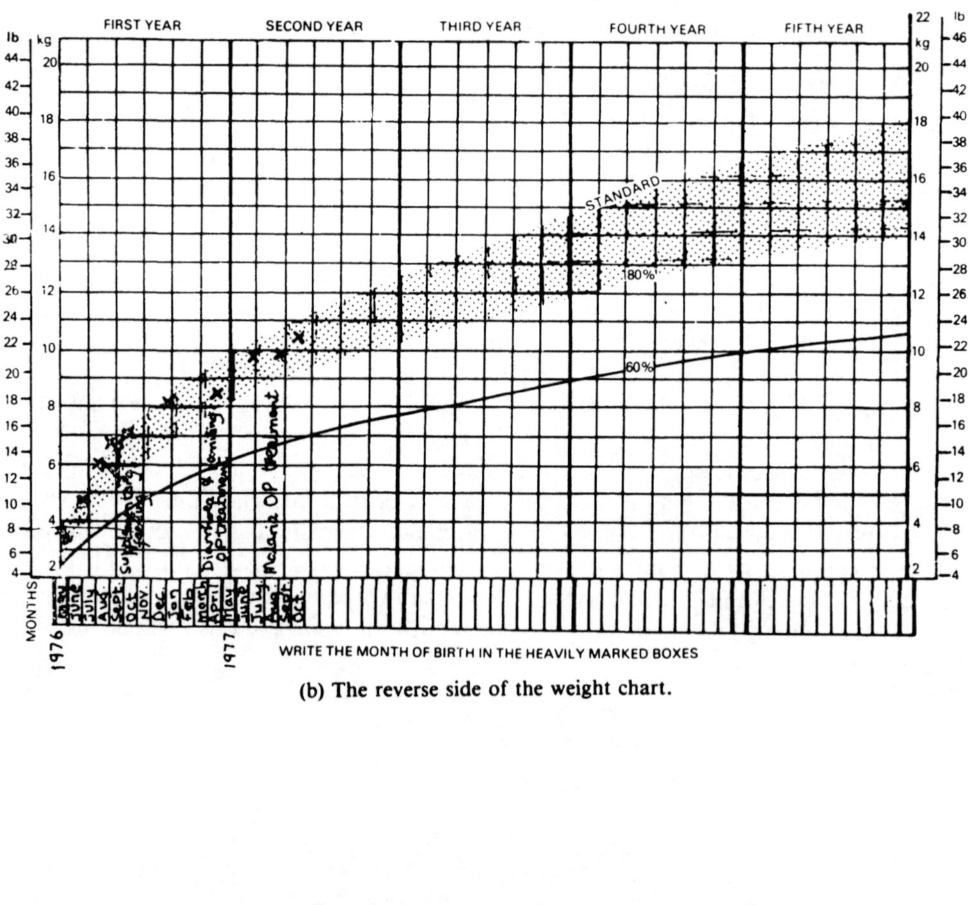

(b) The reverse side of the weight chart.

Integrated MCH Clinics

It may be possible to combine the various MCH clinic into one comprehensive clinic, so that the antenatal and postnatal clinics and family planning, plus the Young Children's Clinic are all conducted simultaneously on the same day and in the same place. This arrangement is ideal for the mother, as she can utilize any of the clinic activities on the same day; she therefore saves time, energy, and sometimes money for transport. Another advantage of the integrated clinic is that it saves staff time by operating all the activities on the same day; and, finally, easy and rapid referral of the mother from one section of the clinic to the other becomes a possibility. This type of clinic may not be possible in a big hospital where there are a large number of patients, but it is ideal in the context of a health centre. It can also be conducted on a mobile basis, provided there is sufficient privacy for the examination of mothers, for giving injections, and for insertion of the intrauterine contraceptive device (IUCD).

Subjects for MCH Clinics

(1) importance of attending the antenatal clinic;
(2) value of other clinics, *viz.* the Young Children's Clinic and postnatal clinics; or if the session is held in an integrated clinic, an explanation of its various activities;
(3) common complaints during pregnancy;
(4) advantages of giving birth in medical institutions; and the concept of mothers at high risk.
(5) care of the umbilical cord, and the prevention of neonatal tetanus;
(6) signs of labour;
(7) danger signs during pregnancy;
(8) dangers of certain types of traditional medicine;
(9) family planning;
(10) diet for the pregnant and nursing mother;
(11) immunization;
(12) value of breast feeding;
(13) weaning diet;
(14) kwashiorkor: cause and prevention;
(15) diarrhoea disease: cause and prevention;
(16) common helminthic infections and their prevention;
(17) home nursing for some common diseases in children;
(18) home accidents and their prevention;
(19) malaria: cause, prevention, and treatment;
(20) personal hygiene and general cleanliness in the home;
(21) preparation for the arrival of the newborn; and
(22) others, depending on the commonest local problems.

Fig. 40.2 **Suggested arrangement for an integrated MCH clinic in the context of a health centre**

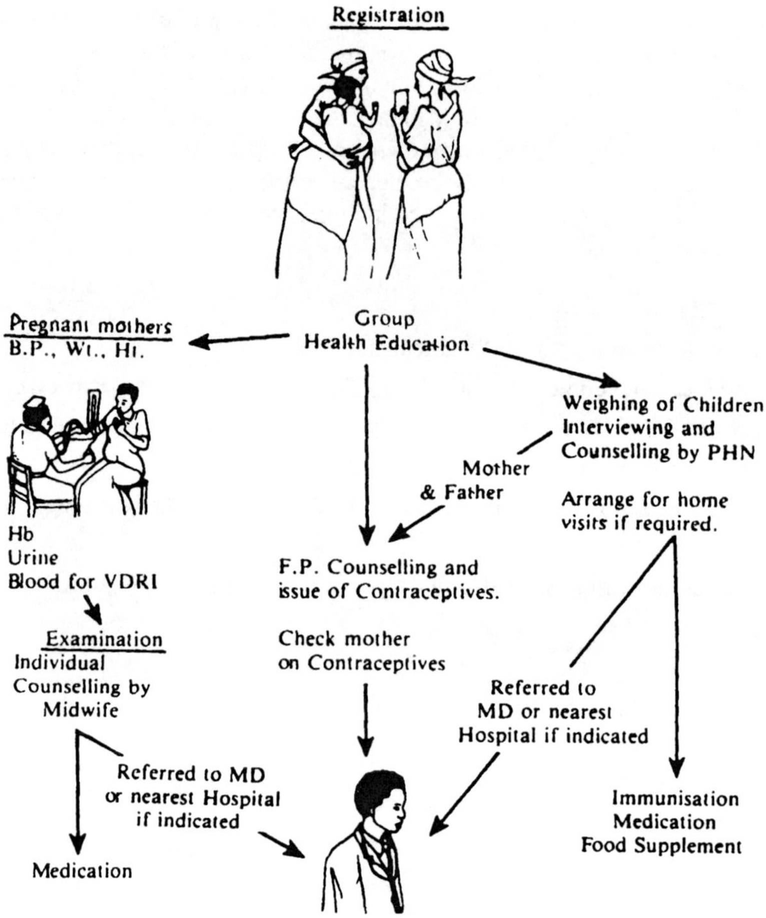

Immunization

Immunization is a very important function of the MCH clinic. Priorities for immunization vary from country to country, and may vary from time to time in the same country, depending on its current problems.

Table 40.5 gives a priority list of diseases against which immunization can be carried out in MCH clinics which will apply very well to most tropical developing countries.

Table 40..5

Diseases	Vaccines
1. Tuberculosis	BCG
2. Diphtheria, tetanus, and whooping cough	DPT
3. Poliomyelitis	Trivalent polio vaccine (oral)
4. Smallpox	Vaccinia
5. Measles	Measles vaccine
6. Tetanus	Tetanus toxoid

Immunization Schedules

There are numerous immunization schedules. Table 40.6 gives a simple, easy-to-remember schedule, and applies very well to developing countries.

Other Child Health Services

There are children with special types of problems that require special services. Examples of these include the following:

1. Orphans or Abandoned Children

Such children need to be looked after in children's homes initially, while in the meantime a suitable home either with a relative or with foster parents is being found.

Most babies' homes would like to keep a newborn baby up to a year or a year and half. Some unfortunate children for whom a suitable home cannot be found may stay for much longer periods.

At present these homes are run by various voluntary organizations, but have support and assistance from the government. Examples of these organizations are the Child Welfare and Adoption Society and various church-organized babies' homes.

Table 40.6

Time	Vaccine	Routine
Pregnancy	Alum absorbed tetanus toxoid injection at 4-6 weeks interval for 2 dosses	IM
Subsequent pregnancy	Booster if 2nd dose of 1st series is completed less than 40 months earlier	
Birth	BCG	Intradermal by tuberculin syringe or Dermojet
6 weeks to 2 months	DPT first Polio first BCG if not given at birth	IM Oral
3 month	DPT (2nd) Polio (2nd)	IM Oral
4 months	DPT (3rd) Polio (3rd)	IM Oral
5 months	Smallpox (vaccination)	Intradermal multiple puncture technique
6-9 months	Measles	Subcutaneously
16-22 months	*1st booster DPT Polio	IM Oral
5 years	2nd booster Dt or TT Polio Smallpox vaccination	IM Oral Intradermal multiple pressure technique

* This period should be 12-18 months after completing the last dose or short of the initial series.

Note: A combination of diphtheria, tetanus (DT) or tetanus toxoid alone is recommended at this state.

Besides giving a child's immunization record to the mother, it is important that the clinic should keep its own records for the area for the purpose of monthly returns.

2. *Handicapped Children*

These include the deaf, blind, crippled, spastic, polio victims, and others. Various voluntary organizations run services for handicapped children, and some have special schools for them.

References

Jelliffe, D.B. (1970). Diseases of Children in the Subtropics and Tropics, *Vital Statistics*, pp. 13-14. The English Language Book Society and Edward Arnold.

Morley, D. (1963). A Medical Service for Children Under 5 Years of Age, *W. Africa Trans. R. Soc. Trop.* 57,79.

Namboze, J.M. (1964). General Infections in the Newborn with Special Reference to E.A. *J. Trop. Med. Hyg.* 67. 131-3.

— (1974). The Trend of Births and Deaths in the Defined Area of Kasangati Health Centre 1964-1971. *Proceedings of the 1974 Annual Scientific Conference of the East African Medical Research Council, Kampala, on 'The Child in the African Environment'*, p.405. East African Literature Bureau, Nairobi.

Population Programme Assistance AID Dev. Bureau for Technical Assistance Office of Population Washington DC 20523, Dec. 1971, pp. 80, 83, 93, 100, 106.

Stanfied, J.P. (1966). Immunizing the Under Fives. In *Medical Care in the Developing Countries*. (ed. Maurice King). Oxford University Press.

Wallace, H.M. (1971). Patterns and Trend in Infant and Maternal Mortality. *Proceedings of the Conference on the Teaching and Practice of Family Health, Kampala, Uganda. 1971*. p.12. Association of Medical Schools in Africa.

Williams, C.D. & Jelliffe, D.B. (1972). *Mother and Child Health Delivering the Services*, p.41. Oxford University Press.

WHO (1950). Report of Expert Group on Prematurity. *Technical Report Series World Health Organization*. **127.**

— (1961). Public Health Aspect of Low Birth Weight. *Technical Report Series World Health Organization*. **217.**

— Late foetal, Infant, Neonatal and Postneonatal Mortality. In *Statistics Annual 1973-1976*. WHO, Geneva.

— (1963). Report on the Expert Committee of the Medical Assessment of Nutritional Status. *Technical Report Series. World Health Organization*. **258.**

41

Section A

Health Care Delivery for Children of School Age

G.O. Sofoluwe

History of School Health Services

It was only in 1812 that the study by a doctor (Dr James Ware) on the health of school children was recorded. He reported on the eyesight of school children in London and of students at Oxford University. Similar investigations were then stimulated in Sweden in 1840, and in Breslau, Germany in 1866. In 1883 the first school doctor was appointed in Frankfurt-am-Main in Germany; two years later two doctors with a similar role were appointed in Lausane, Switzerland; and in 1888 school medical inspection was started in all the political divisions (called departments) of France. Although the first medical investigation into school health was conducted in Britain, yet the first publicly appointed School Medical Officer in England was only appointed in 1890; but by 1905 eighty-five such doctors had been appointed, and the school health service was organized on a national basis in 1908.

The story will not be complete without mentioning that in Nigeria it was only in 1929, and about the same time in Uganda, that the first full-time preventive medical officers were appointed in the two countries to start maternal, child, and school child health services. It was the late Dr Ladipo Oluwole who started this service in Lagos, Nigeria in 1929. Unfortunately, even though over 50% of children of school age (5-19 years) in Africa do not attend any school, yet Africa has not organized any special health services to cover these children.

General Objectives of the School Health Service

Because children who spend a large part of their lives at school are exposed to a wide variety of environmental influences – physical, emotional, and social, it is important that they should be given health supervision at school, so that early signs of illness in them can be detected and the opportunity can be taken to educate them and their parents to gear their learning to acquiring and living in healthy ways.

These would thus include the following:

(1) to detect early deviations from normal health, especially those which will hinder the child from benefitting fully from his education, such as, for example, eye defects; hearing defects; illness affecting the heart, the kidney, and the musculo-skeletal systems; illnesses affecting the genito-urinary systems, causing emotional, mental and social problems; allergic illnesses, including asthma; and many others;

(2) to maintain all children in an optimum state of health throughout their course of instruction. To treat promptly all ill children, and rapidly restore them to health;

(3) to inculcate in the child healthy habits which he should maintain throughout life and by his own efforts;

(4) to teach the child to be always in harmony with himself, his family, his community, his state, his nation and his world, as well as to submit to discipline and to respect his elders, teachers and all those in authority over him.

It is evident that to meet all the above stated objectives, the child needs to maintain a clean environment; to have adequate nutrition; and to be taught to recognize early signs and symptoms of important physical, mental, and social diseases and health problems.

All the above objectives, however, can only be accomplished by the co-operative efforts of the child, his parents, his teachers and his community at large.

The Need for School Health Services, especially in African Countries

Over 80 per cent of Nigerians are deprived of essential health services such as maternal and under-five child health services, and even of scientific curative, preventive, or promotive health services. Hence up to 1929 one quarter of all the children born in Africa died before they attained the age of one year, whilst another quarter (making a total of fifty per cent) died before they reached their sixteenth birthday.

The majority of those who survived till school age will have been partially or totally blind or deaf from previous attacks of diseases like measles or smallpox or meningococcal meningitis, and a number of other illnesses acquired before the age of five years. Many others would have developed epilepsy owing to the prolonged labour experienced by their mothers, who had no ante-natal or intra-natal supervision by western trained midwives or doctors. Many still have yet undiagnosed heart, lung, kidney, and other diseases; whilst a large proportion will have social problems(due either to the divorce or the separation of their parents or to their being boarded out to relatives or to masters who either pay their parents or house the children in return for housekeeping services). This early experience of social deprivation on the part of these children often leads to emotional problems, loss of moral courage and moral balances, and gross behavioural disorders, which may even culminate in criminal tendencies or offences.

Hence Collis *et al.* (1966) found that as many as forty per cent of dropouts among primary school children in Northern Nigeria, (Zaria, Kaduna, Kano,etc.) were on medical, psychological, emotional and social examination found to have one or more of the defects listed in the above paragraph. Similar findings have been reported in Ghana, Dakar, Nairobi, Kampala, Dar-es-Salaam, Lusaka, and many other African countries.

Recent demographic studies in some villages in Okpebho Local Government Area of the former

Bendel State in Nigeria showed that 18 to 19% of the population is composed of primary school aged children (5-9 years old) and between 12.8% and 19.6% are secondary school aged children (10-14 years old). (The wide dispersion from 12.8%to 19.8% of the age group 10-14 years is due to the presence or absence of secondary schools in or near the villages enumerated.) Thus school age children from 5 to 18 years constitute about 30–40% of the population of most African settlements, cities and villages. They thus deserve priority health attention.

Relatively more accurate data was obtained for the Midwest State, now Edo and Delta states, after the last accepted Nigerian census of 1963. Table 41.1 contains the details; but in summary those aged 5-16 years and expected to be in primary schools (5-10 years), secondary modern schools (10-13 years) or secondary grammar schools (usually aged 10-16 years) in total constituted 29.6% of the total population (2 535 839) in the state in 1963.

Table 41.1

Total population Midwest State Nigeria 1963	=	2 535 839	
aged 5-9 years	=	399 459 or 15.8% of total population	
10-14	=	292 545 or 9.6%	
15-16	=	65 580 or 2.6%	
17-19	=	98 370 or 3.9%	
Therefore the total population for those aged 5-19 years	=	855 954 or 31.9%	
Total number of school children in primary grades I-VI in the State (1963)		369 871	
Secondary modern grades I-III (11-13 years) (1963)		36 957	
Grammar school grades I-VI (11-16 years)		7 904	
Teacher training colleges		3 142	
Technical and Trade schools		1 981	
Total		419 855	= 16.6% of total population

If it is assumed that school age children in Bendel State are aged 5-19 years and numbered 855 954 or 31.9% of the total population in 1963, whilst only 419,855 or 16.6% of the total population was in primary, grammar, teacher training, technical and trade centres or schools in that same year, it can be seen that 51% of those aged 0-19 years were not in schools.

If we narrow down to those aged 5-16 years who were supposed to be attending primary and secondary schools, then only 414 732 or 54.7% of the total 757 584 aged 5-16 years were actually in schools. The remaining 45.3% were not in schools. Accurate results cannot be obtained for primary school aged children in schools, as it was and still is the usual practice to admit even adults to primary schools. However 70 to 80% of primary school children aged 5-11 years attended schools in the state in 1963.

But in actual fact only 414 732(54.7%) of the total 757 784 aged 5-16 years in the state expected to be in the schools up to secondary grammar school level were actually present in the schools, so that as many as 45.35% of school age children were not in schools in the state in 1963.

As almost half the school age children in Africa are not in schools and can therefore not benefit from health services taken to the schools *it is important for African governments to arrange health services for all the children of school age, irrespective of whether they attend or do not attend schools*. This chapter will therefore concentrate on proposing measures to provide a comprehensive health cover for all children of school age both in and outside schools in Africa. As the major constraints usually include inadequate manpower, health facilities, and finance, the chapter will suggest how the present limited health manpower and facilities, could be geared to more preventive services, and be made to serve well defined populations living in well defined areas, would prevent many of the illnesses now crowding our curatively-oriented health service. It would therefore be necessary to heed Dr. Laoye's recommendation to utilize the more generous supply of health auxiliaries, school teachers, and school children to deliver health care not only in schools but also to children of school age outside the schools and in the communities.

Manpower Requirements for a Model School Health Service for Children of School Age in and Outside Schools in Africa

Every African country should appoint at least one school health doctor or physician, who should work out a policy and organize and supervise health care delivery services in and outside schools. He should be a public-health-trained doctor, and should be based at the national Ministry of Health. He should prescribe standards for school health programmes at national, state, and local government levels – even down to political ward levels. Every state or province also needs to appoint at least one medical officer for the same purpose.

An experienced community nurse, or health sisters or nurses who have received training in community health and have long experience (of at least fifteen years) should be appointed to work either at local government, town,village or community level to effect delivery of health care in schools. The school health programmes should be operated on the standards laid down for national, state and local governments, and political ward levels. Lower level nurses or community nurses or community health assistants may be appointed for every school. All school headmasters should undergo a course lasting at least two weeks in health care delivery in schools, and shorter refresher courses at least once every five years.

At least two special teachers, who might be designated school health care delivery teachers, and might be biology or health science teachers, should be appointed in every school and made responsible for health care delivery in schools. In mixed schools there should be at least two female and two male teachers to allow for adequate coverage. These teacher should be given at least a four-week course to equip them for their work and should have refresher courses at least two weeks every five years.

All schools should appoint one health care pupil in every class, or a set of at least four students, one for each week in a month, to undertake health care delivery in the schools. In mixed schools one boy and one girl should undertake such duties weekly.

As some parents may be doctors it might be desirable for the headmaster to solicit part-time services from such doctors, especially those with community health training and orientation. It is expected that within the next decade all doctors in Africa will have community health orientation and practice. Similar assistance may be sought from parents who may be dentists, nurses, health inspectors, welfare officers, etc.

An executive committee of parents should be appointed for every school or group of schools in the district or area. To care for the health of the 45% or so of children of school age not attending schools one of the two suggestions mentioned below might be adopted. A team of four male and four female teachers, specially trained in health care delivery in schools, and drawn from some of the schools in every political ward in either the town or the rural area, assisted by about twelve male and twelve female specially trained school children from the same ward as the teachers, should be set up to run school health services for those out of school. This service should be financed by the local government. An alternative is for the local government authority to run special school health clinics for that group or for the two groups (in and out of schools) together.

All the above statements have utilized the principle of involving the child, the parents, the family, the community, the school teachers, and the pupils to complement the activities of the local, state, national and international health agencies in order to provide a comprehensive school health service for all school age children both within and outside schools in Africa.

Comprehensive School Health Activities

These require that all school children should undergo comprehensive medical examinations on entry to or once in at each of the nursery, primary, secondary or post secondary school levels. Such examination will screen for those with visual, hearing,postural, epileptic, emotional, and mental defects, and all the others listed under the first special objectives mentioned earlier.

Parents might assist such programmes by privately paying for their school children to be medically examined, as detailed in a form which should be prepared for this purpose on a national or state or local government basis.

The visual, hearing, postural, emotional, and intelligence tests might be undertaken by nurses, teachers, and even senior school pupils, who could be specially trained to assist or fully perform the test.

Referral of those with defects needs to be undertaken promptly and directed to the appropriate medical specialists. It is preferable for the students to be conveyed to the medical centre in a group by school transport to prevent truancy and other problems.

Personal hygiene inspection of the teeth, nails, feet, skin, and clothes may be undertaken on a weekly or even daily basis until the headmaster is assured that he has attained as high a level of personal sanitation as is desirable. Such inspection may be undertaken by class teachers, or by class prefects specially taught to perform it.

Persistently dirty or unkempt children may be from families with social problems such as divorced or separated parents, or from among those boarded out or those serving as servants, or reveal some mental or intelligence deficiencies. All such problems should be identified and solved rather than resorting as a punishment for such problems to caning, which should be banned in all African schools.

Environmental Health Inspections

Health superintendents and inspectors might briefly train senior pupils and class teachers to undertake detailed environmental health inspection of the dormitories in boarding houses, classrooms, assembly halls, the water supply, the toilets, including bathrooms and latrines, the refuse dump, the lockers, the bookshelves and the kitchen, including the central kitchens provided for the use of a group of schools. The daily sweeping and cleaning of such areas should be made the responsibilities of school pupils, to ensure that they know how to undertake such tasks in their own homes, both at the time and in the future.

Nutrition and Food Hygiene

The kitchens of food sellers in schools must be examined, and the food sellers medically examined to detect carriers and sufferers from food-borne diseases. One of the main reasons for the low level of education yet attained in Africa might be the long term cumulative effects of malnutrition of the foetus during pregnancy, infancy, and the under-five childhood days, together with starvation during the primary school age. Dr Soleye(now Dr Aina) in 1977 found that over 90% of primary school children in a town in Nigeria had their first meal of the day at 1700 hours (5 p.m.) each day – i.e. most came to schools without breakfast, and had no money to purchase lunch at school. Many of the children were therefore forced by hunger to rush at the few who had money to purchase meals. Those who had the money to purchase food were in turn forced to spit into the food to prevent crowds of their colleagues from carrying off the food, which is hardly enough for the purchaser. Thus the nutritional status of most of the school children in Africa leaves a lot to be desired, and has serious effects on their mental as well as moral capacities.

Some successful experiments in supplying balanced nutrition to school children have been pioneered in Africa. These include the Lagos, Nigerian experiment which built one or two central school kitchens from which school meals are prepared and served to individual schools; UNICEF, Lagos state and the Federal government assisted the scheme. It was only partially successful. Also the Food Specialities Company and the De Facto Bakery in Lagos, at the instance of Professor Sofoluwe and Mr Simpson of the Food Specialities Company (previously named Nestlés Products) developed a loaf of bread costing less than 10 kobo (₦0.10), and containing beans, minced meat and flour, which was scientifically proved to provide all the nutrient requirements for school age children. The bread was smeared with margarine and taken with water. As it was served in the class rooms the expense of building and equipping school kitchens was avoided. Unfortunately for one reason or another the system has not yet been widely adopted in practice.

More recently, the Comprehensive High School in Aiyetoro, Mayflower School, Ikenne and the African Church Comprehensive High School, Ikere - Ekiti (all in Nigeria) have developed a scheme whereby all the school pupils grow all their foodstuffs, process the foods, and cook and serve them. In the same schools the children alsô built their classrooms, dormitories, latrines, and bathrooms, and reared poultry, kept a piggery and a few head of cattle and sheep, and became self-sufficient in food supply. They also learnt to entertain themselves by drama, drumming, concerts and plays; and the 800 pupils in the Ekiti school at least graduated from the school having been fully trained in growing, processing and serving their own foods, as well as in building and maintaining their own houses and sustaining their own independent existence by their own efforts – a total education indeed.

Such children and schools could thus provide food for the high-risk groups such as the pregnant, the under-five children, the unemployed, orphans, and other physically, mentally, and socially deprived persons in the community.

The solution to the problems of food hygiene and providing balanced nutrition for school age children in Africa must include making the children grow, process, prepare, cook, and serve breakfast and lunch in the school. They should also be made to inspect and maintain food hygiene in order to prevent food poisoning.

Social Problems

Truancy, indiscipline, bullying, pilfering and other criminal tendencies or offences among school children may be an indication of social problems among their parents and the community as a whole.

Experienced nurses, welfare officers, child guidance officers, psychiatrists, headmasters and senior teachers could be taught to diagnose such conditions and take appropriate remedial measures with the parents of such children.

Recreation

Every child should be made to discover the sports, or recreation, or hobbies best suited to its physical and other capabilities. Every child should be actively taught to keep a sound mind in a sound body. Thus mental fatigue or breakdown will be actively prevented, or at least minimized.

Health Education

The six to twelve, or even twenty-one, years of school days up to university level should be spent in making the school child learn how to live a normal life physically. Hence he or she should be able to undertake basic life activities such as building or repairing or painting houses, repairing water closets, keeping and maintaining gardens, cooking food, ironing clothes, and other such activities.

Excursions should be undertaken to soap making,cloth making, and food factories, to building construction industries, water works, sewage works, refuse depots, markets, and other public places concerned with meeting man's daily needs.

Health education at school level should be practical and the pupils should be made to produce articles practically. The girls should at domestic science classes be encouraged to keep a home practically and to undertake the household chores for at least one week in every school year. This should continue even up to university level. At university level the engineering students should be stimulated to invent gadgets which would improve and promote full environmental health.

Mention of treatment has been left so late because careful planning will limit treatment to emergencies and unpredictable illnesses only. Medical examination on entering any level of school will have revealed the sickly ones, who will then be under strict supervision with the aim of eliciting signs early and undertaking immediate treatment. And immunization for communicable diseases including tuberculosis, tetanus, poliomyelitis, diptheria, mumps, German measles or rubella, and meningococcal meningitis will reduce the prevalence of communicable diseases to manageable levels within the school. While environmental health inspections will prevent food poisoning, endemic illness, worms, anaemia, malaria, and rabies, this last one by keeping the school free of stray dogs and immunizing all pet dogs.

Antisnake venoms should be kept in school compounds even though bush clearing, keeping flower borders well-trimmed, and the keeping of pigs near and in school poultry-runs will keep down the snake population in schools.

Sick parades should be held as often as is desirable, if necessary daily, to facilitate early diagnosis and treatment by the special health teacher or pupils or nurse for the school.

First Aid

The health teachers and pupils recommended for such duties should undertake first aid courses at the Red Cross, the St. John Ambulance Brigade, or at hospitals and other such agencies, and obtain a proficiency certificate. There should be first aid boxes in almost every classroom and in the school clinic if there is one.

Sick Bays

It is essential for all schools to have provision for sick bays where ill patients can be seen by the health teacher or school nurse and kept under observation pending referral to hospital or being sent back home. Sick bays can also be used for isolating cases of communicable diseases.

Referral to hospital should ideally be undertaken by the most senior health teacher or nurse. A school ambulance may be provided for a group of schools in a political ward or district, or by the central ambulance agency, in cases where such a facility has been planned or provided for in African countries.

School Health Records

Good record keeping is the sure foundation to maintaining a first class health level in schools– ideally it is desirable to have the ante-natal, intra-natal, post-natal and under-five child health records of each of the school children in one folder, or merged together on one record card. Thus the health records from the womb to the primary, secondary, and even university stages will have been successfully monitored and integrated.

Registers of defects – visual defects, defects of hearing, epilepsies, asthmatic attacks, emotional, social, mental, and other defects listed earlier – will help direct attention to those children who require closer medical attention, and will thus minimize emergencies.

Monthly health bills or school health reports should be submitted to a school health committee, which may be chaired by the headmaster or the senior health teacher. The committee should include representatives of the school children, the teachers, the parents, the Ministries of Education, Health and Social Welfare, and other representatives of the community, and, where appropriate, the proprietors of the school – for many schools in Africa are now privately sponsored, whether by missions or by the community or private persons. Refresher courses and seminars may be organized for members of such committees by the state education authorities.

In conclusion, we should stress that it is important for educational authorities in Africa to provide all schools with modern hygiene facilities such as water closets, wash hand basins, kitchens, dining halls, sick bays and adequate ventilation.

Various methods for financing the health amenities should be carefully worked out, including involving the school children in building and erecting such facilities, while the government supplies the necessary equipment.

As a clean environment always promotes clean habits, thoughts and actions, the practical involvement of school children in such programmes will reduce the high prevalence of diseases among children of school age in Africa.

References

Hobson, W. (1975). *The Theory and Practice of Public Health* (4th ed:) Oxford University Press.

Laoye, J.A. (1976). *Principles and Practice of Health Education* Macmillian Education Limited, London.

Llwelyn Roberts and Kathleen Shaw (1958). *A Synopsis of Hygiene* (Jamieson and Parlunson) (11th ed). Churchill, London.

Meredith Davies, J.B. (1975). *Community Health, Preventive Medicine and Social Services*. Concise Medical Textbooks. Baillere Tindal, USA.

Section B

The School Health Service

D.A. Ogunmekan

The school health service is a continuation of the health service of the pre-school child from the maternal and child welfare centre.The aims and objectives of the school health service are directed towards an early detection of defects through a programme of periodical medical inspections of school children, a follow-up service, teaching of the staff of the school to detect such defects; whenever possible to minimize the chances of spread of communicable disease and to protect the children from hazards which may cause injury, disease or disability to them.

It also aims at providing a healthy environment to the school child and confers a knowledge within the capacity of his understanding in the principles of healthy living so that the knowledge that he acquires is communicated through the medium of the school child to the parents, thereby educating the parents themselves.

The functions of a school health service include the following:

(1) Regular observations and screening of all children. Early detection of defects in early childhood that can adversely affect both the child's present physiological functioning and his later educational and social adjustment.

In countries with well established child health services, developmental screening is directed towards detecting children with developmental abnormalities at an early age as possible. In developing countries the school health service may be the first contact of the children with the community's orthodox health care system. This unavailability of periodic developmental screening examinations to all pre-school children has great implications for the school health service.

Routine medical inspection was introduced partly to identify previously unrecognized defects in school children. In fact, it provided a screening programme for school children long before screening became fashionable (McKeown & Lowe, 1974). Ideally, each child should be examined at school entry, and on leaving primary school or on leaving secondary school.

In developed countries, the value of the routine medical examination has been queried by Norman (1960), Didsbury (1964) and Horner (1966) and there is increasing use of selective type of examinations and of screening techniques. The importance of diagnosing ailments at school entrance examinations is that they can be dealt with promptly. Defects found at school leaving examination should be referred to the appropriate centre for continued management.

Visual acuity should be tested and if indicated the child should be referred for further testing to be repeated when the child is older if he is too young on school entry. Similarly, audiometry is important to detect any defects in hearing and it may have to be repeated at a later age if the child is too young on school entry. It is important to detect partial deafness and total deafness. If the child's hearing can be corrected with hearing aids and he can cope in a school for normal children, this should be encouraged. Otherwise he should be sent to a school for deaf children.

(2) Ascertainment of children with handicaps which necessitate special educational treatment arrangements.

(3) Provision of certain curative and specialist services and referral to specialist clinics e.g. dental if necessary.

(4) Communicable disease control which is done by prophylactic immunization e.g. tetanus toxoid.

(5) Cleanliness e.g. examination of pupils and control of outbreaks of communicable diseases.

(6) Environmental sanitation which includes inspection of school buildings, lighting and ventilation, sitting arrangements, toilet facilities and availability of playgrounds.

(7) Nutritional defects can be corrected by advice on dietary habits and provision of a balanced diet to school children. There should be regular examination of cooks and all food handlers who provide the school meal service. Any person found to be a carrier of any disease which could be transmitted to the children should not be employed.

(8) Health education is essential to impart knowledge of health and disease to the school child which will be useful not only to himself but also to his parents.

(9) Children should be taught about accident prevention both in the school and at home.

(10) Inclusion of training of teachers in health matters in their curriculum of training is an important factor in a programme of school health.

(11) Special surveys and investigations may be carried out in the school health service.

In most developed countries, some school age children suffer the effects of chronic malnutrition and the multiple infections in early childhood. Oduntan (1973) found that the major health problems of school children in developing countries such as Nigeria were related to malnutrition, multiple infections and trauma. Ogunmekan (1973) found high rates of intestinal parasitic infections among school children in Nigeria, the commonest of which were *Ascaris lumbricoides*, hookworm and *Trichuris trichura*.

Handicapped School Children

The categories of pupils requiring special educational treatment are defined as follows:

(1) Deaf pupils

(2) Partially deaf pupils

(3) Blind pupils
(4) Partially blind pupils
(5) Mentally handicapped pupils
(6) Maladjusted pupils
(7) Physically handicapped pupils e.g. cripples

The principle of education of handicapped children is to provide the type of training which is appropriate to their disability.

The Blind

The blind children need to attend special schools for the blind, designed with care and foresight in order that they should be ideally suitable for blind children. The education of blind children should start as early in life as possible so that they can learn skills required for their educational requirements and for normal activities of daily living. From nursery schools, these children go on to primary and secondary schools. Those capable of attending post-secondary institutions such as universities or vocational training centres should be encouraged to do so.

In Nigeria, there is a special school for the blind where the pupils undergo the normal primary education. Those who have the ability, go on to secondary schools, where they are taught alongside sighted pupils. Special text books in braille are provided for them and they type out their answers during examinations. If possible, they can also record the lectures on tape.

In some parts of the country, the blind pupils attend normal primary schools and a visiting teacher of the blind goes round to give the pupils assignments and the class teachers of the blind pupils monitor their progress until the visiting teacher comes round again to correct the assignments. This early integration of the blind children with sighted children is important for both groups of children to accept each other. The deaf children who are not mentally handicapped attend special schools for the deaf. It is advisable for these children to start school as early in life as possible.

In the special schools for the deaf in Nigeria the pupils follow the normal primary school curriculum. Those who have the ability go further to post-primary institutions such as vocational training institutions or universities. At the present time, there is no provision for university education for deaf pupils in Nigeria and so they go to institutions outside the country.

The children learn to lip-read and also learn the hand alphabet so that they can communicate with signals.

Physically handicapped pupils who are not mentally handicapped include those who have paralytic, poliomyelitis, or other physical disability and they are unable to attend a normal school. The Atunda Olu School, Lagos, Nigeria, for instance, is for pupils who are physically handicapped. The children follow a normal primary school curriculum. The school has a qualified nurse, a physiotherapist and a visiting doctor.

In spite of their physical or mental disability, some of the pupils who have the ability go on to secondary and post secondary institutions. One should bear the following points in mind when advising parents of a child with cerebral palsy or similar handicap:

(a) that none of the parents is guilty;
(b) that much can be done to help the child;
(c) that an absolute cure is not to be expected and that though the child will never be absolutely normal, he can attain a level of training suited to his ability.

The objective of training the mentally subnormal children is to enable them to develop to the limit of their ability so that eventually they can live with varying degrees of help and supervision. However some of them cannot guard themselves from exploitation by unscrupulous persons and it is these limitations which render them incapable of living independently. The educable mentally retarded children can attend a special school where they are taught the subjects in the normal primary school curriculum and those who have the ability can go to secondary school or vocational training centres.

The educationally subnormal children can be trained to attend to their physical needs and learn some skills by assisting with domestic chores or doing routine tasks in a sheltered workshop. For the maladjusted pupils who suffer from emotional instability or psychological disturbance there should be provision for treatment in appropriate centres. In Lagos, the Child Guidance Clinic caters for such children as well as those suffering from a speech defect not due to deafness or mental handicap.

These children are assessed by a team comprising of a child psychologist, a speech therapist, a psychiatrist and a paediatrician to find out the problem of the children. The management of the children is done by a team of professionals specializing in children's problems.

Some of the children are kept in normal schools and sent to the Child Guidance Clinic once or twice weekly while others attend the Child Guidance Clinic for treatment.

Some children are sent to remand homes which are places where juvenile delinquents are kept temporarily whilst awaiting a court order either because they are offenders against the law e.g burglars or because they need care and protection or because they are beyond parental control. A court order eventually sets them free or sends them to an approved school or places them on probation.

References

Didsbury, B. (1964) *The School Health Service and the Family Doctors*, Lancet, (101-4)

Homer, J.S. (1963) The Intermediate School Medical Inspection. Public *Health London* 77, 291-300.

McKeown, T. Lowe, C.R. (1974). *An Introduction to Social Medicare* 2nd edition. Blackwell

Norman, L.G. (1960). *In Modern Trends in Occupational Health* Edited by Shulling, R.S.F. London, P. 268

Oduntan, S.O.(1973). *The Health of Nigerian Children of School Age (6-15 years)* M.D. Thesis, University of London.

Ogunmekan, D.A. (1973). "A Comparison of Combantrin with Antepar and Alhopar in Helminthiasis in School Children in Lagos, Nigeria. *West African Medical Journal* 22, 3 47-48.

42

Contraception

Muriel Oyediran

History

Mankind has always been concerned with the problem of fertility and as far back as 1850 B.C., contraceptive recipes were found in papyri in Egypt. These recipes were for use as pessaries or vaginal douches.

Many other contraceptive folk methods were used throughout the world, such as fumigation of the female genital area by squatting over a fire on which various herbs were sprinkled, or by brewing and drinking various herbal teas. Talisman and amulets were also worn as contraceptive measures.

Abortion, which is still practised today, was also often resorted to and in some communities, in times of extreme hardship, infanticide was resorted to as well.

As more information regarding the human body and its functions was gathered, coitus interruptus was practised. By the 17th and 18th centuries, the caeca of sheep and goats were treated with lye and used as condoms until the advent of the vulcanization of rubber in 1833–44. Once rubber was discovered, it was a short step to the manufacture of rubber condoms, in commercial quantities, followed by cervical caps (seldom used nowadays), and vaginal diaphragms.

Intrauterine Contraceptive Device

The use of an intrauterine device was first documented by Dr Richter in 1909, when he placed a ring of silkworm gut in the uteri of women requiring contraception. Dr Grafenberg, in 1929, also used silkworm gut and rings of silver wire as IUD's. The first International Conference on IUD was held in 1962 and with the discovery of inert plastics, the modern era of the IUD was underway.

The plastic devices are made radio-opaque by the addition of barium sulphate and the most popular and commonly used IUD was the Lippes loop. However the Lippes loop has been withdrawn from the market and the newer copper containing devices have now superseded the plain inert devices. However the copper devices at present have to be replaced every 3–4 years. Progestin impregnated devices are also available.

Mechanism of Action

Although the effectiveness of the IUD in preventing pregnancy is 95–98%, their mechanism of action is not clear cut, however some of the more commonly suggested mechanisms are:

1. Increased mobility of the ovum in the fallopian tubes so that the ovum reaches the endometrial cavity too early in its development to be able to implant. At the same time, the endometrial lining has not had the necessary length of time to mature, to thicken and to become secretory for implantation to be able to occur.
2. Local foreign body inflammatory response to the presence of the IUD causes lysis of the blastocyst or prevents implantation.
3. Mechanical dislodgement of the implanted blastocyst from the endometrium.
4. Increased local production of prostaglandins which inhibit implantation.
5. Biochemical alterations in the endometrial lining by inhibition of the enzymic activity (such as carbonic anhydrase) which affects the ability of the blastocyst to implant.

The intrauterine device must always be inserted after performing a thorough gynaecological examination to exclude abnormalities of the genital tract.

Contraindications to Use

1. Active, recent, or recurrent pelvic inflammatory disease; however an IUD can be inserted 6 months after successful treatment of pelvic inflammatory disease.
2. Known or suspected pregnancy.
3. Severe fibroids with abnormal uterine shape and gross uterine enlargement.
4. Cervical or uterine malignancy.
5. Abnormal uterine bleeding (until the cause is identified and treated).
6. History of ectopic pregnancy.
7. Impaired coagulation time.
8. Valvular heart disease.
9. An IUD may be inserted 3 months after an uncomplicated caesarean section.

Side Effects:

1. Heavier and longer menstrual periods of up to 2–3 days longer than usual for possibly the first 3–6 months after insertion. Any heavy bleeding that lasts for longer than 10 days should be regarded as abnormal and should be reported for management.
2. Intermenstrual bleeding or spotting which usually stops, without treatment, a few months after insertion.
3. Lower abdominal cramps and backache are associated with dysmenorrhoea. Pelvic infection may be suspected if the abdominal pain is severe and associated with a purulent vaginal discharge and fever.

Complications

1. Most expulsions occur within the first 6 months after insertion and it is possible for repeated expulsions to occur. If this occurs then the IUD is not the contraceptive of choice.
2. Translocation of the IUD can occur where the threads of the IUD are not visible, but the IUD is still in the fundus of the uterus. If this is the case, the IUD can be removed fairly easily when necessary.

3. Perforation of the uterus by the IUD can occur, in which case the IUD is found in the pelvic cavity on X-ray. Removal, if necessary, has to be by operative procedure.
   There is a greater risk of pelvic inflammatory disease (PID) in women using the IUD. However the infection can be treated with the IUD in place. Sometimes the PID is caused by a sexually transmitted disease such as gonorrhoea or chlamydia trachomatis and this must be kept in mind so that appropriate investigations can be carried out to establish the correct diagnosis and to give the necessary treatment.

Hormonal Contraception

The oral contraceptive popularly known as 'the pill' has been introduced into family planning programmes since 1960. It is of four types:

1. The combined tablets contain the same amount of oestrogen and progestin in each tablet.
2. The sequential tablets (rarely used now) contain 14 tablets of oestrogen only, followed by 7 tablets of oestrogen and progestin.
3. The tri-phasic tablets which contain varying amounts of oestrogen and progestin in 3 different dose combinations per month. These are advantageous because they follow more closely the physiological hormonal fluctuations which occur in the normal menstrual cycle.
4. The mini pill contains progestin only and causes irregular bleeding.

In Nigeria, the most commonly available tablets are the combined ones. Each packet contains 21 tablets of the hormonal preparation, however some manufacturers make packets of 28 tablets containing 21 hormonal tablets and 7 placebo or iron tablets. In the method of use, 21 tablets are taken on consecutive days and then there are 7 tablet free days during which time withdrawal bleeding will occur (mimicking the menstrual period).

If the preparation contains 7 placebo tablets these are taken instead of having 7 tablet free days. The same withdrawal bleeding will be experienced.

Some other hormonal preparations are:

1. The long acting injections such as Depo-provera and Noristerat.
2. Progestin releasing IUD's.
3. Hormonal vaginal rings.
4. Hormonal implants.

Mechanism of Action

The main action is to suppress ovulation by inhibiting the secretion of the gonodotrophic hormones (follicular stimulating hormone and luteinising hormone) from the pituitary gland. This suppression is effected by the high levels of oestrogen and progestin maintained by the daily intake of the pill. The pill also causes an alteration in the consistency of the cervical mucous, making it thicker and more impenetrable to sperm, as well as altering the endometrial lining.

Contraindications to Use

1. *Thrombosis:* Any woman who gives a history of having had thrombotic episodes of any kind should on no account use the pill. Although the risks of developing thrombotic episodes, while on the pill, have been reduced by the low dose oestrogen pills, which are the only pills available now, studies have shown that the risks of developing cardiovas-

cular disease increase in women who are hypertensive, obese, diabetic, are over 35, and smoke heavily.

2. *Liver disease:* Women who have chronic liver disease or have had hepatitis recently or give a history of cholestatic jaundice during pregnancy should not be on the pill. The pill is metabolized in the liver and if there is severe liver damage this may affect the breakdown of the pill causing higher levels of the hormones to be present and thereby increasing the side effects of the pill.
3. *Cancer of the breast or the reproductive system:* Although the pill does not cause breast or genital cancer, it must not be given to any woman suffering from these cancers. Oestrogen dependent breast cancers can spread more rapidly and the presence of endometrial cancer and adenocarcinoma of the cervix are also complete contraindications to the use of the pills.

Hypertension

The pills can sometimes unmask hypertension and cause a woman whose blood pressure was normal, to rise to hypertensive levels. It is therefore a contraindication to start any woman who has a blood pressure of 140/90 and above, on the pill. If a woman does develop a rise in blood pressure up to 140/90 after being placed on the pill she should be taken off it immediately. In some cases the blood pressure subsides but occasionally the rise may persist, requiring further treatment.

Chronic Disease

Oral contraceptives can be given to women who are receiving treatment for leprosy, malaria, and schistosomiasis. Sickle cell disease sufferers should not be placed on the pill. Although studies do not suggest that the pill can cause crisis to occur, patients on the pill often report an apparent increase in the episodes of crisis they experience while on the pill. Diabetics should not be placed on the pill because the alteration in carbohydrate metabolism which occurs may alter their insulin requirement. In addition diabetes is a risk factor in the development of thrombotic episodes in combination with the pill.

Migraine and Depression

A woman giving a history of migraine attacks may find that her attacks are more severe and more frequent while she is on the pill. Women who have had or who are under treatment for psychiatric illness, especially depressive illness, should not be prescribed the pill as it can affect the mood and cause depression.

Relative Contraindications

Very obese women may find that using the pill causes an increase in weight. If the weight increase is greater than 2 kg and is progressive, then it is appropriate to change her to another form of contraception.

Lactation may be reduced substantially if the pill is used in women who have just started breast feeding. It is therefore advisable to delay giving the pill until lactation is well established at between 3–6 months. By that time the child may be in the early weaning stages and therefore has an alternative intake of food, apart from just the breast milk.

Side Effects

These are usually minor and can be managed. In many cases all that is needed is re-assurance.

1. *Breakthrough bleeding*

   This may sometimes be persistent and is often caused by a patient either forgetting to take her pill regularly at the same time of day or forgetting to take them daily. It can be managed by having the woman take two contraceptive pills per day for 2–3 days.

2. *Scanty menstruation*

   The pill can cause a period to be dark and scanty and in some instances amenorhoea can occur. If a period is missed the pill should be stopped until pregnancy is excluded, as there is a high rate of patient failure in the Nigerian environment. It is not advisable for the pills to be taken in early pregnancy because of a risk of possible congenital defects.

3. *Vaginal discharge*

   Occasionally women on the pill experience increased vaginal discharge which is very often found to be caused by candida albicans (moniliasis). This is due to the fact that there is a reduction in the acid barrier provided by the vaginal secretions and therefore organisms and yeasts such as monilia have a better chance of growing.

4. *Headache*

   This may occur in some women especially towards the end of a cycle of pills. Care must be taken in getting a history to distinguish it from a normal tension headache or migraine.

5. *Pregnancy symptoms*

   In the first few months of use of the pill some women experience nausea, vomiting, abdominal distension, weakness, breast tenderness and enlargement and this may lead them to believe that they are pregnant. These symptoms and signs usually disappear spontaneously at around 3–4 months, once the body has adjusted to the new hormonal levels.

6. *Weight gain*

   A weight gain of 2–4 kg may occur with the pills, however a greater weight gain may require to be investigated and may result in the pill being stopped.

7. *Libido*

   This may be affected and some women may complain of a decrease in libido. On the other hand some women find that once the fear of pregnancy has been removed, their libido increases substantially.

The Long Acting Injectable

The compound used as long acting contraceptives are Depo provera (medroxy progesterone acetate) and Noristerat (norethindrone enanthate). These are given intramuscularly every 3 or 2 months respectively.

The injections act by suppressing ovulation and they also cause eventual atrophy of the endometrial lining leading to amenorrhoea. As they do not contain any oestrogenic compound, they are unlikely to cause thrombosis. However, in view of the fact that once the injection is given there is no way of counteracting the effects, it is usual to apply similar criteria used for the pills, for contraindications of use.

There is no evidence that the long acting injections cause cancer in humans or that they can contribute to the spread of cancer. In addition they do not cause liver diseases but, as they are metabolized in the liver, care must be taken in evaluating their use in women with a history of liver disease.

There is also no proof yet that they unmask hypertension, but if anyone on the injectable does develop hypertension, she should be placed on another form of contraception.

Finally, the major disadvantage of the injectables is that they cause complete disruption of the menstrual cycle, which can result in heavy prolonged bleeding, or irregular bleeding with spotting or complete amenorrhoea. It is therefore important that careful counselling is given to women using the injectables.

Progestin Releasing IUD's

These were introduced in the 1970s and allow for a local delivery of the hormone. The progestasert is a T-shaped device containing 38mg of progesterone which is released at a controlled rate for a year. It has the effect of suppressing the normal cyclical changes in the endometrium, making implantation of a fertilized ovum impossible. The main disadvantage is that it has to be replaced yearly and there can be frequent intermenstrual bleeding and spotting.

Hormonal Vaginal Rings

These rings are circular tubes containing hormones, which are inserted into the vagina in the area of the cervix. One type, which prevents ovulation, releases both oestrogen and progestin. The second type is a ring that releases low levels of progestin only which is thought to prevent pregnancy by action on the cervical mucous and the endometrium.

The two methods of use are:

1. The progestin only ring is kept in the vagina for three weeks at a time and is removed for one week during which time withdrawal bleeding occurs.
2. The combined hormonal ring is kept in the vagina for three months.

Possible side effects are the development of a vaginal erosion or vaginal irritation.

Implants

The implants are made of silastic, either as hollow capsules filled with progestin or as solid rods impregnated with the hormone. They are approximately 2–4 cm long with an outside diameter of 2.4mm.

The implants are placed under the skin with a trocar using a local anaesthetic and a small incision of 5mm is made for the removal which is also done under a local anaesthetic.

The hormone most often used is levonorgestrel and the release of the hormone takes place over a period of 5 years.

Possible side effects are infection and the possibility of keloid formation if repeated insertions and removals are done at the same site.

Other Forms of Contraception

Lactation and Sexual Abstinence

In many cultures child bearing practices involve sexual abstention for varying periods of time, usually related to the length of time needed for breast feeding and the completion of the weaning period.

Although return of ovulation is delayed when a woman fully breast feeds her baby, the time at which return to fertility occurs will vary from woman to woman and the precise time of return to fertility may be difficult to assess. It is therefore important that once sexual relationships are started, the woman must be placed on an effective and appropriate form of contraception or the husband must use the condom.

Barrier Forms of Contraception

These act by forming a barrier between the sperm deposited by the male in the upper vagina and the cervix and uterus.

The condom, which is used by males, consists of a thin rubber sheath which is rolled over the erect penis just prior to coitus. Care must be taken after coitus to remove the condom and discard it without allowing any spillage to occur in the vicinity of the vulval area. The modern condoms are coloured, lubricated for greater sensitivity, and must be used only once and then be discarded.

The diaphragm, unlike the condom, must be fitted by a doctor or nurse to ensure the correct vaginal fit. The diaphragm is dome shaped and is made of rubber and comes in different sizes. After each new delivery a new fitting must be made to ensure that the diaphragm will be effective.

Prior to coitus, the diaphragm is placed in the vault of the vagina where it covers the cervical mucous. It must be left in place for 6–8 hours after the last coitus, before being removed. After removal, the diaphragm should be washed with toilet soap and water and kept in a clean container until the next use.

The diaphragm can be left in place for up to 24 hours at a time after which it should be removed for washing and for personal hygiene. Both the condom and diaphragm can be used in conjunction with spermicidal jellies or creams to increase their effectiveness.

Spermicidal Agents

These consist of vaginal creams, jellies and foams which are inserted into the vagina (using a special applicator) shortly before coitus. The spermicides should be inserted not more than 30 minutes and not less than 5 minutes before coitus. If coitus is repeated again, a fresh application should be made.

The vaginal foams are the most effective of these methods and are usually used alone, unlike the creams and jellies which are commonly used with the condoms and diaphragms.

Rhythm Method

This method is based on the normal physiological menstrual cycle. A woman who has a normal 28-day cycle is most likely to ovulate between the 10th – 18th day of her menstrual cycle. By avoiding coitus during that week she is not likely to become pregnant. However it has been shown that the rhythm method is not a very efficient method of contraception as there is a very high failure rate.

Another way of calculating the fertile period in women whose cycles are irregular, is to subtract 18 from the number of days in the shortest menstrual cycle, for the first potentially fertile day, and for the last fertile day, subtract 11 from the longest menstrual cycle.

The Billing's Method is a variation on the rhythm method where a woman abstains from coitus during the period of time in her menstrual cycle that she produces a tacky cervical secretion, which is an indication of ovulation.

Sterilization

Both male and female sterilization can be performed. In the male this is called vasectomy and in this operation the vas deferens are cut and tied to prevent the sperm being released through the vas deferens into the urethra, during ejaculation. The operation is a minor one and can be performed under a local anaesthetic.

In the female, the modern methods of sterilization involve the use of sophisticated equipment. The laprascope can be used through the abdominal route or the culdoscope, by the vaginal route. The fallopian tubes are either cut and tied or cuterized with diathermy.

The advantage of these newer operative procedures, is that the patients do not require to be hospitalized for more than a day or two. In some cases the sterilization can be reversed; however the success rate of complete reversal with pregnancy resulting varies with the experience of the surgeon and is still very low.

Abortion

Abortion, as such, is not a form of contraception. However in many countries it has been legalized and has been made a much safer procedure so that some women tend to regard it as an alternative to regular contraception rather than as a back up to failed contraception.

The usual methods of performing legal abortion are by:

1. Menstrual regulation where negative pressure is applied to a catheter attached to a syringe, which is placed in the uterus, and the endometrial lining is sucked into the syringe. This procedure should be performed within six weeks of the last menstrual period.
2. Vacuum suction is another method which is used for pregnancies of 6–12 weeks.
3. Saline injection into the amniotic sac of the foetus, is used for pregnancies up to 16 – 24 weeks. This causes premature labour with expulsion of the foetus.
4. Prostaglandins are also available for use to dilate the cervix and cause expulsion of the foetus.
5. Dilation and curettage is one of the older methods of performing abortions in pregnancies of less than twelve weeks, however one of the possible complications is perforation of the uterus.

Frequent resort to abortions can cause problems such as pelvic infection and secondary infertility and the effective use of efficient and safe forms of contraception is to be preferred.

References

Billings E. & Westmore A. (1982) *The Billings Method,* Richard Clay The Chaucer Press Ltd., Bungay Sufolk.

Family Planning Methods and Practice: Africa. Centre for Disease Control Atlanta, 1983.

Fryer P. (1967) *The Birth Controllers.* Transworld Publishers Limited, London.

Kleinman L. Ronald (ed.) (1980) *Family Planning Handbook for Doctors.* International Planned Parenthood Federation 5th Ed.

Porter Cedric W., Waife Roland S. & Holtrop Hugh R. *The Pathfinder Fund USA,* 1983.

43

Student and Staff Medical Services

Adebola Ore-Olorun Erinoso

Definition

Student and staff medical services refer to the type of medical services delivered for the benefit of students and staff in a tertiary educational institution such as the polytechnics, colleges of education, or the universities, whether state-owned or federal-owned. Such students are under continuous mental stress for their academic studies and need special medical attention, care and advice.

Objectives

The objectives of an African health service for tertiary institutions are as follows:

(i) to provide a comprehensive community health service for the students and staff;

(ii) to provide a comprehensive health service including food hygiene and, prevention of all forms of accident;

(iii) to provide ample social welfare and social development services;

(iv) to advise on adequate nutrition both for students, and more especially for the junior staff members and their families. To offer health education to all, including senior and junior staff, and especially pregnant women and the under-five children of the junior staff;

(v) to provide a student health counselling service directed mainly towards preventing diseases to which students and staff of tertiary institutions are particularly liable, such as mental and nervous breakdown, venereal diseases and also to encourage all students to study hard, play well and relax fully at all times;

(vi) to provide advice, immunization, and the necessary health examinations for all travellers, especially for senior officials and academic staff who may have cause to travel abroad either as consultants, or on a course or during the annual leave;

(vii) to co-ordinate and integrate the institutional health services with those of neighbouring government and private health clinics in the further promotion of a comprehensive health service for the entire staff and students of tertiary institutions. This is necessary because many students and staff who are not offered intramural accommodation often reside in rented houses near and around the institution.

The Promotion of Family Health

The staff medical services at any tertiary institution should extend to the wife and children of all the members of staff i.e. both senior and junior.

This is to minimize the time wastage of a lecturer taking members of his family to one of the nearby hospitals. In the past, even if a staff member had 12 children, they were all entitled to receive free medical services. However, since the commencement of SAP (Structural Adjustment Programme for our economic recovery) only one wife and four (4) children are treated free of charge, e.g. at the University Health Services in Ibadan and The Polytechnic, Ibadan. If there is a second wife and other children, i.e. more than 4 in number these others are treated as bill cases i.e. the member of staff is billed to pay for their treatment. This system has been adopted by the University Health Services too.

Children of staff members are usually treated free of charge only when they are under 18 years of age. However, between the ages of 19 and 25 years if the dependent is still in a higher institution of learning, he is still allowed to continue to utilize the medical services free until he is out of the institution, and is either gainfully employed or independent.

Special Health Problems in African Tertiary Institutions

As there is poor coverage of basic health services, inadequate health manpower, equipment and financial resources for building health facilities in African countries, well over seventy per cent of the students, junior staff members and their dependants may never have had any medical examination in any form in their lives before being admitted to, or employed in an African tertiary institution. As a result, the compulsory pre-entry and pre-employment medical examinations for students and staff respectively often reveal a variety of pathologies. In addition the attendance at out-patient clinics of new students and staff, especially in newly established African tertiary institutions, tends to be high.

The high out-patient attendance often misleads newly established African tertiary institutions to relax their efforts to enforce a policy of compulsory pre-entry and pre-employment medical examinations; and this sometimes results in premature deaths of brilliant young academicians and students from diseases such as acute renal failure, diabetic coma, and other rapidly fatal conditions which could have been detected earlier.

Some institutions do not insist that the Chief Medical Officer or Director of institution health services possesses specialist qualifications and adequate experience in public health. Such unqualified personnel therefore often prove ineffective in advising or assisting the chief officers of the tertiary institutions (vice-chancellors, rectors, registrars, as well as the governing council members) to undertake health planning on campus; to provide health institutions or rented houses for staff and students; to prescribe healthy housing standards; or to provide clean potable water, balanced diet, welfare facilities, and other essential health services for the Institutions.

Some still do not include professionals and experts in public health on the relevant committees.

It is essential that the senior officials in tertiary institutions, who are often non-medical, should trust senior community health staff to advise them and their committees on the active practice of integrated health, and not merely run a curative medical service directed to nothing better than the simple prescription of drugs.

Medical Examination

Four types of medical examination can be performed within the institution.

(i) Pre-admission Medical Examination

This relates to all new students in the institution. The medical examination is comprehensive and includes the measurement of the students' weight and height as well as testing of their visual acuity by Snellen's chart, urine examination for albumin and sugar. A physical examination is done and a chest x-ray is taken. Formerly Mantoux test or Heaf test was done to exclude tuberculosis, but the reagents are now very scarce and extremely expensive in the country.

It is mandatory for every student to be certified medically fit by the attending physician before being registered in the faculty. This is to ensure that a disease like tuberculosis is not spread amongst the students.

(ii) Pre-employment Medical Examination

All appointments including the renewal of contract appointments are normally subject to medical examination. Only those certified fit are allowed to take up any appointment.

(iii) Periodical Medical Examination

It is done occasionally or on request to ascertain that no medical problem is being overlooked.

(iv) Post-illness Examination

This examination is undertaken for students or staff who have been involved in a protracted illness e.g. a serious road-traffic accident, a psychiatric problem or any other severe debilitating illness.

This is to ascertain if the student can still cope with his studies or if the member of staff is still capable of working or if he needs to be re-deployed to another unit or department.

Sick Leave Certificate

When a staff member is incapacitated from duty through illness, he should present himself to one of the staff doctors at the health centre for examination, treatment and obtainance of an appropriate certificate for excuse duty or light duty as the case may be.

The sick certificate issued is often in triplicate form:

(a) One copy is sent to the Establishment for the confidential file of the staff member;

(b) The second copy is sent to his Head of Department;

(c) The third copy is retained at the health centre for his medical records.

Sick certificates obtained from neighbouring hospitals or hospitals outside town where such a member of staff is hospitalized must be submitted within 48 hours to the Chief Medical Officer/ Director of Medical Services for countersigning. This is usually sent with the relevant medical report.

Refund of Medical Expenses

In the past, authorized prescriptions or investigations not available at the health centre were usually refunded if undertaken elsewhere.

When students or staff members are referred to neighbouring hospitals for admission, the expenses are refunded if the Medical Officer authorizes it and the funds are available.

Today, most medical bills arising from such referral cannot be refunded by the majority of tertiary institutions.

Health Education

This can be undertaken daily during consultation, or occasional lectures can be given to the student body and staff using audio-visual methods, e.g. films on venereal diseases, immunization, sex education, sanitation, etc.

Treatment Outside Nigeria

The Vice-Chancellor or Rector on the recommendation of the Director of Medical Services or Chief Medical Officer or of a Medical Board, may authorize the reference of a case for treatment outside Nigeria provided the Director or Medical Services or the Medical Board, as the case may be, is satisfied that such treatment is not available in the country.

Medical Board

If a staff member is unable to resume work when his authorized sick leave is exhausted, a report of the Medical Board will be obtained. The Medical Board will be composed of the Director of Medical Services as chairman and one or two medical officers as members, out of which one should be, as far as possible, the doctor who is treating the person concerned.

Orientation for Fresh Students

At the beginning of every session, a lecture is delivered by the Director of Medical Services to all freshmen to acquaint them with the medical services available in the institution and to take them on a tour of the (Medical Department) Health Centre.

Tips for Good Health

1. *Meals:* Students are encouraged to take *three* balanced meals a day and not substitute snacks and a drink for lunch. Today in some institutions, students eat only one or two meals a day due to financial constraints.
2. *Sleep:* It is desirable to have a six hour sleep per night. This refreshes one and relaxes the brain.
3. *Exercises:* Engage in these daily. These can be breathing exercises, walking, jogging, skipping, swimming, table tennis, lawn tennis, badminton, netball or football.
4. *Drugs:* Avoid drug abuse and misuse; it could lead to physiological complications. It is not desirable to mix orthodox medicine with alternative medicine. It can be harmful.
5. *Smoking and Alcohol:* Smoking causes lung cancer. It can cause chronic lung problems and a painful death. It is desirable to avoid it. Excessive alcohol intake may cause yellow eyes and a swollen tummy full of fluid. Remember, if you drink, don't drive and if you drive don't drink!
6. *Venereal Disease:* This is still common in our environment and AIDS is the latest scourge in this line. The disease has no cure. So, please keep to one sexual partner. It is safer.
7. *Cleanliness:* Cleanliness eliminates skin diseases like eczema, ringworm, ticks, head louse, etc. Efforts should be made to wash towels and beddings every week and underwear every day.

Medicare Available

(a) Daily consultation by doctors.

(b) Giving of daily injection by the nurses.

(c) Dressing of wounds daily, except on Sundays.

(d) *Pregnant female students* After missing a second period, the student should report to the doctor, so she can commence ante-natal care. She is usually referred to a nearby hospital for confinement.

(e) *Hospitalization:* Any students or staff requiring admission into a hospital should be referred for treatment.

(f) *Family Planning:* Various methods of family planning are available – from the condom to the use of the intra-uterine contraceptive device.

(g) *Immunization:* Students and staff or their families can be immunized against cholera and yellow fever when they are travelling abroad. Staff children have immunization facilities against the six communicable diseases namely polio, diphtheria, pertussis, tetanus, measles and tuberculosis.

(h) *Home and Hospital Visits:* Students or staff members who are very ill or are hospitalized are visited in their homes or in hospitals by the health sisters who give their progress reports.

Medical Statistics

During the 1988/89 session a total of 29,242 patients were seen. The statistics attached shows the number of attendance at the Health Centre, The Polytechnic, Ibadan, Oyo State – Annexure I.

During the same period, the type of cases the students presented at the Health Centre, The Polytechnic, Ibadan is shown as Annexure II utilizing the International Classification of Diseases.

Annexure I

Attendance At The Polytechnic Health Centre, Ibadan, Oyo State From 1st October, 1988 - 30th September, 1989

MONTHS	STUDENTS	SENIOR STAFF	SENIOR STTAFF DEPENDANT	JUNIOR STAFF	JUNIOR STAFF DEPENDANT	CORPERS	BILL CASES	MEDICAL EXAM.	IMMUNIZATION	TOTAL
October '88	113	140	531	405	920	5	101	15	23	2,235
November '88	279	432	924	433	558	1	104	217	22	2,970
December '88	186	180	430	383	476	5	88	577	26	2,352
January '89	405	179	515	375	412	2	89	710	23	2,710
February '89	444	113	377	292	360	5	67	334	48	2,040
March '89	418	225	301	346	641	3	26	115	57	2,132
April '89	446	196	435	367	471	6	31	140	53	2,145
May ' 89	625	221	565	485	498	-	65	29	55	2,543
June '89	356	251	618	502	653	13	69	25	89	2,575
July '89	276	183	627	545	593	11	43	11	61	2,350
August '89	539	235	561	593	658	4	68	07	63	2,728
September '89	055	302	578	750	620	18	71	33	65	2,462
									Grand Total	29,424

Annexure II

Infections and Parasitic Diseases	Neoplasm	Endocrine Nutritional and Metabolic Diseases and Immunity Disorders	Diseases of Blood and Blood Forming Organs	Mental Disorders	Diseases of the Nervous System and Sense Organs	Diseases of the Circulatory System	Diseases of the Respiratory System
001 - 139	140-239	240 - 279	280 - 289	290-319	320-359	390-459	460-519
M.F 751 Otitis 20 Drancuntiasis 15 Chickenpox 3 Conjunctivitis 22 Carbum 35 Dental Caries 12 Whitlow 10		Dysmen 25 Avitaminosis 25	Sickle cell 3	Neurosis 41	Tension Headache 20 Neuralgia 10 Arthralgia 15 Glaucoma 5 Myopia 20 Hypochrondiasis 1	Hypertension 25 Anaemia 5	U.R.T.I. & Coryza 140 Asth. 15 Pneum 10 Kock's 5 Tonsillitis & Pharyngitis 30
868		50	3	43	71	30	200

Diseases of the Digestive System	Diseases of the Genito-urinary System	Complications of Pregnancy child-birth and the Puerperium	Diseases of the Skin Subcutaneous Tissue	Diseases of the Musculo-Skeletal Systems and connective tissue	Congenital Anomalies	Certain Conditions Originating in the Perinatal Period	Symptoms Signs and Ill-defined Conditions	Injury and Poisoning
520 - 579	580 - 629	630 - 676	680 - 709	710 - 739	740 - 759	760 - 779	780 - 799	800 - 999
E.N.T. 122 D.U. 25 Helm. 32 App. 111 Haemorrh 10 Gingivitis 10	G.U. & U.T.I 33 Dysuria 20 P.I.D. 2	Cycsis 11	Cellu. 30 Derm. 75 Allergy 25 Furunculosis 25 Skinsepsis & Uriticaria 26	Myalgia 55 Carbun. 35 Arthritis 10			P.U.O. 2	R.T.A. 20 Snake Bite 1 Human Bite 1
Total 310	55	11	181	100	0	0	2	2

44

Occupational Health Services

G.O. Sofoluwe

History

Ramazzinic, born in 1641, is internationally acclaimed as the father of occupational health in the world. He was the first to document accurate observations of the diseases, hazards, and toxicity experienced by persons undertaking different occupations. His treatise still remains a guide for all workers in the field of occupational health.

Industrialization, which has revolutionized the world, also brought in its train social problems of almost unconquerable dimensions. As men at different periods of their lives seem to manifest different levels of tolerance to the various physical, chemical, and biological stresses to which they may be subjected, the scope of occupational health has gradually been extended to include anthropometry, ergonomics, environmental monitoring, and toxicological and welfare services.

Africa is the latest arrival into the industrialization programme and consequently has the youngest and in many cases the most ineffective occupational health programmes. It has however a splendid opportunity to correct the mistakes of the earlier industrialized nations. The Ministries of Labour in some African countries should be congratulated for blazing the trail of occupational health services on the continent through their Factories Inspectorate Divisions.

Similarly the International Labour Organization (ILO) and the World Health Organization (WHO) and many bilateral agencies have contributed both technically and financially to the development of the occupational health services in Africa.

The principles of running an effective occupational health practice in Africa will therefore be described here for the guidance of young physicians.

Occupational health services include the promotion and the maintenance of the health of all workers. Formerly the largest industries and the mines were the only ones provided with occupational health services, but nowadays such services are being developed in large, medium, and some small-scale industries.

Medical Examinations and Occupational Health Screening

The first line of defence in the prevention of occupational diseases and accidents, and in minimizing hazards and toxicity, consists of the series of medical examinations which can be carried out on prospective part- or full-time employees. These include *pre-employment medical examinations* which aim to ensure that the prospective employee is medically fit to work in any of the multifarious units or departments in the establishment. A minor argument exists about whether such examination benefits the worker or the employer. In Africa, where unemployment is rife, employers, especially those from countries with underdeveloped occupational health services, still tend to underestimate the importance of such examinations, and prefer to eliminate their sick, and especially their chronically ill worker in order to replace them with others from the abundant labour market of the unemployed.

Pre-placement medical examinations: A partially blind person might be employed as a lift attendant in a brewery, he certainly could not be employed as a sighter in the same brewery. Whereas a sickler might be employed as a clerk by an airline, he almost certainly could not be employed as the pilot of a jumbo jet. Pre-placement medical examinations, therefore, aim to fit workers in different jobs in terms with their health status.

The new terms of 'occupational health screening' is now made to refer to the two types of medical examinations mentioned above. As industrialization and scientific inventions increase, the scope of such medical examinations is steadily getting widened, refined, and assessed to cut down cost and enhance productivity. Therefore special codes for the medical examinations of airline pilots, drivers, and compressed air workers, for example, have now been drawn up and embodied in legislation in developed countries. The United Nations agencies also assist by drawing up codes for these and other similar aspects of occupational health practice for voluntary adoption and implementation by member countries. An up-to-date and valuable publication which scientifically assesses the value of occupational health examinations has been published by the United Kingdom Society of Occupational Medicine, entitled *Health Screening*.

Periodic Medical Examinations: In cases where people engage in hazardous occupations, periodic medical examinations, including special tests and environmental monitoring, are conducted regularly so as to remove the worker fully or temporarily from the work environment if he is succumbing to the hazards or toxicity arising therefrom. For example, workers exposed to lead, mercury, noise, asbestos, fibres, atmospheric pressure, gravity, or ionizing radiation are subject to periodic medical examinations, which have now been codified in many countries of the world. Professor Atherly has directed attention to the need for regular assessment of one such codified periodic medical examination in one of his papers entitled 'Occupational audiometry-its place, functions and evaluation'. He accurately assessed the value, cost, and effectiveness of periodic audiometry for workers exposed to noise. African physicians therefore need not merely undertake such a system of medical examinations for its own sake, but need only do so when it is of value to the employees, employer and the nation. There are also special medical examinations of workers for establishing invalidation, and for obtaining other social security benefits such as workmen's compensation, disability pensions, and so on.

Ergonomics and Anthropometry

Earlier workers in the field of occupational health had demonstrated the importance of making the job suit the physical, mental, and biological make-up of man; and this has led to the development of the occupational health sub-specialties of anthropometry and ergonomics.

Anthropologists make detailed studies of the physical, mental, and biological make-up of man; while ergonomics, including machine designer, engineers, and industrial psychologist, utilize the derived knowledge to design machines, machine controls, and the vast array of industrial tools and home equipment.

Sofoluwe (1967) conducted a survey on how far ergonomic principles were applied in a representative sample of industries in Lagos, the erstwhile capital of Nigeria. He showed that there was a lot of ignorance on the use of the in-built ergonomic principles in the imported tools and machines: for example, the tailors in a textile factory suffered chronic pain in the back and the knee joints owing to their failure to adjust the seats of their sewing machines to their anthropometric measurements. It was also found that some imported machinery had been designed for the anthropometric measurements of industrialized nations, and did not include any device to adjust them for the smaller Africans. A brewery lost hundreds of bottles of brew until the conveyor belt was adjusted six inches lower, to the eye level of the sighters. Urgent research on ergonomics, anthropometry, machine design, and industrial psychology are now needed in Africa.

Environmental Monitoring for Physical Hazards, Chemical and Radiation Toxicity

Man has been exposed, for example, to heavy metal–leads, mercury, etc., for centuries before their deleterious effects were discovered. Earlier means of control, treatment, and prevention had therefore consisted mainly of biological monitoring, including testing for lead and mercury in urine, blood and other body fluids. Judicious interpretation of these results has developed to such a point that thereafter accuracies could only be enhanced by simultaneous interpretations of the results of biological and environmental monitoring. In some developed countries, up to about twenty to thirty years ago, workers could be compensated if they had more than certain quantities of toxic materials such as lead in their blood, urine, etc.; and this constituted the sole evidence of their having been poisoned during their work. More refined modern methods, including continuous environmental monitoring for lead at all the different points at which the workers have been officially engaged in working, now produce clear evidence as to whether the worker was or was not been exposed to dangerous quantities of the toxic substance in the course of his employment. It has thus now become possible for the employer to claim no liability on the grounds that the worker must have been exposed to toxic materials outside his place of employment. In fact, it is now possible to trace lead brought home on the clothing of workers; and hence strict regulations have been enacted covering the provision of protective clothing, washrooms, changing rooms, etc., to limit the spread of toxic materials to the homes of workers.

Fortunately, engineers, chemists, and machine designers have introduced automatic and easily manipulable equipment to monitor the effects of (i) physical hazards such as heat, inadequate ventilation, radiation, light, colour, humidity, atmospheric pressure, noise, vibration, and static electricity; (ii) chemical and toxic effects; and (iii) biological effects from, for example, allergens from plant and animal sources, atmospheres impregnated with vegetable fibres, and so on.

An effective occupational health physician in Africa, irrespective of whether he is employed in a big industry, where both an occupational health hygienist and a doctor specially responsible for human and environmental monitoring, or in the numerous small industries, would do well to keep abreast of knowledge in this field and apply it judiciously to enhance productivity and promote comprehensive health in his workplace.

As many big new industries are sited in newly inhabited areas, the African occupational health physician has to include environmental health duties. Thus he will advise management on town and village planning; on housing, water supply, sewage and refuse disposal, and drainage; and on food hygiene, and measures against soil, water, air, and other forms of pollution; and on other environmental sanitation measures. He may have to advise on the development and maintenance of recreational facilities; and on appropriate 'keep fit' exercises. In multi-million naira projects of industries, consultants are usually employed to design the environmental health projects, and the occupational health doctor has only to maintain them. The doctor is usually assisted by health superintendents and his sanitary team.

First Aid, Emergency, Routine Curative Treatment, and Nursing Facilities

The majority of industries in Africa (with the notable exception of those large industries which merely establish branches in Africa, while the parent organization remains based in Europe and America) merely employ physicians on a part-time basis to conduct pre-employment examinations and treat employees on demand. Such doctors are referred to as 'retainers'. They are usually private or public sector practitioners, including university physicians. The companies obtain tax relief for their expenditure on such services. Unfortunately, as the majority of such doctors are not trained, the present practice is almost entirely curative. The majority of the physicians now employed do not visit the industries, and are not competent to assess or to correct the numerous hazards and toxicities to which the workers are exposed; and, worse still, they are not able to undertake environmental health monitoring. In short, most industries in Africa have not realized the importance of and the benefits accruing from employing physicians with training and experience in occupational health. Governments hitherto have not felt concerned enough to regulate such practices by enforcing the International Labour Organization (ILO) Recommendation 112. African universities through their medical, engineering, and nursing schools could thus assist the government by sponsoring training programmes for all doctors, nurses, managers, personnel officers, and engineers, and all health and health-related officials in all working places – to include not only industries, but hospitals, shops, and other appropriate fields for the practice of occupational health – so that they could all be stimulated to implement the recommendations.

However, adequate provisions for first aid in every unit of the industry, and clinics run by nurses, physicians, physiotherapist, radiographers and auxiliaries, are the minimum requirements for the establishment of any occupational health service in all working places in Africa. Scientific manpower studies are also required, to advise on the numbers of staff required per population of workers per industry.

Good record-keeping is the backbone of a successful occupational health practice in Africa; and all industries should be assisted to keep useful health records.

The occupational health physician should be able to relate smoothly and effectively with management, shop floor supervisors, workers, trade unions, safety officers, and interested parties outside the factory, such as, for example, universities, government hospitals, medical associations, Ministries of Labour and Health, and other public, private and voluntary organizations and welfare agencies.

The occupational health service should have first class facilities for undertaking resuscitation and emergency treatment, and for the evacuation of the injured to hospitals. The physician should make a preliminary visit to the workers (before he starts work) to list the processes which will be liable to generate emergencies or dangerous occurrences, and compile a schedule or drill for dealing with such possible emergencies.

It is necessary here to mention that Africa has added sales promotion to the scope of occupational health nursing, as many drug firms and food factories employ nurses as sales promoters and representatives. Thus they sell and advertise milk and food products, as well as cosmetics, etc., some of them retaining as part of their duties the well-organized normal occupational health duties of an occupational health nurse in developed countries.

Occupational nurses in Africa constitute the first, and in many cases, the only health-team members engaged in many enterprises, even including large-scale ones such as dams, construction companies, and breweries, which are often unsupervised by any doctor whatsoever. Radwanski, Pickering and Sofoluwe successfully initiated refresher courses for occupational health nurses in Lagos, Nigeria in 1970; and Sofoluwe similarly introduced occupational health courses in Lusaka, Zambia in 1973; while Oleru and Olugbile also ran similar courses in Ibadan and Lagos in 1978. These courses were specially adapted to African situations. There is now a need to extend such training courses to retainer physicians, full-time occupational health physicians, hygienists, engineers, safety officers, auxiliary health workers, ergonomists, industrial psychologists, physiotherapists, and the other occupational health team members previously mentioned.

Safety and Accident Control and Prevention in African Industries

Prevention of accidents in industries employing more than twenty persons was pioneered by the Factories Inspectorate Divisions of the Ministry of Labour in all English- and French-speaking countries in Africa. Details of the programmes can be read in the proceedings of the 1968 Lagos 'International Symposium on Occupational Health in Developing Countries', edited by Wassermann & Sofoluwe.

Factories inspectors, who were usually civil, mechanical, electrical, or other engineers, visited industries regularly to ensure that all safety regulations detailed in the Factories Acts (modelled on the 1945 Acts in Britain and France) were obeyed. They also educated employers, workers and all concerned on the prevention of accidents. National Industrial Safety Council, composed of representatives of management, and trade unions and the Factories Inspectorate of the Ministry of Labour are formed to regularly discuss and formulate policies, and to educate management and workers on safety measures. Regular seminars and conferences are held, and periodicals and journals are published whose objects is to create an awareness that will minimize the rate of accidents at work.

In 1968 the Nigerian Ministries of Labour and Health and the University of Lagos, with assistance from both the International Labour Organization and the World Health Organization, and in co-operation with the Permanent Commission and the International Occupational Health Association sponsored the Lagos International Symposium on Occupational Health for Developing Countries. Representatives from nearly all the African countries attended and read papers. The developed countries in America and Europe were also well represented. The proceedings of the 1968 symposium (which are still obtainable from the Department of Community Health, College of Medicine, Universities of Lagos, Nigeria) documented in details all aspects of the then existing occupational health services in Africa, and fully described the formulation of policies and the problems encountered in all parts of Africa and the developed countries.

In summary, safety and accident control and prevention in African countries need to include the following measures: notification of all accidents and dangerous occurrences to whichever of the Ministries of Labour, Agriculture, Forestry, or Mines is appropriate; the formation of safety committees and the appointment of safety officers in all industries; education of employers, management, employees, trade union officials, and everyone involved in industry; research by doctors, engineers, industrial psychologists, etc., from universities and related institutions on the active prevention of accidents in all workplaces; drills based on scientifically accurate data for dealing with those accidents which will nonetheless inevitably occur, and with the evacuation of those affected to treatment centres; appointment of first aid officers both on the shop floor and in clinics, as well as the provision of comprehensive first aid equipment in all industries; provision of safety libraries, including data on existing knowledge on accident prevention and on the promotion of comprehensive safety in all undertakings including officers and transport industries, and also good records on accidents and dangerous occurrences, which should be kept both by the workplaces and by the factories inspectorate statutorily charged with keeping such records, with the ultimate objective of preventing such accidents in the future.

Rehabilitation

African countries are now gradually developing rehabilitation agencies and building rehabilitation facilities. The limited existing facilities are linked with orthopeadic services. They include limb-fitting and maintenance units; physiotherapy units; and rehabilitation facilities for the blind, deaf, and physically or mentally crippled. They are still far from being comprehensive, and the provisions differ in extent in the different countries.

The African occupational health physician needs to have accurate knowledge of the existing rehabilitation facilities. The physician should also be able to arrange both medical and vocational rehabilitation for all workers under his care.

Welfare Service

The African occupational health physicians and nurses, as well as personnel managers and public relation officers and consultants, should be able to provide the wide spectrum of welfare services which are required for Africans who have been removed from relatively stable villages to face the great variety of social problems in the cities and settlements where industries now exist.

Adequate liaison with the government and private or voluntary welfare agencies are essential for the purpose. Thus the Chief Occupational Health Physicians on plantations, dams, oil rigs and refineries, universities, and other industries sited in new settlements would also need to serve as Chief Social Welfare Officers in those places, which often in effect constitute 'new towns' in Africa.

Provisions for the child in need of care, for marriage guidance, and for juvenile delinquents, for schemes to settle matrimonial problems and prevent divorce and separation, a need to be made by the African occupational health physician. It must however be stressed that as African industries provide Africans with much needed employment, they should also provide simultaneously a variety of welfare services which assist the employed to provide the basic necessities of life for their relatives and extended family members. Thus a close study of an oil palm research station in

Nigeria, with a population of workers and their relatives of about 700, revealed that all the workers – both senior and junior – provided welfare services for their aged parents, nephews, nieces, cousins and many other groups of extended family members. It is essential therefore that all industries in Africa should include adequate provisions for this in their policy for the provision of housing, schools, and health facilities. The Nigerian Tobacco Factory in Ibadan, Nigeria, stimulated by its trade union, granted financial services to the wives, children and extended family members of their employees at a cost – a scheme partially paid for by the employees, but heavily subsidized by the employer. The management was well rewarded with a drastic reduction in sickness, absence and a much increased productivity.

Government regulations exist for the provision of funds for pensions, superannuation, and workmen's compensation, and for National Provident Funds, etc. The African occupational health physician needs to have accurate knowledge of these, and should liaise with the personnel officer in inducing management to extend such provisions beyond the minimum provided for by the government.

Occupational Health Legislation

To date only rather limited legislation exists in Africa in the field of occupational health. The big industries and employers of labour in Africa, however, often operate the stipulations of the existing occupational health legislation in the developed countries in which they originate to the benefit of African countries. Many African countries assent to the Occupational Health Recommendations and Regulations and the other stipulations of the International Labour Organization (ILO), WHO, UNIDO, and other United Nations agencies. Occupational health physicians in Africa need therefore to keep abreast of such occupational health legislation, regulations, and codes of behaviour as are stipulated by the United Nations agencies and enforced in the developed countries of Europe, America, and Asia, especially as they need to supervise the health of many nationals from such countries who are now employed in African industries.

Health Education for Occupational Health Development in Africa

The low level of technological development in African countries makes it very expensive to obey health legislation. For example, an employer was quite prepared to pay for the manufacture and instalment of a guard to his machinery, although there was no such machinery available for purchase, nor was there any agency or unit in that African country which could manufacture it. Thus the cost of importing such guards, and of course the delay which would be necessitated in their use would create conditions for accidents, injuries, and deaths in some industries.

Thus active and comprehensive health education facilities are needed for employers, employees, trade unions, government ministries, and the entire public, including the workers' families, to inform them of the hazards, toxicities, and other health problems encountered in workplaces.

Employers, employees, and voluntary agencies such as Chambers of Commerce, as well as government-sponsored National Industrial Safety Councils, Trade Union Schools, Universities, Colleges of Technology, and Schools of Agriculture and Forestry are resource centres for health education and information in the field of occupational health. The African occupational health physician could also usefully subscribe to the International Labour Organization's 'Abstracts of occupational health and hygiene', as well as join his local society of occupational/health physicians or other similar societies in the African countries, Europe, or America, or subscribe to the publications of the Permanent Commission and the International Association of Occupational Health to keep abreast of occupational health development in his special field.

Special Industries of Particular Importance to Africa

African occupational health physicians need to be very conversant with the hazards, toxicity and other health problems existing in the occupations peculiar to the continent. These include the following:

(1) traditional or subsistence farming, undertaken by over eighty per cent of Africa, especially in the villages; the newly emergent large mechanized farms and other agro-based industries;
(2) plantations – for example, cocoa, oil palm, rubber, coffee, tea and sugar cane plantations;
(3) forest reserves, tree felling and saw mills;
(4) mines – for example in Nigeria tin and coal mines, in Zambia copper, lead, and zinc mines, in Ghana gold mines, in Gabon radium and manganese mines, and in Zaire diamond mines;
(5) oil drilling, production, and refineries:
(6) associated manufacture of chemicals from oil and oil products;
(7) textile mills, breweries, and printing factories;
(8) hydro-electric dam constructions;
(9) transportation industries – airways, railways, water and road transport, etc.;
(10) building and road construction industries; and
(11) small-scale industries within and outside industrial estates.

These are only a few of the hundreds of groups of new industries now in operation in Africa. Fortunately, the ILO encyclopaedia and other ILO publications exist, which have detailed the possible hazards and toxicity which are involved, or which may be encountered in the above listed occupations. The headquarters of firms engaged in similar operations in Malaya, in other parts of Asia, and in South America have publications on similar problems, as well as on measures taken to combat them. The African occupational health physician needs to subscribe to such publications. He also needs to document his observations accurately, to further add to existing knowledge on the prevention and control of such problems.

Occupational Health and Health Promotion in Africa

Sofoluwe (1965) made a survey of traditional industries in a small town of 30 000 population in Nigeria and found that all the industries manufactured essential facilities for meeting basic health needs and for promoting health. They included soap industries to promote personal hygiene; food factories such as a corn mill, etc., to provide essential calories and meet food requirements; carpentry for housing and furniture provision; well-diggers for water supply; and weavers to provide essential clothing and a few luxury items.

A similar survey made in Lagos, Nigeria, revealed that the majority of industries there in fact endanger health, and often flood the country with potential teratogens and carcinogens.

Sofoluwe had also in two other articles advocated that industrialization in Africa needs to be geared to promote better health in the continent. Thus for example, poor housing is responsible for producing over 180 diseases in Africa; and remedying this situation will require that industrialization be geared to providing a self-contained housing unit for every one in Africa at a cost all can afford. Fortunately, this is being accomplished by the establishment of many low-cost prefabricated housing units in Nigeria, Kenya, Zambia, and many other African countries, as well as by a new edict in Nigeria which makes it mandatory for industries employing over 500 workers to build or provide houses for their workers. Free land is being offered by the government as an incentive to the achievement of this policy.

There is also a need for African countries to establish high-powered, multi-disciplinary inter-agencies, committees or commissions to accurately promulgate policies for ensuring that all or almost all manufactured articles are made in such ways as will best contribute to solving the prevalent health problems in African countries. The United Nations Industrial Development Organization co-ordinates the activities of ILO, WHO, and other United Nations agencies for assisting African countries in gearing their industrialization programmes to meeting each country's basic health needs.

Training Facilities in the Field of Occupational Health in Africa

African occupational health physicians should strive to be well prepared for their services, assist in sponsoring training programmes for their health team members, and be conversant with available training schemes and programmes for health and health-related professionals and auxiliaries, such as, for example, engineers, occupational hygienists, safety officers, personnel officers, trade union officials, etc.

For Physicians. There is as yet no institution in Africa south of the Sahara sponsoring specialist courses for occupational health physicians. Refresher courses and seminars, however, have been sponsored by some universities and societies of occupational medicine in some African countries. Some African universities include didactic and practical postings in occupational health in their medical undergraduate courses.

Nurses. Occupational health nurses' associations have co-operated with Lagos and Ibadan Universities in Nigeria and in Lusaka, Zambia to run refresher courses for practising occupational health nurses in those countries. There is a need now to start certificate courses, as well as regular refresher courses and short courses.

Engineers. Safety courses are now being gradually introduced into the curriculum for civil, mechanical, and electrical and electronic engineers. The University of Mauritius has successfully pioneered such courses, and special courses on environmental and industrial health are now incorporated into the degree programmes for engineers in that country.

Health Inspectors. The Inspectorate Division of the Ministry of Labour organizes regular seminars, symposia, exhibitions, etc., on safety.

A Trade Union School in Lagos, Nigeria, and perhaps similar bodies in other African countries, includes lectures on occupational health in the courses for the unions' members.

There is an urgent need to expand the scope of occupational health training courses in Africa. Many occupational health physicians and establishments, however, successfully organize first aid courses for their safety officers and for trade unionists and others. Red Cross Societies and St. John's Ambulance Societies have greatly helped in running such courses.

Overseas Courses

All African occupational health workers should try to obtain a copy of the special booklet compiled by ILO which lists under different countries the different occupational health courses existing for physicians, nurses, engineers, occupational hygienists, safety officers, personnel officers, and other occupational health team members.

As those from English-speaking African countries tend to go to Britain and the USA for such courses, intending applicants could also seek up-to-date information on such courses from the National High Commissions or Embassies of those countries, or from senior African occupational health physicians and nurses.

45

Occupational Health

G.U. Oleru

Introduction

Occupational (Industrial) Health

Occupational health is the discipline that promotes the physical, mental and social well being of man in the workplace by ensuring through *anticipation, evaluation and control* that the workplace, exposures and machines are at defined acceptable risk levels or optimum states that do not produce observable impairment in the health, productivity and efficiency of the worker.
Occupational health stands on the tripod ANTICIPATION, EVALUATION AND CONTROL.

Anticipation

The work environment, apart from being different from the natural or ambient environment is always in a flux, it is always changing. The changes can be brought about by:

(i) man changing his work-schedule as in shift duty,
(ii) changes in production or manufacturing process and/or the
(iii) introduction of higher levels of noise, radiation , heat or chemicals occasioned by wear and tear of machinery and inadequate maintenance and by human error or judgement.

The changing environment in the workplace would subject the worker to a considerable amount of stress. Man's homeostatic mechanism can cope with some of this stress; others may impose immediate (acute) and long term (chronic) effects whose manifestations may not be apparent even long after the exposure has ceased. It is this knowledge that the worker is constantly exposed to stress and that every stress imposes a consequence on man that informs ANTICIPATION in occupational health. It is common sense to anticipate that every exposure in the workplace has a probability of producing an undesirable effect, no matter how marginally adverse that effect may be.

Evaluation

Evaluation in occupational health is predicated on the existence, either observed or anticipated, of a background state, in the case of human condition or the level in the case of physical or chemical stresses. Evaluation determines whether there is a measured shift from the background state or level and whether the shift is of sufficient magnitude to call for measures to control and forestall an adverse consequence (health damage) manifesting itself in the worker.

The background data required in evaluation are usually obtained through:

(i) a comprehensive preplacement (not routine medical examination) screening of the prospective worker and

(ii) assessment of starting levels of exposures, stresses, and machine efficiencies in the workplace.

Control

Control in occupational health (hygiene) involves taking steps to forestall further shifts in workers' state, exposure levels or machine condition that could be productive of an adverse consequence for the workers. Control measures in occupational health are usually targeted at the personnel, the process and /or the machinery in the workplace.

Occupational Health: Its Practice (Occupational Hygiene, Occupational Medicine) and its Scope

Given the different competencies required – those of assessing health risk factors (biological, chemical and physical) and of assessing workplace machinery and operating efficiency – occupational health is multi-disciplinary.

It involves medicine, biology, chemistry, physics, biochemistry, ergonomics, engineering, psychology and sociology, to name a few.

Occupational health is *occupational medicine* when the practitioner is a physician engaged in the assessment and management of clinical conditions emanating from the workplace.

It is *occupational or (industrial) hygiene* when the practitioner is a non-physician but is engaged in the monitoring, assessment and control of biological, chemical and physical health risk factors in the workplace.

It is ergonomics when the focus of the practitioner is on the association of machine design with human comfort and efficiency.

Its Scope

The organogram in (Fig. 45.1) shows the scope of occupational health, its functional units and the intrinsic and vital links between the various functional units. The individual units lack relevance and credibility if they are not linked to each other. For example, an industrial health clinic would lack relevance and credibility in occupational health, if its main function is to treat symptoms devoid of data on the type, level of chemical or physical or psychological agents that produce the symptoms in the individual patients. Furthermore, the clinic cannot adequately assess the severity of the symptoms if the facility for biologically estimating the absorbed level of the agent is lacking.

Fig. 45.1: **Organogram For The Functional Units In Occupational Health**

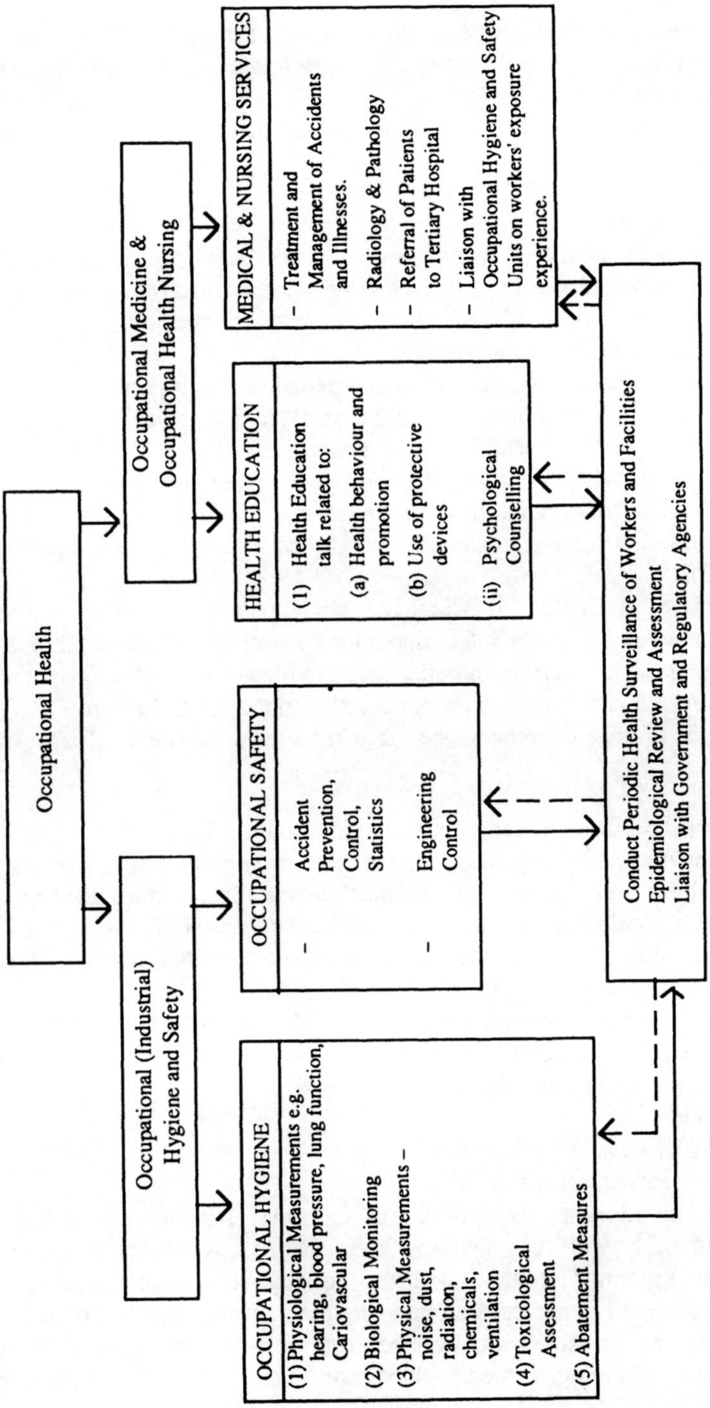

Many industrial clinics in developing countries treat only symptoms. They have no relevance to occupational health; they neither evaluate nor control; even their anticipation of health consequences of exposures in the workplace is questionable. They are not informed on the type and actual levels of exposures in the workplace. Many lack even such basic screening tools as spirometers and audiometers.

Occupational Surveillance

A critical component of occupational health is surveillance. Since experience or exposure in the workplace is in a flux, the health service dedicated to the workplace, has of necessity, to be dynamic and investigative. The dynamic and investigative posture is achieved through surveillance.

Surveillance involves the following processes:

(i) Understanding and anticipation of risks associated with particular exposures in the workplace. Understanding of the risks associated with exposures is achieved through literature search. A useful starting point is the Index Medicus which provides references on published works. Other important reference sources are: *The International Register of Potentially Toxic Chemicals,* a journal devoted to information on hazardous chemicals published by the United Nations Environmental Programme (UNEP).

(ii) Environmental Health Criteria Series documents published by the International Programme on Chemical Safety under the sponsorship of UNEP, ILO, and WHO.

(iii) *The Occupational Health Guideline* series published by the Occupational Safety and Health Administration – the United States Department of Labour.

To facilitate the use of these references, one has to know the exact chemical names of the agents used in the workplace.

Preplacement or Preoperational Record and Benchmark Levels

The existence of preplacement or preoperational data on significant parameters concerning individuals and facilities is critical for a surveillance scheme. The data would serve as reference points for longitudinal assessment of both personnel and facilities in the workplace. Familiarity with threshold limit values (TLV) for the various agents in the workplace is also critical for a successful surveillance scheme,

Although the TLV vary with time and country, depending on the toxicological data available, they serve as useful bench marks to monitor exposures in the workplace to ensure that they do not reach levels that can produce acute effects in the exposed worker.

Follow-up of the Worker

The follow-up of the worker is achieved by:

(1) Personal monitoring through the use of dosimeters that help establish time weighted exposure of the worker to radiation, noise, dust, chemicals and so on.

(2) Biological monitoring that establishes the internal exposure (internal dose) of the worker to chemical agents. The internal dose, recently absorbed or already stored in the body can be established by measuring levels of the chemical agents or their metabolites in biological media, blood, urine, hair, expired air, adipose tissue, saliva, etc.

(3) Physiological assessment of respiratory, cardiac or auditory function of the exposed worker to identify what the shift exposures in the workplace have produced in these functions.

The Influence of Economic Factor on the Scope and Practice of Occupational Health

An analysis of the industrial performance of developing countries published by the United Nations Commission on Trade and Development (1986) showed growth in only eight industrial sectors and these were mainly in light manufacturing or assembly plant operations as per example: food products (4.1%), beverages (5.6%), tobacco (8.0%), wearing apparel (3.9%), leather and its products (6.5%), footwear (3.4%), printing and publishing (3.0%), and miscellaneous – petroleum and coal products (3.7%).

The proportion of the population employed in these industries and therefore at probable risk of exposure showed a corresponding shift of between –3.8 and 3.0 per cent. The unemployment and underemployment rates in 1982, when the report was compiled, were between 50 and 60 per cent for Africa.

Estimating the adult, productive population of Africa at about 35% of the entire population of about 800 million, there are about 280 million people who face occupational health risks arising from agriculture, manufacturing, construction, mineral exploration and exploitation, petroleum and other energy sources (uranium) exploitations.

To this number must be added a quarter (100 million) of the children's population engaged in employed labour.

If Nigeria's example serves as the archetype, the characteristics and magnitude of risks faced by the 400 million employed population of Africa are multiple and varied and have not been clearly defined.

The commitment to occupational health is low, the inescapable consequence being parasitic, endemic diseases and severe infrastructural and social deficiencies. The industrial clinics in Nigeria are restricted to the management of endemic diseases – malaria, diarrheal, etc. to the almost total exclusion of occupational health problems.

It is not surprising to find cases of fibrosis in some industries being passed off as tuberculosis and the services of the affected worker dispensed without compensation.

Nigerian workers are seldom provided with protective devices and when they are provided with them, they hardly ever wear them. A study of Nigerian textile workers who wore no ear muffs and were exposed to noise levels of between 90 and 115 dBA showed a threshold shift that increased with duration of employment and ranged from 2.17 dB to 11.67 per year of employment after adjustment for age. A similar group of American aerospace workers exposed to similar levels of noise, but protected with ear muffs, showed no perceptible hearing change.

The organized trade unions are of little assistance to the industrial worker. Their leadership is ill educated and mostly unaware of the short or long term consequences of the exposures their members suffer. Protective devices and better working conditions have low priority among their articulated concerns.

The attitude of government to occupational hygiene is that of benign neglect. There are no regulations on exposure levels in Nigeria. The Industrial Safety Act of 1955 which was revised in 1987 does not address the level and nature of exposures in the workplace or the health damage that can emanate from them. It is concerned with accidents on the factory floor. It offers no sympathy to a coal miner for instance, who during 20 years of service in the mines has had no accidents, no trauma and not even bruises, but yet develops debilitating coal workers' pnemoconiosis. The miners' exposure hazards are not addressed nor are his future health needs anticipated.

The revised Act also lacks enforcement capabilities. The Factory Inspectorate Division of the Ministry of Labour, vested with the statutory responsibility of enforcing the act is poorly equipped, and poorly staffed. It has about 24 factory inspectors for a nation of over 120 million people and over 40,000 factories, giving factory definition as a workplace employing at least 25 persons.

The industries themselves evade responsibility for excessive exposures in their factories by employing casual or transient or migrant labourers in hazardous operations. When regular workers are engaged in hazardous exposures, they are offered dietary supplements (like milk) or they are bought over, as in the case of workers in the acid fume filled anodizing section of an aluminium plant, with a lump sum terminal payment of a years' salary in lieu of medical coverage or compensation.

Education and Research Programmes

Nigeria has eleven medical schools and none offers a diploma or a degree course in occupational medicine or hygiene. The University of Lagos is the only one offering a semester long course in occupational health in its Master of Public Health programme.

The bulk of the physicians who supervise industrial clinics have no speciality training in occupational medicine and most of them have only had a few course exposures to occupational medicine in the process of degree programmes abroad.

Keeping track of the exposure of the worker in Nigeria is a daunting exercise. Many workers are lost to follow-up when they leave the workplace. Both management and the unions maintain no permanent records on the worker. Compensation programmes are usually limited to accidental injuries and not to exposure-induced physiological disabilities.

Disease registries are rare and are plagued by lack of computerization and incomplete diagnosis and registration. These factors coupled with the long latency periods that characterize occupationally-induced diseases (few industries in Nigeria are more than 25 years old) limit occupational health research to monitoring exposure levels and manifestations of probable occupational diseases. Etiological studies are difficult if not impossible at this stage.

Conclusion

Exposures in Nigerian industries are excessive and unregulated. Granted the current low priority given to occupational health and the rapid industrialization of the Nigerian economy, occupational exposures are likely, before the year 2000, to pose severe additional health problems before the investments on primary health care and infrastructural developments can put a lid on endemic and communicable diseases.

References

Oleru, U.G. (1980) A Comparison of the Heating Level of Nigerian Textile Workers and a Control Group. *American Industrial Hygiene Association Journal* 41, 283-287.

Oleru, U.G (1989): "The Neurological Effects of Exposure in a Nigerian Paint Factory" *Journal of Occupational Medicine* (In Press).

Savell J.F. & Toothman E.H. (1987): Group Mean Hearing: Threshold Changes in a Noise Exposed Industrial Population Using Personal Hearing Protectors'. *American Industrial Hygiene Association Journal* 48, 23-27.

United Nations (1986) *Trade and Development Report* 1986. UNCTAD/TDR/16, Pub. No 86. II D.5

46

Occupational Safety and Health in Africa and the Role of the International Labour Organization (ILO)

M. Mokrane

With the industrial progress and the increased emphasis on agriculture, hazards in the workplace are also changing in Africa. The need for a more integrated approach is generally recognized, and an increasing number of countries try to incorporate occupational safety and health in their development plans. In spite of efforts made by African countries to improve occupational safety and health conditions, however, the situation remains acute and is even worsening in some respects on the African continent.

Statistics of occupational accidents and occupational diseases are rarely available in Africa, and it may be said that these accidents and diseases are grossly under-reported because of a lack of reporting practice, training and technical knowledge. While it may be risky to compare accident rates between countries, the information that is available indicates that the probability of being a victim of fatal accidents may be for an African country several times higher than in an advanced country. There are reports that the number of occupationally injured persons increased faster than the labour force. Despite the virtual absence of reliable statistics on occupational diseases, there is no doubt that these diseases are common and often serious.

It is important to promote effective occupational safety and health services in all the African countries. Particular attention is drawn to the role of legislation, extension of available services, participation of managers and workers and training and information.

Occupational Safety and Health Conditions

Industrial Enterprises

The transfer of technology has contributed to an increase in machinery and productivity. However, it has also introduced new occupational hazards; dangerous processes, continuing use of chemicals of which the toxicity is known (such as solvents, asbestos, vinyl chloride) as well as of new chemical products (such as various fertilizers, pesticides, herbicides), heat, noise and vibration, paced or repetitive work, night and shift work and occupational stress.

While many large, modern enterprises in developing countries have high safety standards, there are widespread problems of safety and health with imported machinery, guarding, maintenance and training. Large industries which are branches of multinationals have better conditions, but usually not as good as in the home country. It happens that processes and equipment designed to be used in safe conditions in industrialized countries are not adapted or can even be dangerous in developing countries because of local conditions as regards the physical, psychological and social environment. Sometimes new machines do not have the same safety standards as those required in exporting countries.

The problems are quite often of organizational nature. Safety guards are sometimes removed in an attempt to increase output. Few measurements are done in the working environment to assess the implementation of standards and to monitor the health of workers. It is often found that safety and hygiene provisions are not always implemented by workers and there is some reluctance in wearing individual protective equipment, where available. The need for such equipment is often mentioned but can sometimes be hardly fulfilled because such equipment cannot be found on the market at the national level.

Safety and health committees, often provided by law, are not always established and, when such is the case, they are rarely operational, due to a lack of training in occupational safety and health and their duties.

A medical service often exists within the enterprise but its activities are predominantly curative for the worker and his family. The physician, overloaded with curative tasks, is not in a position to devote time to the surveillance of occupational hazards; in addition, his training does not prepare him for preventive action to protect the health of the worker in specific and practical working conditions. Thus, pre-employment and periodic medical examinations, if carried out, do not consider the relationship between the fitness of the worker and the specific hazards of his occupation.

Generally, poor working and living conditions also make workers more susceptible to occupational accidents and diseases. In conclusion, occupational safety and health conditions need to be improved by concerted efforts of implementing rules and regulations and raising an awareness of social partners. There is a basis for further development but this needs a more definite intervention of employers' and workers' organizations in order to inform and provide safety and health education to workers who are directly concerned by the improvement of working conditions and environment and by the promotion of their health.

Small and Medium-sized Enterprises

The economic role of small and medium-sized enterprises is more and more widely recognized by governments, but they are in a precarious situation because of their limited financial capacity.

These small enterprises where family and personal relationships are predominant as compared to labour relations, are scattered over the whole national territory. Many of them are not registered with social security or factory inspectorates, and it is generally difficult to secure sound working conditions. Equipment and methods of work are often old-fashioned. The work is performed under bad conditions without minimum welfare facilities such as drinking water, hygiene, rest-room, etc.

Medium-sized and particularly small enterprises may not be covered by regulations and they are not submitted to inspection or control of the workplace. Generally, there is no health surveillance. Thus, hazards in the working environment and harmful agents constitute a continuing risk which may endanger health and sometimes the lives of workers.

The fact that employers do not have much experience, that they have only a limited financial capacity and that workers are precariously employed explains that dangerous and unhealthy practices persist. The high percentage of seasonal and temporary workers aggravates the situation.

It seems important to provide support to these enterprises in finding and implementing practical improvement measures. Experience in many countries show that simple and low-cost measures may increase the productivity and bring about a measurable level of safety and health of workers. These are for example: machine guarding and maintenance, better organization of work, better supervision of workplaces, information and education of employers, supervisors and workers, disciplines and implementation of instructions, etc.

Agriculture

In agriculture, work is generally arduous and depends on the weather and the seasons. Transfer of technology has brought benefits but they have not always reached the more primitive rural areas. The work of the agricultural worker and his family life are closely connected. The whole family, man, wife and children, are often involved in the work. There is heavy reliance on the work of women who have the additional task of cooking, housekeeping and child rearing. All the family members are subjected to various hazards. In addition to occupational hazards, inadequate or polluted water supplies, insects, snakes and the harsh environment contribute to the widespread problem of ill health.

For the most part, agricultural workers are dispersed in remote rural areas and are not easy to reach by those attempting to provide services or to exert legislative control. However, the homes of the agricultural workers, the bases from which they set out and to which they return, are usually grouped in village communities. While it is clearly impossible for the providers of services to make contact with the agricultural worker at the place of work, he is nevertheless accessible in the community. There are certain advantages of making contact through the community, making self-help within the community a possibility. It is advisable to include provision of occupational safety and health services into the arrangements for primary health care, or at least to establish a close co-operation with the health services.

Agriculture in a number of countries is characterized by an influx of migrant or part-time labourers. Some occupational problems then become seasonal ones. The provision of any occupational health service for these itinerant workers creates particular difficulties and special provisions have to be made for them.

The Informal Sector

The size of the informal sector in African countries can be considerable, particularly in those countries where the percentage of urban labour force is high.

Street vendors, home workers, village craftsmen, providers of small services such as shoe blacks and car washers, as well as small-scale tradesmen on the edge of the manufacturing and construction industries are all regarded as being within the informal sector. The spectrum is wide and to some extent it overlaps the ground occupied by small enterprises so that one is indistinguishable from the other.

What has been said about conditions of work in small industries can be said with equal validity about conditions in the informal sector. There are, however, those involved in this sector who have no fixed workplace and others whose workplace is their home. The latter, largely women and children, suffer the dual hardship of following two occupations, home-making and earning money for a livelihood and of working in the spaces which serve the twin purpose of living accommodation and workshop. Some of the resulting health problems have been well recorded but more systematic fact-finding needs to be done about occupational ill health in this sector.

A major problem in attempting to provide an occupational health service for people working in this sector is that of locating and identifying them. In many cases the enterprises flourish on the fringes of the law, evading planning and building regulations, or being in ignorance of them. In many cases, the employers may simply wish to keep the authorities at arm's length. Correspondingly, many governments have made little provision for regulating the conditions of employment of workers outside the organized sector due to the smallness of their staff and facilities. As people in this sector are outside the established administrative structures and in some cases prefer not to alter the state of affairs, it is doubly difficult for those structures to support the provision of services for which they were not designed.

Many of the constraints described as applying to small enterprises apply likewise to the informal sector – lack of capital, lack of knowledge of simple accountancy, lack of knowledge and training, and illiteracy. Training in the avoidance of occupational ill health and the provision of better working conditions can rarely be provided through formal government channels. Community-based, multidisciplinary efforts seem necessary for penetrating and improving working conditions in the informal sector.

One feature which is common to agriculture, small industries and the informal sector, is the absence of any significant organizational representation of the workforce. There is thus no internal pressure for improvement in working conditions and there is no internal structure or communication network by means of which information can be circulated to workers.

Occupational Safety and Health as an Emerging Issue

More governments are becoming aware of the economic and social importance for improving working conditions and environment and promoting workers' health as well as of the necessity to integrate them to the priority actions of the plan of the development.

This awareness is growing progressively among the employers' and workers' organizations even if their actions in this field remain limited because of the lack of material resources, information and training.

The regulations on occupational safety and health exist in all African countries. Certain countries have revised their legislation with a view to covering the new industrial activities and ensuring better protection of workers. In general, the national authorities try to have sufficient means so as to permit labour inspectorate to achieve their missions particularly in the field of occupational safety and health. Special attention is paid to their training in this field.

In many countries, prevention-oriented units within social security institutions develop activities for preventing occupational risks such as: control and surveillance of the enforcement of regulations; financial measures such as loans, subsidies, decreased or increased contributory fees; collection of information and statistics; reporting and notification of occupational accidents and diseases and investigation after fatal or serious accidents.

Meetings and other workshops are organized at different levels in order to disseminate information and exchange experiences involving safety and health practitioners.

At the enterprise level, occupational health services and safety committees are progressively established. In certain countries, radio and TV spots on occupational safety and health are broadcast regularly, and attempts are made to produce films showing good safety and hygiene practice.

In many countries in Africa, awareness is thus growing that conditions of safety and health at work can be improved by establishing a coherent national policy and promoting practical measures.

The Role of the ILO

Being conscious and preoccupied of the urgency of this situation, member states of the ILO in Africa reaffirmed on several occasions their wish to promote an occupational safety and health policy.

In 1977, in Abidjan, the ILO Regional African Conference expressed its strong support to the International Programme for the Improvement of Working Conditions and Environment (PIACT) launched in 1976 by the ILO and invited African countries to use facilities available within the framework of technical co-operation programmes of the ILO. In 1983, in Tunis, the ILO African Regional Conference examined the question of 'working conditions and environment' which was placed on its agenda and adopted the resolution which specifies the action to be taken to promote occupational health and safety at work.

The International Programme for the Improvement of Working Conditions and Environment (PIACT), was designed to 'promote and support' activities of member states in these fields. With the limited resources available to it, PIACT has developed significant promotional activities in the African region. Full details on activities carried out between 1976 and 1981 are contained in the report submitted to the Tripartite Advisory Meeting of the Evaluation of the International Programme for the Improvement of Working Conditions and States. Activities carried out in 1982 included several missions by the Regional Adviser (bringing the total of countries visited – often more than once – to nearly 30), the visit of a multidisciplinary team to Angola (bringing the number of multidisciplinary team visits to Africa to five) and the organization of a national tripartite seminar in Niger (the fifth to be organized in an African country), a course at the Turin Centre, including field visits to France and Algeria, for 21 governments, employer and worker participants from French-speaking African countries on policies and principles for the improvement of working conditions and environment and a Tripartite African Workshop on Labour Inspection as a Means of Improving the Working Conditions and Environment for French-speaking countries.

Multidisciplinary team missions and national tripartite seminars have been instrumental in helping countries to overcome a failure to consider workers' well-being, as was pointed out by an African government participant in the Tripartite Advisory Meeting on the Evaluation of PIACT, who underlined the importance of PIACT in generating awareness of the problems of working conditions and environment. Against austere economic backgrounds, it is particularly important – and particularly difficult – to generate such awareness. It can be said that PIAC has to some extent succeeded in promoting a concern for the improvement of working conditions and environment in a number of African countries, but a lot more remains to be done in this connection.

Multidisciplinary team missions and national tripartite seminars have also encouraged tripartite participation in decision-making and the setting up or revival of standing tripartite machinery to oversee the formulation and implementation of policies. This is also important: the tripartite approach to the solution of problems in the field of working conditions and environment cannot be over-emphasized since joint action by government, employers and workers is almost always necessary for the definition and implementation of realistic programmes.

Training activities have also made a significant contribution: courses and workshops, such as the ones mentioned earlier, and individual fellowships have provided opportunities for participants to analyze the individual strengths and weaknesses of their national systems, and there is evidence that on their return to their country they have imparted ideas and enthusiasm to colleagues and have initiated activities.

ILO's action to support the activities carried out by member states has been equally significant.

As regards standard-setting, a landmark was the adoption in 1981 of the Occupational Safety and Health Convention (No. 155) and Recommendation (No. 164). These new comprehensive instruments lay down for the first time internationally recognized standards aiming at the formulation, implementation and periodic review of a coherent national policy on occupational safety and health and the working environment, in the light of national conditions and practice and in consultation with employers' and workers' organizations. These new instruments, which have been designed with a view to introducing the degrees of flexibility necessary for wide implementation, will no doubt go a long way towards encouraging member states to promote the progressive application of new and far-reaching measures at the national level.

The new standards on occupational health services (1985) will be of great help to African countries, where such services need to be developed and strengthened.

Throughout the 1980s, the strengthening of occupational health services which take account of various work-related hazards has become an increasing focus of attention. The multidisciplinary approach, widely accepted in the 1960s and 1970s, has further evolved in the 1980s. The trend was visible particularly in the following three aspects: the gradual extension of occupational health services to different working populations including those in small enterprises and agriculture; programmes to combat hazards due to new and transferred technologies; and active participation of employers and workers.

The Occupational Safety and Health Convention, 1981 (No. 155) and its accompanying Recommendation (No. 164) which reflect the new development prescribe the progressive application of comprehensive preventive measures and the adoption of a coherent national policy, while establishing the responsibility of employers for making work and equipment safe and without risk to health and the duties and rights of workers. These instruments stress that occupational health services are entrusted essentially with preventive functions and are responsible for advising employers, workers and their representatives on maintaining a safe and healthy working environment and on the adaptation of work to the capabilities of workers as well as on roles, best use of resources and co-operation rather than on administrative structures that can be flexible.

This development is in accordance with a growing awareness that better working conditions and a safe and healthy working environment are a positive contribution to national and community development and a measure of success of economic and social policy. Experience in many countries shows that improved organization of safety and health programmes can reinforce a link between the conditions in which work is done and the quality and quantity of production.

As a result, an increasing emphasis has been placed internationally on action-oriented programmes that can cope with various health-affecting factors. The transfer of technology and various new technologies have also drawn attention to this aspect. Experiences within the framework of the

ILO's International Programme for the Improvement of Working Conditions and Environment (PIACT) indicate that concrete improvements can be made when appropriate organizational support is given in a flexible manner with a view to enabling people to identify local needs and carry out practical solutions. While the latest achievements of occupational health services are significant, much remains to be done in adjusting the services so as to meet the 'local' needs of different working populations.

In this regard, the following three aspects will require particular attention: (a) adjusting the services to local needs; (b) providing opportunities for applying practical improvements rather than establishing administrative models; and (c) organizing workplace activities aimed at immediate solutions.

Work on the safe use of asbestos, which culminated in the adoption of new standards in 1986, will also be of great interest to a number of African producing countries, as well as the standards of safety and health in construction, 1988.

Studies and research have been pursued and the dissemination of ILO and national research findings has been stepped up. The International Occupational Safety and Health Information Centre is extending its network of national centres and has now about ten in African countries: the International Occupational Safety and Health Hazards Alert System now has competent bodies in more than 100 countries that are to be part of the System, more than 30 of which are in Africa. The dissemination of information and experience through congresses and symposia has been pursued, and whenever possible fellowships have been awarded within the framework of the ILO's technical co-operation programme to enable African specialists to attend such meetings.

Technical co-operation activities focused mainly on countries' needs in the specialized field of occupational safety and health, included training as well as the development of legislation and regulations and the strengthening of factory inspectorates or occupational safety and health institutes.

In African countries, the workers whose working conditions most need improvements are also those whom it is most difficult to reach. There is a need to design more effective means of intervention, particularly for small enterprises and the unorganized sectors. Effective delivery systems need to be developed in a purely African context. This illustrates the need to encourage the development of African approaches to the problems of working conditions and environment, relevant to the local physical and socio-cultural environment. Such factors as the climate and distances, national structures and traditional customs will have a bearing on national approaches. The ILO tries also to collect and disseminate information on major features of African programmes as well as to promote inter-African co-operation and develop national capabilities which can contribute to regional self-reliance.

Following these conclusions, practical activities have been developed in 1988-89 with a view to promoting a coherent policy in occupational safety and health, to strengthening the occupational health services and to training the health occupational personnel as well as the workers and their representatives. Among these activities, we may point out the Subregional Workshops on occupational safety and health in Algeria, Ghana, Malawi, United Republic of Tanzania; National Tripartite Seminars and Consultancy in Algeria, Angola, Benin, Burkina Faso, Cameroon, Congo, Djibouti, Ethiopia, Gabon, Togo, Tunisia; Training Courses and Fellowships in Benin, Burkina Faso, Mauritius, Malawi, Rwanda, Senegal, Somalia; and Technical Co-operative Projects in Morocco, United Republic of Tanzania, and Zimbabwe.

These PIACT practical activities and technical co-operation projects will be pursued in the 1990-91 Programme and Budget in the framework of the orientations developed in the Medium-Term Plan 1990-95 with a view to extending progressively occupational safety and health to all workers particularly for the less accessible working populations. The priority areas are training and education and the provision of information and exchange of experiences.

Notes

1. A similar course for English-speaking African participants had been organized in 1980.
2. A similar workshop for English-speaking countries was held in 1981.
3. Coppée, G.H. "Les contributions de la médecine du travail à la santé au travail – l'approhe de l'Organisation internationale du travail", in *Revue francaise des affaires sociales* 1989; 43 (1): 45-74.
4. Directorate of Labour Inspection of Norway, ILO, WHO. Education and training policies in occupational safety and health and ergonomics – International Symposium. Geneva: International Labour Office, 1982.
5. ILO. Improving working conditions and environment: An International Programme (PIACT). Geneva: International Labour Office, 1984.
6. International Labour Conference 70th Session 1984. Report V(1), Occupational health services. Geneva: International Labour Office, 1983.
7. Jarvisalo, J.; Kalimo, E.; Lamberg, M.; Rantanen, J.; eds. *Occupational health as a component of primary health care.* Helsinki: National Board of Health, 1986.
8. Kogi, K. "Occupational safety and health in small enterprises; training needs, in *East African Newsletter* 1988; 88/3: 4-7.
9. Kogi, K.; Sen, R.N. "Third World ergonomics", in *Int. Rev. Ergonomics* 1987; 1: 77-118.
10. Tripartite Advisory Meeting on the Evaluation of the International Programme for the Improvement of Working Conditions and Environment (PIACT): Review of activities (1976–81) and future orientation (Geneva, ILO, doc. TAMPE/1982/1; mimeographed). See in particular Appendix II.

47

The Health of Forestry Workers

E. Babajide Lucas

Forestry is one of the most strenuous and hazardous occupations. Most forestry operatives suffer serious disorders of their musculo-skeletal systems, after only a few years of working. Organs such as the eyes, ears, lungs and the heart are also adversely affected. The relatively high level of manual operations of forestry work in Africa makes workers there more prone to the degenerating ailments. In view of the dangers being posed by the diminishing of the world's forests, the health of forestry workers should be of great concern. Forests supply many with basic fuel; they provide raw materials for producing sawnwood, pulp/paper, etc. Forests' amenity and cultural values have for long been recognized in black Africa. The devastations brought about by the Sahellian droughts of the 1970s have now made many to be aware of the forests' roles in soil protection, amelioration of climate and improvement of agricultural productivity. In the public health sector, forests in several areas of Africa provide a safer place to dump garbage. They also provide what Poore (1967) described as a 'buffer against epidemics, pests and diseases affecting both man and his domesticated plants and animals'.

The type and nature of forestry activities, the working conditions and living environment of workers and the tools/equipment employed are important factors that influence workers' health. Other factors include the degree of training of workers, and the concerns shown by governments and employers in the plights of forestry workers. All these factors should be duly considered before any viable programme for improving the health of forestry workers can be drawn up.

Forestry Activities

The primary activities undertaken by forestry workers can be grouped into six:

(i) Aerial survey of sites earmarked for establishing forestry plantation.

(ii) Engineering works – design, construction and maintenance of roads, culverts/bridges and labour camps; maintenance of machinery etc.

(iii) Establishment of tree nurseries.

(iv) Site preparation, tree planting and tree crop maintenance in the form of tending, thinning, de-limbing etc.

(v) Protection of forests against fire, pests and log thieves.

(vi) Tree exploitation and primary conversion of logs in the forests, using mobile mills.

It is only nursery work that requires low-to-medium level energy input, of the activities listed. While a bus driver in a township route requires between 8 and 10 megajoules per day of energy expenditure in his work, Lehman (1962), Strehlke (1979) and some other researchers have recorded average daily energy expenditure in forestry work of between 12 and 20 megajoules. Almost all of the activities listed require workers to be in the standing posture during work. The effects of work strains on forestry workers are discussed under diseases and accidents suffered by forestry workers.

Living Environment and Working Conditions of Forestry Workers

Forestry operatives in Africa normally live in camps within the forest area or in nearby villages. The most productive forests are in East, West and Central Africa. These forests span from the swampy, coastal regions to the slopes and peaks of the mountains. The temperature under shade may rise in some areas up to 50^0C and may be as low as 0^0C on the mountains. During the harmattan season (in the derived savanna), cold, dry wind blows at a speed approaching 40 metres per second. Reports from some African countries indicate that the hostile forest environment contribute greatly to the discomfort and poor health of forestry workers. The ergonomic concept of work-place design which is greatly improving the well-being of factory workers is not feasible in forestry. In the African rain forest, the sheer denseness of the forests with numerous undergrowths, heavy tree buttresses, stilt roots especially in the mangrove swamps etc. make work-place design impossible.

Although forestry camps are evacuated during the rainy seasons, off-season rains frequently meet workers in camps. These camps are usually badly overcrowded, with the attendant spread of communicable diseases. Camp structures do not provide adequate protection from dangerous animals such as snakes, bushcows and crocodiles. Both the camp and the village dwellers are frequently short of food and other amenities. This makes workers use untreated stream water (or water from dug wells) for drinking and bathing. Foraging for food, workers occasionally fall victims of food poisoning from varieties of cassava, yam, beans and mushrooms.

Equipment, Tools and Machinery

Machine tools in use for clearing are generally the heavy tractors and similar equipment. These are supplemented by chain saws and by manually held tools such as axes, matchets and handsaws. Some elements of mechanization (using chain saws) are also introduced to log felling and exploitation. For most other operations, manual tools are preponderant. These manual tools contribute to the heavy work strain suffered by forestry workers. The mechanical tools, when in use, constitute accident hazards and cause some specific diseases. These are discussed later.

Training of Forestry Workers

Usually, no formal training, other than giving experience on-the-job, is available for forestry operatives who have to undertake the brunt of the physical work. Because of this, dissemination of safety and health rules to this category of staff is inhibited.

Attitude of Employers

Employers of forestry workers all over the world do not generally accord adequate consideration for the provision of safety and health gadgets for their workers. Studies carried out by people both in the developed and the less developed countries indicate this.

Attitude of Governments

Governments are the major employers of forestry workers; private sector employment is largely confined to wood exploitation and processing. Governments however do not view forestry workers the same way as factory workers. Regulations similar to factory laws are not available generally for forestry workers. With practically no laws specially directed to protecting the health of forest operatives and with no monitoring system for their welfare, these workers are almost entirely at the mercy of their employers.

Common Diseases among Forestry Workers

Diseases are responsible for many more forestry man-day losses than accidents in most of the African countries with intensive forestry practice. Unfortunately, employers and even workers do not always adequately link these diseases with the type of occupation: at least not as dramatically as in the case of accidents.

The hostile climate of the tropical African forests frequently causes conditions such as headaches, dizziness, heat stroke, and cold and chest ailments. There are many instances of workers labouring several hours under intense sunlight, with a temperature above 40°C and relative humidity approaching 100%. Essential body salt and water are then lost through perspiration, and if these are not replaced promptly exhaustion and heat-related ailments are experienced. The glare of the sun itself and its varying illumination as the clouds move along the sky, damage the eyes of some forestry workers. In the mountainous areas, the cold seasons are usually severe, while in the derived savanna, strong, cold, dry winds blow during the harmattan seasons, leaving most workers with ailments such as lung complaints, nose bleeding, dried skins, and general discomfort. Numerous communicable diseases such as tuberculosis spreads in the overcrowded and unhygienic camps. Malaria is an ever-present scourge. Diseases associated with water such as guinea worm, typhoid and schistosomiasis are common. In Nigeria, Oseni (1968) reported that in some camps, as much as 50% of the workers may be affected by filariasis. Bilharziasis and other tropical diseases abound. Cuts and bruises are readily infected leading to cellulitis and at times, tetanus.

Trees and other forest plants cause a variety of health problems for forest workers. A few of these and the ailments they cause are listed in Table 47.1. One of the most common is the injury inflicted on forest workers by thorns on plants that they pass by, while walking through the forests. Stinging plants are few but they not only cause discomfort, but also cause the need for hospitalization of forest workers occasionally. *Mucuna* spp is particularly unpleasant and was used by natives at warfare and civil uprising. Felling and log conversion within the forests are particularly unhealthy, since facilities such as wood dust extractors are not feasible in the forest. Pit-sawing has now virtually disappeared. This used to be the worst activity as far as energy expenditure and ingestion of health-imparing wood dust are concerned. The list in Table 47.1 is not near being exhaustive. There are numerous other health-imparing plants species in the African forests. Fortunately, some of the older serving forest workers are able to identify some of these plants and caution their less-experienced colleagues.

Table 47.1
A Few of the African Plant Species which can Impair the Health of Forestry Workers

Plants which may have thorny boles	Stinging plants	• Silk cotton plant: the fibres irritating human body	Plants with pollen/slash/ wood dust that aggravate asthma and similar condition	Plant whose slash/wood dust cause dermatitis	Plant whose slash emits sickness inducing odour	Plant whose slash causes blindness	Plant whose parts cause death if ingested even in small quantities
Acacia spp.	*Mucuna spp.*	*Ceiba pentandra*	*Albizzia zygia*	*Cholorophora spp.*	*Croton megalocarpus*	*Anthostema spp.*	*Erythrophloeum spp.*
Bombax spp.	*Urtica*		*Autranella congolensis*	*Diospyros spp.*	*Combretodendon spp.*		
Ceiba pentandra			*Baillonela toxisperma*	*Mansonia altissima*	*Dialium dinklagei*		
Dalbergia melanoxylon			*Casearia buttiscombel*	*Pterocarpus spp.*	*Guibortia spp.*		
Erythrina senegalensis			*Croton megalocarpus*	*Tieghemella sp.*			
Fagara zanthoxyloides			*Gonioma kamassi*	*Turreanthus africana*			
			Pterocarpus spp.	*Vitex doniana*			

Diseases also result from work strain and use of equipment. The very hard manual work involved in lifting, pulling and generally manipulating excessive weights, wielding axes, cutlasses etc require heavy energy expenditure as earlier noted. This is made worse by the standing posture in practically all forestry work. The musculo-skeletal system of forestry workers is generally badly affected. The commonest complaint among the workers is backache; and progressive damage to the vertebra column. Joints all over the body are affected. Heart diseases are common. In some forestry workers, an average initial heart-rate of 77 beats per minute was found to increase to over 130 and these high rates are maintained for the long hours of work. Enlarged hearts have been observed by physicians treating forestry workers. Chain saws now in use in many areas also contribute to diseases suffered by forestry workers. The vibrations induce 'white finger' diseases, pathological reactions to excessive noise from the chain saws and inhalation of the exhaust fumes from the chain saw engine are common.

Accidents in Forestry Work

Forestry work is very prone to accidents, even in the more developed countries where many safety features and controls are available. Accidents in forestry work in Africa would have been more common and serious but for the lower level of mechanization of operations. The common types of accidents with tools and equipment are matchet/axe cuts and occasionally cuts from chain saws. Accidents on the heavy clearing and exploitation equipment (tractors, etc) are infrequent.

Accidents that are brought about by the nature of work and the environment include being struck by falling trees, lightning, attack by wild animals and getting trapped in forest fires. These are more frequent and serious than accidents caused by tools and equipment. There are many fatalities recorded for people hit by falling trees during exploitation or other forestry activities. Although there are standing rules in many areas, that camps be constructed away from tall trees, this is not always feasible, and lightning strikes at camps occur occasionally. Snake bites and snake spitting onto worker's eyes are common. Effective anti-snake serum is quite scarce in camps and village hospitals. Animals such as bush cows, crocodiles etc. occasionally attack workers. During the dry seasons, some forests are cleared by burning, to give way for new planting. This is common although some countries have legislated against the practice. There are instances of workers getting trapped in such fires.

One of the major problems is the poor communication from the forest site to the towns where health facilities are better provided. The difficult terrain and the limited transportation facilities available cause serious delays in taking the injured to hospitals, while first-aid facilities in camps are usually quite limited.

A Programme for Improvement

A five-point programme for improving the health of forestry workers in Africa is prescribed. These are:

(i) provision of essential facilities;
(ii) training of forestry workers;
(iii) intensification of relevant research;
(iv) getting governments to show more concern; and
(v) publicizing the deplorable health situation of these workers for the awareness of the public.

Noting that facilities are generally inadequate all over the area, it is necessary to produce a checklist of facilities and to specify those that are mandatory. These are facilities for preventive and first aid measures. Water and a means of sterilizing it by boiling or solar disinfecting should always be available. Salt should also be readily available and those working in hot sunny weather should be encouraged to take salt water periodically. Protective wear for the eyes, ears, head, etc whenever applicable, should be mandatory. A first aid box with facilities for dealing with cuts, snake bites, etc should also be mandatory. Motorcycles are perhaps the most feasible means of conveying the sick to nearby villages and from there, buses can take him to a hospital in the town. This is because motor cars are hardly available in some of the forest sites and the lorries in use are too cumbersome in the forest terrain. It should be mandatory to consider the camps as semi-permanent shelters rather than 'temporary' ones. This is by improving on their structural integrity.

The training of workers in the use of the various equipment and in operations should not be confined to on-the-job basis. Training should be extended to basic ergonomic principles, accident prevention, first aid etc. These used to be handled on an *ad-hoc* basis by the ILO and UNIDO in the past. It is necessary that this assistance be revived.

Research needs are inter-disciplinary in nature. Social scientists should research into the pattern of life and travails of forestry workers. Forest scientists should prove the extent that the poor health of forestry workers has impeded afforestation and how these have affected the environment and reduced the available wood resources. Engineers should study the various operations and tools in use in order to design and produce tools that are ergonomically more satisfactory. The economics of the fast turn-over of competent forest workers who are incapacitated in their early lives and have to depend largely on relations should be analyzed and documented. Medical scientists should collate information about peculiar ailments of forestry. They should collaborate with foresters to look at the flora and its health implications to those exposed to them. Appropriate treatments at camp level for various ailments should be devised. These are all fertile areas of research that have been scarcely exploited.

Governments should be urged to provide basic legislations and to set in motion inspection and enforcement machinery. It should be recognized that forestry workers (many of them government employees) are part of the labour force for which the government has ultimate responsibilities, just as they have for factory workers.

Publicity is a tool for exposing socially unacceptable situations. Feature articles in popular local dailies are necessary to periodically bring to focus the importance of forestry work to survival and the very poor state of health of forestry workers and the causes. Such exposures should aim at raising public opinion to prevail upon employers and governments to effect changes for the better.

Concluding Remarks

Forestry workers, who are providing vital services for the survival of people, are unable to provide efficient services because of their poor working conditions and their poor health. This situation will continue to adversely affect afforestation until it is contained. Environmental disorder such as erosion, desert encroachment and soil infertility will continue to plague the African continent until the working conditions of forestry workers have been improved.

References

Abeli, Willbard S., (1979). A Survey of Ergonomic Aspects in Tanzania in, Van Loon, J.H., Staudt, J.F. & Zander, J. (ed.): *Ergonomics in Tropical Agriculture and Forestry*. Centre for Agricultural Publishing and Documentation. Wageningen. Pp. 115-118.

Austen, D., (1974). *Heat Stress and Tolerance in Two African Populations*. Ph.D. Thesis, Pennsylvania State University, U.S.A.

Axelson, O., (1974). *Heat Stress in Forestry Work: An Attempt to Evaluate the Physical Work Capacity of Forest Workers Influenced by a Hot Climate*. Food and Agriculture Organization of the U.N., Rome.

Buchbeger, J., (1983). Health Consequences of Forestry Work in the *Proceedings of an International Seminar on Ergonomics Applied to Forestry*. Pp. 223-230. Vienna and Ossiach/Austria.

Dada, S., Lucas, E.B. & Olorunniwo, F.O., (1989). A System Approach to Planning and Control of Tree Harvesting in the Tropical High Forests in, Pritchard, M.A. (ed.) *A System Approach to Forest Operations, Planning and Control*. Forestry Commission Bulletin 82. H.M.S.O., London, Pp. 147-153.

Fox, R.H.(1953). *A Study of the Energy Expenditure of Africans Engaged in Various Rural Activities*. Ph.D. Thesis, University of London.

Giordano, G. (1973). 'Les Emplois et les Applications des Bois Tropicaux' in; *Properties, Uses and Marketing of Tropical Timbers*.

German Foundation for International Development in Collaboration with F.A.O. DOK 688. A/a DSE III IT/8/83. West Berlin. Pp. 23-30.

Grandjean, E. (1982). *Fitting the Task to the Man. An Ergonomic Approach*. Taylor and Francis Ltd., London.

International Labour Organisation (1981). *Occupational Safety and Health Problems in the Timber Industry*. I.L.O., Geneva.

Jambawai, Samuel Musa (1979). 'The Forest Worker's Tool and Safety in Sierra Leone' In, Van Loon, J.H., Staudt, F.J. & Zander, J. (eds.): *Ergonomics in Tropical Agriculture and Forestry*. Centre for Agricultural Publishing. Wageningen. Pp. 119-120.

Lucas, E.B. (1983). 'Factors Preventing Wider Commercialization of Nigerian Trees' *Forest Products Journal* 33 (5): 64-68.

Oseni, A.M. (1968). 'Health of Forestry Workers'. In *Proceedings of an International Seminar on Occupational Health for Developing Countries*. Lagos. Pp.485-497.

Poore, Duncan, (1976). 'The Value of the Tropical Moist Forest Ecosystems and the Environmental Consequences of their Removal'. Paper Submitted to the Committee on *Forest Development in the Tropics*. FO: FDT/76/8 (g) Food and Agriculture Organization of the U.N. Rome.

Strehlke, B. (1979). 'Tropical Work and Working Conditions in Forestry', in, Van Loon, J.H; Staudt, F.J. & Zander, J. (eds) *Ergonomics in Tropical Agriculture and Forestry*. Centre for Agricultural Publishing and Documentation. Wageningen. Pp. 39-44.

Tomanic, S & Majaac, M. (1983). 'The Strain Experienced by Workers during Cutting and Primary Conversion of Wood' in the *Proceedings of an International Seminar on Ergonomics Applied to Forestry*. Vienna and Ossiach/Austria Pp. 52-57.

United Nations Industrial Development Organization, (1983). Occupational Safety and Health in Wood and Wood Products Industries. *Sectoral Working Paper Series* No. 9. UNIDO, Geneva.

48

Section A

Occupational Toxicology

George U. Oleru

Estimating the Population, the Exposure Sources and the Risks

An analysis of the industrial performance of developing countries published by the United Nations Commission on Trade and Development (1986) listed eight leading industries with growth rates of 4% to 8% as follows:

Food products	..	..	4.1%
Tobacco	..	..	8.0%
Leather and fur products	..	..	6.5%
Printing and publishing	..	..	3.0%
Beverages	..	..	5.6%
Wearing apparel	..	..	3.9%
Footwear	..	..	3.4%
Petroleum and other energy resources			5.0%

The proportion of the population employed in these industries and therefore at probable risk of exposure can at best be an estimate, in the face of inadequate information on employment statistics. The productive adult population of Nigeria is about 32% of the nation's 120 million people. To this number must be added a quarter (or 18 million) of Nigeria's children population to obtain a good estimate of 50 million as the population at risk to occupational exposures. The risks the worker faces vary with the nature, size and capital base of the industries concerned.

The Traditional Indigenous Industries

For the workers engaged in the usually small scale traditional or indigenous industries, the risks are those arising from:

(i) Metal fabrication – black smithing, bronze works where the prominent exposures are welding fumes, metal fumes, coal dust, heat and ultraviolet radiation. Metal fabrication in many parts of Africa dates back to over 500 years as the artifacts from the Benin, Ife, and Nok cultures indicate.

(ii) Textile production – weaving and dyeing – producing exposure to cotton dust, chemicals and dyes.

(iii) Wood processing – including logging, saw milling, carpentry, carving.

(iv) Quarrying and mining – producing exposure to silica and trace metals.

(v) Agriculture – with rapid population growth the traditional 'slash and burn' subsistence farming has given way to intensified land cultivation involving the use of pesticides and fertilizers.

(vi) Cosmetology – including hair dressing – producing exposure to chemicals, alkali and dyes to predominantly female workers engaged in the occupation.

The risk groups in the small scale indigenous industries

(i) are usually small and unstable.

(ii) experience unregulated and probably acute exposures.

(iii) use local primary health care as the main or only health care contact. The primary health care system lacks the capability to screen and investigate or manage the peculiar occupational health problems these workers present. It has no capability for chemical safety, or toxicological assessment.

The Large Scale Industries

The large scale industries in Africa are generally multi-national and have assets that far exceed those of many nations. They employ vast arrays of chemicals, materials and processes that threaten not only the health of the workers but also of the general environment.

The workers in the large scale industries are sufficiently large and stable and constitute 'epidemiological cohorts' with good follow-up prospects via pension schemes, worker compensation, or provident fund scheme.

Secondly the exposures in the large scale industries are regulated in many countries and are measurable over a range of values that can produce identifiable dose-effect associations.

Table 48.1 gives a glossary of types of industries in Nigeria, the exposures encountered and the population at risk in both small and large scale holdings, and some epidemiologically determined outcomes.

Table 48.1
Industry Types, Exposure and Risks

Industry Type	Exposure Hazards	Risk Population		Epidemiological Outcomes
		Large Scale	Small Scale	
Food products including bakeries	Wood Smoke, heat PAH, NO_2 SO_2, CO, burns	3,000	60,000	Bladder cancer gastric cancer bronchitis asthma and, infertility
Beverage	Noise, grain dusts, lead	20,000	2,000	Deafness, asthma and encephalopaty
Wood and cork-product	Pentachloro – biphenyls wood dust, glue, noise, solvent	20,000	40,000	Leukaemia, asthma, respiratory tuberculosis, behavioural and neurological problems
Plastic foam	TDT, vinyl chloride	40,000	–	Asthma, liver cancer, brain and lung cancer
Iron and steel including metal fabrication	Silica, ferrus oxide, lead, NO_2, CO_2, H_2S, solvents, heat noise, UV radiation	50,000	6,000	Cardiovascular cancers of liducy, bladder civilusis, hypertension, infertility and deafness
Health care	Viruses, bacteria, radiation, chemical, shift duty	80,000	3,000	Infertility or reproduction failure, AIDS TB, depression, abortion

The Routes of Exposure and Determinants of Passage of Toxic Substance

The routes by which occupational exposure makes an impact on the human system are:

(i) Tropical or subcutaneous – through which fat soluble substances or lipids and solvent enter the circulatory system through the skin. Substances that have been identified as readily absorbed through the skin are analine, hydrogen, cyanide, phenols, some hormones, mercury and benzene.

(ii) Inhalation – the route through which particles and vapour impact on the human system via the respiratory tract.

(iii) Ingestion – the route through which substances are present in food, particularly xenobiotics, foreign bodies, that have no nutrient value, enter into the human system through the gastro-intestinal tract.

(iv) Bodily and organ impaction – the route by which physical agents like radiation, vibration, noise, electromagnetic waves, and heat impact on the human system via the whole body, ear drums, or gonads and initiate adverse effects in the human system.

Fig 48.1

The Routes of Exposure of the Human Body to Agents in the Occupational Enviroment

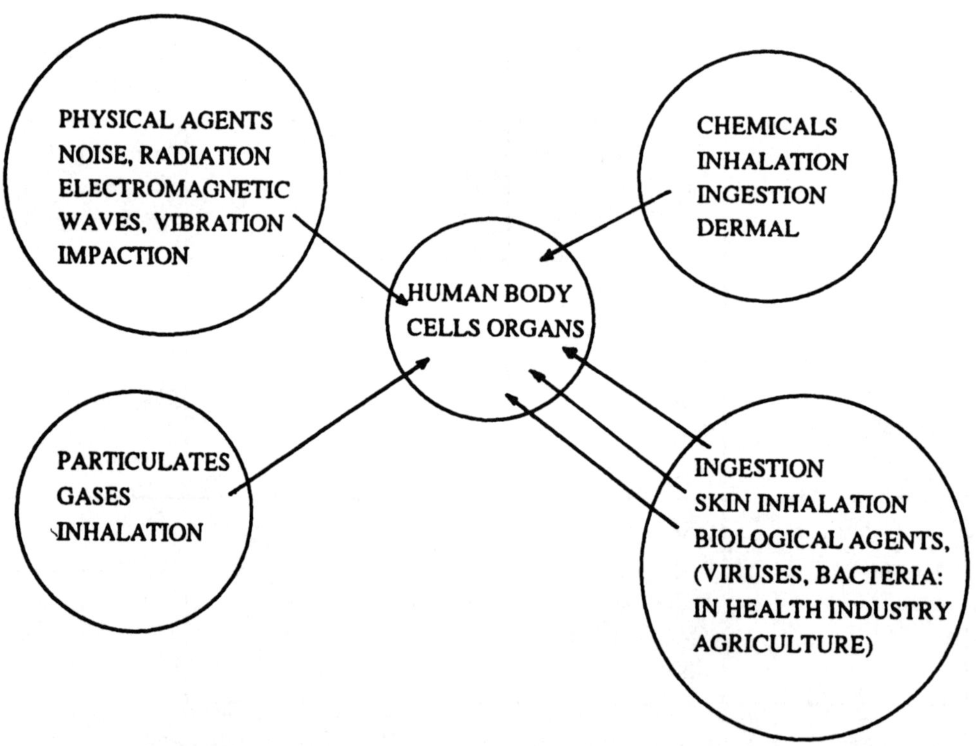

The passage of the inhaled, ingested or subcutaneously absorbed substance through the human system is not free. It is regulated, by a host of factors including the physiology and cell composition of the target sites, the morphology, physical and chemical characteristics of the exposure agents themselves. The determinants of passage for occupational agents are the skin, cilia, mucus membrane, enzyme composition of cells, particle size, velocity and shape.

For an agent that enters the system subcutaneously, an intact skin can restrict or prevent its passage. However, solvent, greases and other chemicals that are fat soluble can easily permeate through the skin to the circulatory system if the skin is unprotected. Hand gloves and protective clothing offer good protection against subcutaneous agents. In addition, they offer protection against contact dermatitis agents like, cement dust, metals, like ricket, some lipids and solvent.

The skin also offers some protection against low energy radiation, as encountered in medicine. However, the protection offered is not adequate hence medical personnel dealing with radiation, X-rays and isotopes, are required to wear lead shields or aprons for further protection.

For inhaled substances, the muco-coliary membrane of the respiratory system in addition to particle size, velocity and shape are the key determinants of passage.

The mucous membrane moistens the inhaled particles, increase their mass and thereby reduce their velocity. The cilia on these muco-ciliary membranes as well as walls of the respiratory system offer an obstacle to the movement of the inhaled particles and either trap them or diminish their momentum, thereby considerably reducing their penetration of the system. The wafting movement of the cilia also pushes back the incoming particles to the upper respiratory system for them to be retained there and ultimately expelled by sneezing or other means.

There are five mechanisms for particle transport through the respiratory system and these are interception, impaction, sedimentation, diffusion, and electrostatic precipitation. The most important of these are impaction, sedimentation and diffusion.

In the ciliated, warm and moist nasal passages, particles with aerodynamic diameter greater than 1mm (micrometer) deposit by impaction on the nasal hairs and at the bends in the nasal path ways and by sedimentation; particles less than a tenth of a micrometer (0.1mm) deposit by diffusion.

Particles in the nasopharynx, oral passages and larynx i.e. the nonciliated large airways, are either carried to the oesophagus and swallowed or wafted to the upper respiratory system by mucus belt arising from the trachea.

In the tracheobronchial region, the large degree of tubination greatly reduces the air velocity. At low velocities, the particles are deposited in the tracheobronchial region by sedimentation and diffusion in contrast to impaction in the large, upper air ways. Soluble particles are cleaved through the bronchial blood flow.

In the alveolar zone where gas exchange takes place, the insoluble particles deposit by sedimentation and diffusion. The particles deposited in this region are removed very slowly and may have clearance half lives of several years.

The importance of the size and shape of the inhaled particles in determining their toxicity is illustrated with the case of asbestos. The carcinogenicity of inhaled asbestos is dependent on both the shape and dimension of the fibres, with a critical length/diameter ratio being at least three to initiate carcinogenesis. This critical ratio involves all repairable chrysotile and amphibole fibres with a length of more than 5mm and a diameter of less than 3mm. Asbestos particles with diameters between 0.1 and 0.2mm are the most carcinogenic.

Metabolic Transformation

Once non-nutrient 'foreign compounds' or xenobiotics cross the body's first protective barrier via inhalation, ingestion or subcutaneous absorption, the body's systems, especially the liver, kidney, gastrointestinal tract and lungs metabolize them, make them more polar (water soluble) and hence more quickly eliminated from the body.

The factors that influence the metabolism of xenobiotics in the human system are:

(i) Genetic composition – The genetically determined G6P6 deficiency in man is said to determine man's reaction to solvent and also ozone.

(ii) Age – At birth,the metabolizing enzymes are not fully developed, so neonates and infants are affected by much lower levels of exposure than adults. The exposures can emanate from work clothes which the parent may take home.

(iii) Route of exposure – Active substances taken subcutaneously are likely to exert some active and toxic affects, as they enter the circulatory system promptly and exert immediate effect.

(iv) Chronic exposure – Chronic exposure to drugs can result in decreasing response to a chemical agent as a result of decreased sensitivity to the agent or increased rate of metabolism.

(v) Other factors – The other factors that could affect the metabolism of chemicals are sex, stress, temperature, humidity and diet.

The metabolism of foreign compounds occur in two phases: In phase I, the compound is oxidized, reduced or hydrolyzed which results in functional groups being exposed or introduced into the molecule of the exposure agent. Other phase I reactions include deamination, dehalogenation, ring formation, and ring breakage.

In phase II reaction, the product of phase 1 is conjugated (by condenzation reaction) with an endogenous metabolite such as glucoronic acid, sulphuric acid, or amino acid to produce a less lipid soluble and polar compound.

The two-phase metabolism can be illustrated with benzene. In the first phase, benzene is oxidized to phenol

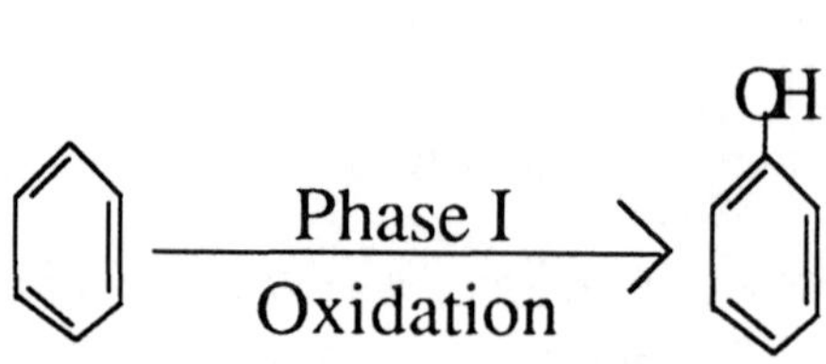

Fig. 48.2(a)

The phenol produced in phase I is transformed in phase II reaction by conjugation to phenyl hydrogen sulphate and phenyl ß–D–glucuronide

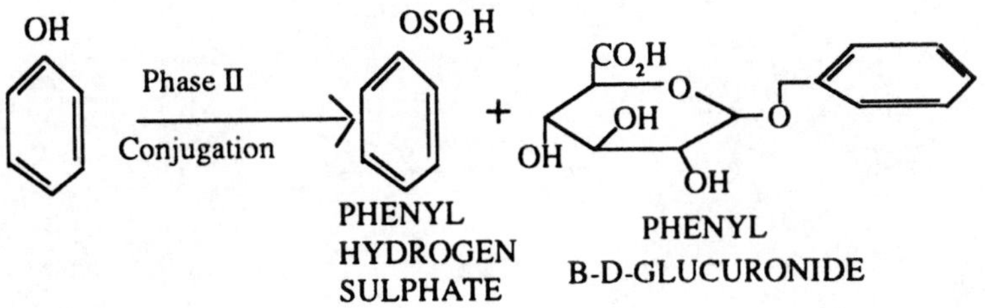

Fig. 48.2 (b)

In some cases metabolism may not be in two phases. It may occur only through one phase.

Not all compounds are metabolized. Substances which are readily absorbed from the intestine, such as highly polar compounds or highly volatile compounds are rapidly excreted or expelled from the lungs with expired air.

Substances which are both not polar and metabolically inert and not readily excreted are stored or sequestered in fatty tissues, kidney or bone marrow. Examples of these compounds/or elements are:

(i) hexachlorobenzene which is sequestered in the fatty tissue.

(ii) cadmium which after undergoing some metabolic transformation is bound to the thiol protein group in the kidney cortex and stored there.

(iii) lead, also after undergoing slight metabolic transformation to lead triphosphate is stored or sequestered in the marrow of the long bones which is estimated to hold about 50% of the body's lead burden. In the bone marrow, lead retards the maturation of red blood cells, producing stippling of red blood cells and anaemia.

Lead also inhibits the synthesis of haemoglobin by interfering with δ– aminoleulonic acid and coproporphyrin III, two important substances necessary for the formation of haemoglobin. In lead poisoning the excretion of coproporphyrin increases from the normal range of 0.5 to 1.5 mg/litre to about 9.18mg/litre.

Undesirable Adverse Consequences of Metabolism

Although the main objective of metabolic transformation is to make absorbed, inhaled or ingested substances less toxic, polar and quickly excreted, that end-point is not always attained. Some substances that are relatively innocuous, may be made toxic during metabolic transformation. The process is called intoxication or lethal synthesis.

Examples of lethal synthesis or intoxication are given in Fig. 48.3.

Lethal Synthesis

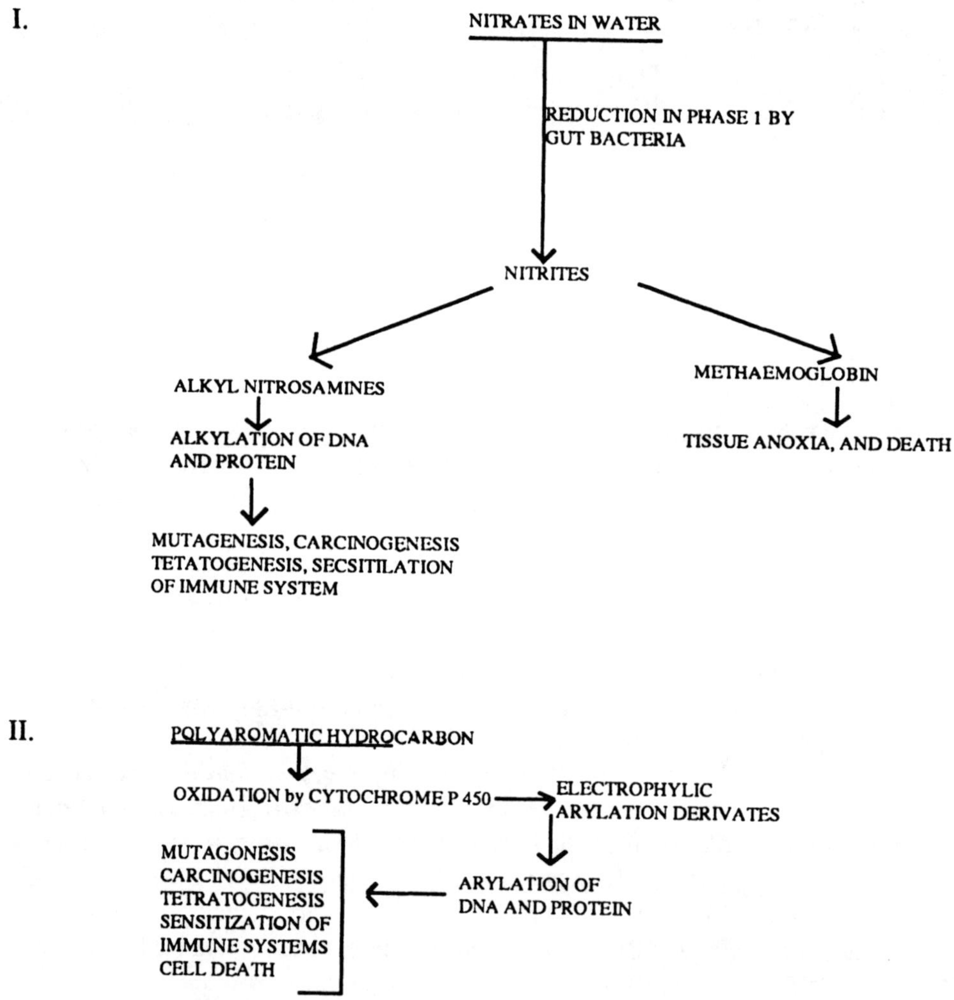

III.

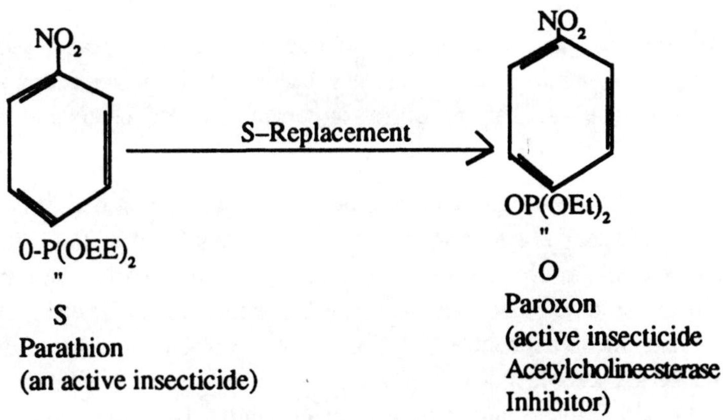

Fig. 48.3 **Examples of lethal synthesis**

Immediate, Local Effects or Acute Toxicity

If the 'xenobiotic' is not metabolized and eliminated, it could exert a toxic effect. The effect could be immediate (acute) or long term (chronic) depending on the level of exposure, durability and duration of contact with the body.

Substances which exert acute toxicity include pesticides, organic solvents, acids, metal fumes, trace metals, and so on. The acute effects are systemic and often involves the central nervous, respiratory and reproductive systems.

Neurotoxicity (Pesticides, Solvents)

A number of occupational agents affect the central nervous system and the most prominent of these are pesticides, solvents and lead.

Pesticides: There are two major groups of pesticides, organophorous and chlorinated hydrocarbon pesticides. Both groups of pesticides impair the central nervous system by impeding neurotransmission.

Neurotransmission is effected by the hormone acetylcholine. At the end of neurotransmission acetylcholine is hydrolyzed to choline (Ch) and acetic acid. The hydrolysis is an enzymatic reaction mediated by the enzyme acetylcholine esterase (AChE). Pesticides directly inhibit the flow of acetylcholine, and consequently neurotransmission is not broken. This may lead to shock and paralysis. acetylcholine esterase remains unutilized in the body and the level of serum cholineesterase is taken as an index of the severity of the poisoning.

Lindane is one of the most widely used insecticides with a broad spectrum of activity against various pests like flies, lice, fleas, ticks and mites. It is also used as a household preparation in shampoo, and creams or lotions against scabies and pediculosis.

The symptoms of lindane poisoning in man include headache, muscle pain, nausea, vomiting, anaemia, hypertension, convulsion, renal failure, acidaemia, respiratory failure with cyanosis and death. Acute CNS poisoning by lindane has produced peripheral neuropathy, encephalopathy and death.

Lindane has several names including gamma-hexachlorocyclohexane, gammalin, gammalin 220, aficide, agrocide, lendox, lintox etc. and because of its acute neurotoxicity it has been extensively used by Nigerian fishermen to effect large catches, consequently poisoning marine life and human populations.

Organic Solvents: These are a group of volatile compounds or mixtures that are relatively stable and exist in the liquid state at temperatures of approximately O° to 250°C. The common organic solvents are classified as aliphatic hydrocarbons, cyclic hydrocarbon, aromatic hydrocarbon, halogenated hydrocarbon, ketones, amines, esters, alcohols, aldehydes and others.

Organic solvents are used for extracting, dissolving, or suspending materials such as fats, waxes, and resins that are not soluble in water. The removal of the solvent allows for complete recovery of the solute. Organic solvents are also used in paints, adhesives,glues, coatings, and decreasing and cleaning agents and in the production of dyes, polymers, plastic textiles, printing ink, agricultural products and pharmaceuticals. Over 50 million tons of organic solvent were produced in 1984 alone and about 10 million workers were exposed.

The acute neurotoxic effects of organic solvents are narcosis, anaesthesia, CNS digression, respiratory arrest, unconsciousness and death. Others include impaired psychomotor function as measured by reaction time, manual dexterity, coordination or body balance.

Some epidemiological studies have shown significant neuro-behavioural defects in workers chronically exposed to organic solvents. Some of the defects include reversible subjective symptoms like fatiguability, irritability and memory impairment. Impaired intellectual function including decreased concentration ability, memory and learning ability was also prominent among chronically exposed workers. Solvent abusers have been reported to suffer, in addition, structural CNS damage.

Apart from being neurotoxic, some organic solvents like benzene, carbon tetrachloride, trichloroethylene, and 1, 1, 2, 2 tetrachloroethane are carcinogenic while others like 2–methoxyethanol and 2 – ethoxyethanol and methylchloride are genotoxic or reproductive hazards.

Pulmonary Toxicity

Pulmonary toxicity is difficult to recognize because of the delay in its clinical onset which may be as long as 15 years in silicosis or 30 years in asbestos related lung cancer. Even the nocturnal symptoms associated with farmer's lung do not appear until about 6–8 years exposure to mouldy hay or grains.

Occupational pulmonary disease (toxicity) can be classified according to the pathological mechanisms involved as nuisance, irritant, immunologic, fibrogenic and carcinogenic. The irritant gases affect the upper respiratory system and when inhaled in large concentration induce alveolar damage and oedema. Farmer's lung is caused by exposure to respirable pores of diameters between 0.5 and 3.0mm that require heat and moisture for optimum growth. Workers with farmer's lung present malaise, fever, chills, dry cough, and dyspnea within hours of exposure to mouldy grains.

Genotoxic Effects

Although the fertility and birth rates in developing countries, particularly Nigeria, are reportedly high, there are still many cases of wasted conception. The search for the cause has invariably focused on women. In Nigeria, many a marriage is not contracted unless the woman has proved her fertility and carries to the altar a near term pregnancy.

The cause for reproductive failure in Nigerian families is equally likely to be found in the men, given the fact that:

(i) some workplace exposures of men are known precursors of abortions, infertility and congenital deformities.

(ii) nearly only men are engaged in industrial productions in Nigeria, that carry the candidate mutagens and teratogens. See Table 48.2. Some of genotoxic agents that affect the male reproductive system are given in Table 48.2. These agents produce organic dysfunction by either (i) damaging male germ cells causing mutation and/or infertility, (ii) anatomical lesions in spermatogenic tissue, and (iii) loss of libido and impotence.

Many of the agents that produce infertility in males are also capable of inducing spontaneous abortion in the unexposed sexual partner. Anaesthetic gases, vinyl chloride, chloroprene, and several other hydrocarbons produce infertility in males and spontaneous abortion in their unexposed wives.

Table 48.2

Occupational Toxicants of the Male Reproductive System

Toxicant	Occupations
Alkylating agent	Chemical & Drug Manufacturing
Anaesthetic gases (nitrous oxide)	Medical, dental: veterinary medicine
Cadmium	Ore smelters, battery workers
Carbon disulphide	Viscose rayon manufacturers, soil fumigators
Carbon tetrachloride	Chemical workers, dry cleaners
Diethylstilbesterol (DES)	DES manufacturers
Chloroprene	Rubber workers
Ethylene oxide	Hospital sterilizers
Hair dyes	Cosmeticians
Lead	Ore smelters, battery manufacturers, police
Manganese	Ore smelters, welders
Vinyl Chloride	VC/PVC manufacturers and processesors
Elevated CO_2	Brewers and chemical manufacturers
High temperature	Bakers, glassblowers foundry and oven workers
Microwave	Radar operators, repairmen and air crew
X-Radiation	X-ray technicians, nuclear specialists, radiologists and radiotherapists

The maternal factors that have an adverse impact on reproduction, are those that impair the function of ovaries to produce the correct balance of hormones necessary for proper implantation of the fertilized ovum.

Foreign substances that pass from the maternal blood stream into the uterine fluid are another cause of reproductive failure or toxicity. The uterine fluid provides the preserving and nutrient environment for the fertilized ovum as it passes through the uterine tube to the uterus.

Substances which have been isolated in uterine fluids and which are capable of genotoxic effect are caffeine, nicotine, continine, isoniazid, salicylate, barbitol, thiopental, DDT, trace metals particularly, lead and copper emanating from the intrauterine devices worn by women.

Although some substances may not enter the uterine fluid and interfere with implantation, they could still affect reproductive outcomes if encountered at the gestational stage. The impact of any particular agent is dependent on the dose of the agent and stage of gestation.

Some of the agents known to produce adverse reproductive outcomes when encountered in pregnancy and the occupational environments in which they are encountered are shown in Table 48.3

Table 48.3

Agents that could have Adverse Reproductive Outcomes when Encountered During Pregnancy

Agent	Occupational Environments
Alkylating Agents	Drug workers and manufacturers
Anaesthetic gases	Operating room personnel
Arsenic	Agricultural workers
Benzene	Chemical workers, gas station attendants
Carbon monoxide	Police women, toll booth operators
Chlorinated hydrocarbons	Dry cleaning, laboratories
DES	Drug manufacturing
Dimethyl sulfoxide	Laboratory workers
Dioxin	Agricultural workers
Infectious agents	Hospitals, health care industry
Iruising radiation	Medical radiation, nuclear power plants
Organophosphates	Pesticide handlers
Polychlorinated	Electrical power
Biphenyls	Generation; microscopy

Cardiovascular Disease and Workplace Exposures

Although the etiology of cardiovascular disease is well documented, the identified factors, particularly the social risk factors account for only 50% per cent of the disease prevalence or incidence. The etiology of cardiovascular disease is multifactorial. The fact that current etiology accounts for only 50% of the disease prevalence suggests that the search for causes should shift to other risk factors, especially occupational.

Some of the difficulties in linking occupational exposure to cardiovascular disease arise from the following:

(i) there is no distinctive work-related pattern.

(ii) there is no reliable uninvasive test for diagnosing cardiovascular disease in asymptomatic individuals.

(iii) cardiovascular disease shows a predilection for middle aged and elderly individuals.

Despite these difficulties, an increasing association between cardiovascular disease and the following occupational agents have been established.

Table 48.4

Association between Cardiovascular Disease and Occupational Agents.

Carbon monoxide	For miners, acetylene workers Iron and steel workers, carbon black makers, diesel engine operators, petroleum refinery workers, foundry and blast furnace workers.
Carbon disulphide	Dry cleaners, electroplaters, rubber workers, rubber-cement workers, electroplasters, paint workers, preservative producers and, rubber workers.
Cadmium	Alloy makers and jewellery workers.
Cold	Refrigerator workers, out-of-door workers, packing-house workers and computer room workers.
Heat	Bakers, smelters and foundry workers.
Fluorocarbon	Dry cleaners, drug makers, plastic makers,

	refrigerator makers, rocket fuel workers and solvent workers.
Lead	Smelters and battery makers.
Noise	Textile mill workers, petroleum workers, metal workers and lumber workers.
Methylene chloride	Anaesthetic makers, degreasers, solvent workers and stain removers.
Arsenic	Alloy makers, insecticide makers and smelters.

Cancer in the Workplace
Much of human cancer is believed to result from exposure to environmental chemicals. The mechanism of chemical carcinogenesis is not fully known, but studies show that the process may be multi-stage and multi-factional and that some of the chemicals have significant roles in carcinogenesis either as

(i) cancer initiating agents or
(ii) cancer promoting agents.

The properties of the two types of agents follow.

Cancer Initiating Agents
Cancer initiating agents:

(i) are carcinogenic by themselves.
(ii) have activity strictly determined by molecular structure.
(iii) are generally active in more than one tissue.
(iv) have no detectable threshold dose;
(v) require metabolic activation and covalent binding to macromolecules as in phase II metabolic transformation.
(vi) are more active in proliferating tissues.
(vii) induce rapid shift in biologic potential of cells.
A single exposure is often sufficient to initiate carcinogenesis.

Examples of occupational exposures identified as carcinogenic in cancer initiators are shown in Table 48.5

Table 48.5
Chemicals in the Workplace linked to Human Carcinogenesis

Agent	Target Organ	Occupational Groups
Aromatic amines (e.g. Basic Yellow 2)	Bladder	Chemical, rubber, dyestuff production.
Asbestos	Lung, pleora peritoneum	mining, processing shipyard, insulation construction

Benzene	Zymnal gland, lymphoid, bone marrow	Petrochemical, petrol attendants, laboratory attendants
Coke oven emissions	Lungs	Iron and steel foundry, blast furnace workers.
Chromium compounds	Lungs, sinuses, kidney	Metal alloy product, steel, cement and paint workers.
Mustard gas	Lung, connective tissue	Mustard gas production workers, soldiers.
Nickel	Lung, larynx, nasal passages, connective tissues	Electroplating, iron and steel, ceramic storage, battery production and petroleum refinery workers.
Vinyl chloride	Liver, brain, lungs angiosacoma	Plastic (VC and PVC) production; vinyl asbestos tile workers, packing industries.
Soots (aromatic hydrocarbons) tars, mineral oils	Skin Scrotum, bladder, gastrointestinal	Chimney sweeps Petrochemical workers

Cancer Promoting Agents

Cancer promoting agents

(i) are not carcinogenic alone;
(ii) have activities strictly determined by molecular structure;
(iii) produce reversible and have a non-cumulative effect on single or individual exposure. Repeated exposures are required to promote carcinogenesis;
(iv) may not require metabolic macromolecular binding to RNA or DNA for action;
(v) are not mutagenic but may enhance induced mutations;
(vi) induce proliferation in target tissues.
(vii) produce intermediate, progressive stages prior to overt carcinoma.

Examples of cancer promoters are phorbol esters, food additives, steroid hormones, phenobarbitol, cigarette smoke and asbestos.

References

Brown K. & Balmain A. (1986) *Molecular Mechanisms of Chemical Carcinogenesis in Environmental Toxicology and Ecotoxicology*, WHO Copenhagen 1986.

Buckly R.D., Hackney J.D., Clark K. & Posin C. (1975) 'Ozone and Human Blood' *Arch. Eng. Health* 30, 40-43.

Calabresse E.J., Kojola N.H. & Carnow B.W (1977). 'Ozone; A Possible Cause of Hemolytic Anaemia in Glucose 6–Phosphate Dehydrogenase Deficient Individuals' *J. Toxicol, Enviom Health* 2, 709–712.

IRPTC (1988) *'Organic Solvents' IRPTC Bulletin* 40.

Lippman M., Yeates D.B. & Albert R.E.(1980). 'Deposition, Retention and Clearance of Inhaled Particles' *British Journal of Industrial Medicine* 37, 337–362.

Milham S. (1983). 'Occupational Mortality in Washington State, 1950–1979' *USDHS, NIOS* No. 83–116, 1983.

Miller J.A; Battistini V., Cumming RLC *et. al* (1970). Lead and Aminolevulinic Acid Dehydrogenase Levels in Mentally Retarded Children and Lead-poisoned Juckling Rats, *Lancet* 2: 695–698.

Munk, Z.M., Manter, A. (1977) 'Acute Lindane Poisoning with Development of Muscle Necrosis' *Canadian Medical Association Journal* 177, 1050–1054.

Oleru U.G. (1987) 'Respiratory and Non-Respiratory Morbidity in a Titanium Oxide Paint Factory in Nigeria' *Am J. of Industrial Medicine*, 12, 173–180.

Rosenman K.D. (1984) 'Cardiovascular Disease and Workplace Exposures' *Archive of Environmental Health* 218–224.

Schottenfeld D. (1984) 'Chronic Disease in the Workplace and Environment' *Cancer Archives of Environmental Health* 39, 150–157.

Seukoft, I., Hammond E.C. (1968). 'Community Efforts of Non-Occupational Environmental Asbestos Exposures' *Amen. J. Pub. Health* 58: 1658–1662.

Stellman J.M., (1979) Reproductive Disorders on Male/Female Workers. The Effects of Toxic Agents in Reproduction in Occupational Safety and Health Symposia. 1978 NIOSH CINCNNATI 1979.

WHO (1982). 'Recommended Health Based Limits in Occupational Exposure to Pesticides' *WHO Technical Report Series* 677 WHO, Geneva 1982.

UNIDO (1985). *Industry and Development Global Report 1985*.

Section B

Organic Agriculture

Clarence and Cla Hopmann

Organic agriculture is an alternative to conventional (synthetic chemical) farming. The use of strong chemical pesticides, herbicides, and fungicides, has a distinct correlation to many illnesses in farm labourers and consumers of farm products as well. The problem of many food related illnesses and environmental contamination is one which man himself has produced. Technological advances are beneficial, as long as humanity as we know it is not erased in the mean time.

Not only is chemical farming a health problem for humanity, it is a disease for the pocket book too. The high cost of chemical treatments, which are only a temporary solution to a problem, leaves only a small profit margin for a business if any at all. The high cost including the ill effects for the populace and environment is only one thing, immunity of pests to chemical agents is becoming one of the most feared responses of mother-nature to date. An example of this phenomenon was just after 1942 when DDT was introduced in massive amounts around the world. DDT had been touted as a 'miracle pesticide' by Swiss Chemists who hailed the product as the most potent poison of its time.

DDT was advertised as a completely safe compound, conveniently cheap, a super-potent insecticide that would eventually rid the world of pestilence and subsequently, hunger as well. During World War II, it was sprayed in powder form on American troops, prisoners and even civilian population to control lice and cholera. When the war was over it was used by farmers around the world to rid their fields of insects. Dr. Paul Herman Maller, the Swiss scientist who perfected DDT's use as an insecticide, was later awarded the Nobel Prize in 1948.

But by 1957 DDT lost its glitter. New strains of bugs developed, with genetic resistance to DDT. What happened was that over the course of, sometimes, hundreds of generations insects developed enzymes that defaced the toxic elements within the pesticide. Nature was doing its duty. Today in the United States, we lose at least one pesticide a year to immunity. The expanding expense is enormous, to research and to develop a new strain of pesticide now costs in excess of 45 million

U.S. dollars. This has affected the producer as well. The cost of production is steadily increasing as farm commodity prices are falling. The only alternative is to phase out conventional (chemical) farming to a safe, feasible, sustainable agriculture. Organic farmers are true stewards of the earth. A healthy soil produces a healthy plant which produces a healthy person.

Some alternatives to the use of chemicals for controlling pests are IPM (Integrated Pest Management) and organic agents combined with good crop rotational practices. Organic fertilization practices are cover crops, compost procedures and organically produced fertilizers.

49

Sports, Recreation and Games to Fully Promote the Health of Staff and Students in Universities and Colleges in Africa

J.C. Omoruan

Sports, recreation and games are commonly referred to as pastime activities. What these activities are and to what extent they are capable of promoting the health of the individual will be discussed in this chapter.

The important characteristics of games are firstly, voluntary physical activities that are systematically performed. There is always an opposition, for in a solitary or one person game, the player mentally pits an aspect of himself or herself against another. The popular game of Ludo is an example. In games, there are usually rules however simple because there are predictable outcome goals that result in winning, losing or a draw.

Sport on the other hand is generally a highly organized game. The rules are more technical and the organization becomes more complex. It should be noted that in ordinary usage, these words 'Game' and 'Sport' are interchangeable.

Recreation takes place during leisure time. It is an activity and not idleness. It is voluntary. There are passive as well as active recreation activities. Recreation is enjoyed by all irrespective of age, sex, religion, race and state of health. Unlike work, nothing seems to be lost if it is not done. Yet, the reward of recreation is immediate unlike in some forms of work. Generally speaking, recreation helps to 're-create' an individual.

The concept of health we want to consider in this discussion is the one defined by the World Health Organisation (WHO) as 'a state of complete physical, mental and social well-being, not merely the absence of disease or infirmity.' Some people have considered this concept as utopian. This writer does not share this view. Rather, it is a very high goal which is attainable. It is in this light that we will consider the health of the students and staff of the colleges and universities in Africa.

Most, if not all of Africa still belongs to the developing third world. Most of the countries that were once colonized recently gained their independence. To a great extent, most of these African countries only have political independence while their economy and social well-being are still tied to their former colonial administrators. The fact that many of these African countries are at present under military rule also shows that all cannot be well with them. The political instability with poor economy obviously brings stress and frustration which affects the health of the citizens. If developed countries cannot meet all the health needs of their citizens, we should talk less of the developing ones.

Like in other parts of the world, universities and colleges in Africa are communities in the larger communities. Whatever affects the larger community will to a great extent affect members of these universities and colleges. But because these educational institutions are centres for the elites of the society, the students and staff enjoy relatively better health facilities than the rest of the larger community. Apart from health centres and hospitals that are provided for the whole community, these higher educational institutions have in addition, programmes of sports, recreation and games. For the purpose of our discussion, sports and games will be grouped together. In most, if not all African countries, colleges and universities have the sporting and games facilities in the community. There are qualified personnel who administer sports. Some of these institutions have departments or faculties of health, physical education and recreation. It is interesting to note that while in the Anglophone countries, sports administration in higher institutions to a large extent is autonomous, while that in the Francophone is strictly controlled by the Ministry of Youths and Sports.

As has been mentioned earlier, these educational institutions have their own communities who utilize the sporting facilities and equipment that are available. Occasionally, people from outside do make use of these facilities. The programme of sports, games and recreation in these institutions are virtually the same. The differences are in the scope and quality. The first aspect of the programme to be considered is the competitive sports. This again is sub-divided into intramural and extramural sports.

Intramural Sports

This is a programme of competitive sports within the four walls of the institution. The competitions involve all the students and sometimes members of staff. The number of sports to be competed for depends on the available facilities and equipment. The competition could either be inter-faculty, halls of residence or both. In most cases, star sportsmen and sportswomen who are in the 'school' teams are not allowed to participate. The reason is that they have been sufficiently exposed in sports. These competitions are played either on single elimination or on league basis. Students and staff are very keen to win honours for their faculties or halls of residence. Those who are able to make the teams as well as those who could not, find themselves fully engaged. Those who could not make the teams form themselves into 'Supporters Clubs.' They cheer their teams with songs, dances and some other displays. There seems to be another competition among these cheering groups. At the preliminary stages of the sport competitions, members of faculties or halls of residence who are not competing do come out to watch others to assess their strength and weakness. Some sports attract more spectators than others for various reasons. So also do some departments or halls of residence attract very large spectators. The staff members are never left behind. Various cups and trophies donated by some members of staff and other well-meaning people of the community are competed for. This occasion is also used in selecting new star sportsmen and women who will in future represent the institution, state or the nation.

Another unique aspect of these competitions is that staff members have the opportunity of seeing their students from perspectives other than the classrooms or laboratories. The leadership and followership potentials are exhibited by both staff and students and this makes for a better communal living. Each student makes his or her contribution however little. New friends are strengthened. The social and emotional benefits can not be over-emphasized. Students from different disciplines and halls of residence meet to compete to test their strength and weakness. While winners try to control their ecstasy, losers learn to accept defeat and wait for another day. On the whole, the joy and merriment that go along with these competitions leave no one in doubt that the health of the students and staff is greatly enhanced.

Extramural Sports

This programme is mainly for the elite sportsmen and women in the institutions. They represent their institutions, state and even the nation in sports competitions. Wherever possible, the services of experienced coaches outside the institutions are utilized to complement that of the physical educationists. These students have the opportunity to interact with students and people outside their institutions. They take part in such competitions as the West Africa University Games (WAGU), African Games, Federation of International Students Union (FISU) Games just to mention a few. Besides, they sometimes compete in the Commonwealth and the Olympic Games. Members of both the academic and the administrative staff do accompany the teams as officials. Sport competitions at this level are bound to test the physical, emotional and social well-being of the people involved. Individual attention becomes important. In the advanced countries, such students are placed on a special diet all the year round and in addition receive special medical attention. They are on scholarship as well. But in Africa, few scholarships are offered to sportsmen and women. The so-called special diet and medical attention are only available during competitions. Donations from companies that produce beverages like cocoa drink, sugar, milk and the rest are given to these students.

As has been mentioned earlier, these programmes of competitive sports enable students to compete outside their institutions. Sometimes, students travel outside their countries for sports. During these periods, they gain a lot of experience. The standard of environmental sanitation of these other places attract their attention. The quantity and quality of food and in fact the general standard of living seen in the places which they visit have both positive and negative effects on them. Students and staff also have the opportunity to make new friends with people of different races, creeds and educational background. Some of these associations could last a life-time. Many of these competitions have gone a long way to help improve the standard of sport facilities and performance in African countries. Teams from Africa can no longer afford to clad themselves in poor sports dress or look hagard either on or outside the sports arena. The standard of living and personal hygiene of teams from Africa has greatly improved over the years. All these are partly the effect of interaction with other people through sports. Unfortunately, the unstable political situation in many African countries, coupled with the poor and mismanaged economies have not made it possible for colleges and universities to play hosts to these developed countries. This could have been one of the best organs for international understanding. Youths, they say are the leaders of tomorrow. Like other members of the community, sportsmen and women's health is protected by the international regulations for all immigrants to all parts of the world (WHO). And so before athletes and officials travel outside the countries, all the required immunization is done. In fact, all over the world and especially in Africa, all sportsmen, women and their officials who have to travel outside the countries are regarded as ambassadors and are so treated. Hence sports administration in higher institutions of learning in Africa is very closely supervised by the Ministry of Youths and Sports. The health of the students who engage in international sports competitions deserves special concern. There have been occasions when some of these competitors have been disallowed to compete or travel on health grounds. As required by all international sports organizations. each team is expected to have a medical personnel among the officials. Staff and students who engage in sports receive greater and better medical attention than other members of the community. There is no doubt that these special students who have been able to attain such high standards in sports also enjoy the goodwill of the rest of the community.

Recreation Among Staff and Students

Most students and staff in African colleges and universities are indigenes, there are few foreigners. A great percentage of the staff are educated in foreign countries, and so our institutions of higher learning remain great reminders of our colonial experience. These communities of elitist people have lived for a long time in the culture of the colonial administrators. It is only in the academic content and structure that the various independent states of Africa have effected changes. By and large, the people's life style remains foreign. In Africa today, much premium is placed on paper qualifications. These and many other factors have affected recreation for students and staff.

It is said that 'all work and no play, makes Jack and Jill a dull boy and a dull girl.' Our students and staff sometimes take time off to recreate. The outdoor sport facilities and the gymnasia are used. This is not organized and very few participate. For the students, they are married to their books as they cannot afford to lose the most cherished certificates, diplomas and degrees. They can not as well afford to idle away in recreation as they call it. The staff members are no better. The existing staff clubs are mainly drinking places with little indoor games. At the best, a few people play lawn tennis. Even those staff members who were staff sportsmen and women while at school refuse to show any interest. There is a very small number of very dedicated staff members who have contributed a lot to sports. Many staff members have been known to threaten students with failure if the students show a keen interest in sports and recreation. The whole system is not a happy one. With all the benefits one can derive from recreation, there is need for rethinking. The following suggestions are based on experience of some colleges and universities that have attained some measure of success in the area of community recreation, and if adopted will help to improve the situation.

First, there should be the introduction of many indigenous recreative activities including games, arts, crafts, etc. Competition can be arranged to stimulate interest.

Second, since sports equipment is so expensive today, the institutions should try to buy some and rent them out.

Third, there should be an increase of sport facilities with flood lights provided so that they can be used day and night.

Fourth, programmes of intramural sports can also be made to incorporate recreation; and as such, separate staff should be made to administer them.

Fifth, the programme for recreation should cater for the disabled and other special members of the community.

Sixth, a course in practical physical education and sports should be made compulsory for all students.

We have observed that while some attention is paid to sports in our colleges and universities, little or no attention is paid to recreation. It should be noted that even the sportsmen and women need recreation as well. Since recreation takes place during one's leisure hours, our institutions of higher learning have a role to play in preserving the essence of community life through recreation. In a community, people share experiences and learn to cooperate with others. Friends are made for social unity of the group. Barriers which so frequently divide people and retard community efforts are broken in community living. When people are at peace with each other, and are happy, they will lay a foundation for healthy living. Sports, games and recreation surely offer opportunities for healthy living.

PART SEVEN

Public Health Administration and Health Planning in Africa

50

Principles and Practice of Health Services Administration and Planning in Africa

G.O. Sofoluwe

Introduction

Acute health manpower shortage and lack of financial resources have been the main excuses for not sponsoring scientifically based health planning and administration in Africa. This chapter suggests that there are sufficient resources, thus such an argument is not entirely acceptable.

Like the rest of the book, this chapter is directed mainly to medical students, the young medical graduates who will have to work in health-deprived rural areas of Africa, general medical practitioners and community health physicians or primary health care doctors who will be responsible for sections of communities or districts or parts of a political ward in a local government area, whether urban or rural. The conclusions are mainly based on studies carried out by Sofoluwe in the Bendel State (now Edo and Delta states) of Nigeria.

It should be possible before the year 2000 for Africa to achieve up to 60 to 70 per cent coverage or more of at least the following:

(1) ante-natal, intra-natal and post-natal cover for all pregnant women;
(2) infant and under-five child health cover;
(3) essential health cover for primary and post-primary school children;
(4) health screening for working age, middle-aged and elderly persons in Africa;
(5) minimal environmental health programmes, such as town and village planning, food hygiene and a potable chlorinated water supply, refuse and sewage disposal, proper drainage, and the minimizing of soil, water, air, and indoor smoke pollution;
(6) adequate nutrition for high risk groups including the pregnant and the under-five age group;
(7) minimal social welfare and social security benefits;

(8) a comprehensive network of health facilities for meeting out-patient and emergency services;
(9) some limited network of referral centres for high level curative services; and
(10) a scientifically based health plan, administration and management schemes.

The Past Century

Western or scientific medical practice was introduced by Europeans into Africa less than a century ago. Hospital and preventive health services were first provided for the few European civil servants, commercial officers, and for those who could afford them. Bold attempts were made to tackle epidemic and highly endemic diseases. This resulted in the eradication or effective control of yaws, yellow fever, sleeping sickness, smallpox, and, to a limited extent, malaria. Medical field units and *grands endemics* services in Anglo- and Franco-phone African countries respectively were the most rewarding and successful contributions of western medical practice. It was possible for almost every African to have at least one medical examination a year and those afflicted with any of the above-named diseases to receive treatment at least once a year in their own villages.

The further development of health facilities – hospitals, clinics, health officers, maternity centres, and dispensaries – was effected by missionaries, private organizations, clans, communities, self-help groups, and lastly and least effective, the local government councils. As most local government councils could not raise much revenue, health was relatively neglected. Health services, therefore, depended largely on national, regional, divisional, or state administration for finance, equipment and for high-level manpower supply.

Integration Today

Viable Government Areas

The first step towards effecting a more respectable basic health coverage in Africa lies in comprehensive development of viable local government authorities which will be able to raise enough resources for basic health and socio-economic development. Thus, in 1975, for example, Nigeria was divided into about 280 local government authorities which had on the average a population of about 150,000, and only rarely up to 250,000–500,000, living in about one hundred or more square miles in rural areas, and as little as one or a few square miles in the towns; and this is the type of unit which needs to be considered for these purposes. The subdivision of Nigeria to smaller and smaller local government authorities is a continuing exercise.

The second step was the creation of industrial zones to cover two or three or even four such local government areas. The creation of such industrial zones was aimed at curbing the present massive rural-urban drift, with its disastrous social consequences.

Socio-Economic Development and Community Action

The third was the realization that the governmental sector alone could not fully finance the development of basic health services and their socio-economic infrastructure within a reasonable period of time. Hence strong community development sections of the Ministries of Economic and Rural Development were created to provide grants to self-help groups.

Bendel State (now Edo and Delta States) Government in Nigeria has made remarkable achievements in this direction. Thus the then nineteen Local Government Areas in the state had electricity, good pipe borne water supply, good local government roads, primary and secondary schools, rest-houses with their own catering, health facilities, post offices, markets, agricultural projects, high courts of their own, and sufficient high-level manpower for administration, education, and engineering. The community groups and self-help groups have contributed in large measure to the realization of adequate provision of the basic socio-economic infrastructure in the local government areas.

Curative and Preventive Medicine

Hitherto all African countries had been guilty of regarding curative Western medical practice as synonymous with a comprehensive health service, hence over ninety per cent of the expenditure of the governmental health sector has been devoted to curative services.

The governments of the East African countries of Kenya, Tanzania, and Uganda, as well as Zambia have over the past decade or two ago markedly changed to a more positive comprehensive health development, and have achieved a remarkable success of coverage in terms of water supply, healthy housing, and good town and country planning; nutritious food supply and the construction of effective sewage and refuse disposal systems; and the development of a generous network of health centres in the few cities and for a high percentage of the rural dwellers. Professor Fendall of Liverpool University, England, who was formerly Director of Medical Services for Kenya, contributed largely to this remarkable and valuable change of policy.

Ghana in West Africa has also made remarkable strides as the East African countries. Accra – the capital – is a vivid example of the success which could be achieved by sponsoring an integrated curative and preventive health service with an emphasis on environmental health programmes.

Manpower

The Community

Success in health administration and planning in Africa can only be achieved when health is integrated fully with the socio-economic development programmes, and when policy-makers as well as the entire community realize that all their daily activities should be geared to promoting better health for all in the nation.

Special Trainers in New Programmes

A scheme for the use of trainees in the health sector either on a full or part-time basis in the local government authority areas should be initiated. The trainees could be made to provide health services to more remote and hitherto unserved areas.

Current Trainees in Medical and Para-Medical Schools and other Institutions

Assistance could be sought and obtained from nearby training schools of medicine and nursing, and from health inspectors, community development officers, welfare officers and other institutions. A comprehensive health service in the local government authority areas could be manned by trainees.

Kenya, Tanzania and some states in Nigeria are currently adopting the suggested programme. Kenya has in fact effectively teamed up medical students with other members of the health team, including engineers, for undertaking health service programmes in all divisions in the country.

Traditional Doctors

Not much is known about the principles and practice of traditional health services in Africa. Studies hitherto have concentrated on enumerating traditional healers, and the various specialities they practice. A rural community health study in Okpebho Local Government Area in the then Bendel State (now Edo and Delta States) of Nigeria revealed that there tends to be one traditional healer available to every one hundred members of the population. In addition, the healers seem to be either experts in one speciality or undertake general practice.

There is, however, a well developed network and system of referral both within the clan and outside the clan, even to super-specialists who may reside hundreds of miles away from the village. The training of traditional healers is on an apprenticeship basis. Students may travel hundreds of miles away from home for their tuition.

Assessment based on interviews with those healed, and not on a strictly scientific basis, suggest that there is scope for supplementing scientific or western medical practice with traditional midwifery, psychiatry, and orthopaedic medical practice. Traditional medicine is the sole provider of moral and spiritual health for a majority of Africans, including even those who have been fully or partially converted to Islam and Christianity.

The facts stated above, would enhance future health administration and planning in Africa. The huge potential resources that might be released by integrating potential traditional medicine into Westernized medical practice for the full coverage of basic health services within the next twenty or forty years in African countries can no longer be ignored.

Collection of Basic Data and Planning Health Action

Health and socio-economic development in Africa have been planned either without or with inadequate accurate data.

Obtaining accurate statistical data in Africa is a complex process, and is often impeded by the gross instability of the community and high migratory tendencies.

In view of the above discussion, this chapter will concentrate on enumerating the principles for public health administration and health planning at the local government authority (LGA) level only, and on how to obtain accurate statistical data for such an exercise.

A comprehensive local health study as detailed in WHO Technical Report Series No. 194 (1960) should be conducted to obtain accurate information on the following:

(1) ecological features contributory to the endemicity or lack of it of the prevalent or non-prevalent diseases in the community;
(2) resources for the future development of health services;
(3) general manpower resources, especially those which would need to be harnessed for health development;
(4) cultural and other features which could hinder or boost health development;
(5) agricultural, industrial, educational, and other socio-economic resources for health development;
(6) resources for improving health information and data – for example, for establishing health and death registration, etc.; and
(7) traditional resources, existing programmes and others sponsoring a comprehensive social security programme.

This chapter places emphasis on the following basic data:

Geography. It is essential to accurately delimit the ***area*** to be served and all attempts should be made to obtain a good map of the area. The Ministry of Lands and Surveys in all Anglophone African countries would be able to supply a suitable map for the exercise. Up till 1970 Kenya obtained aerial photographs of the entire country every ten years.

The map can be used to obtain a census, and then to plan within the local government areas the siting of basic health facilities so that they are realistic in terms of the manpower available, the population needing health services, and the transport system available.

Mapping. The only existing map of the local government area in one survey was obtained after a month's research from an abandoned former seat of health administration for the area.

Aerial photography has also been utilized in an area where a generous research grant was provided for a university rural community health project. (Here too a useful map had also been drawn by a physician.)

University geography departments are also useful resources for obtaining such maps in Africa.

Census: Even though censuses are expensive, and a lot of political upheavals are associated with census enumeration in Africa, it is extremely necessary to obtain accurate data on total population, with details of the age and sex breakdown.

A population pyramid for the community is a *sine-qua-non* for scientifically accurate health planning and administration.

The writer has, therefore, made various experiments, some of which proved successful, and thus advocates the following measure for obtaining accurate census data in Africa. As most African countries have conducted at least one census count, it should be possible to obtain data on the census enumeration areas (EAs) utilized. The Chief or Deputy Chief Statistician of the Department of Statistics of the Ministry of Economic Development will thus be able to give to the community health physician in charge of the LGA data on boundaries, and perhaps also on total populations, together with age and sex breakdown of representative census enumeration areas (EAs) in the LGA. For example, in Benin City, now renamed Oredo LGA, there are 320 enumeration areas (EAs); but 16 or 32 of these can always be chosen at random to represent the LGA or local government area.

Each EA has about 800 of a population. It should, therefore, be possible to enumerate 16 or 32 such areas and draw up a representative population pyramid of the local government authority (LGA). Dr Fatoba, a Nigerian Youth Service Corps doctor who worked under the direction of the writer, utilized primary school teachers, senior primary school pupils, and literate village heads to obtain accurate census data of 17 villages and 2 towns of the major clan in Okpebho Local Government Area. Thus he enumerated a total population of 34,000 people in and around Ekpoma, the capital of the Local Government Area, and additionally produced an accurate map of the area.

As Duncan of Nairobi has shown, a sizeable proportion of Africans live in settlements of less than 500 population; and it is thus relatively easier to obtain census enumeration of such small settlements in Africa than it would be in areas where larger settlements are common. University of Benin medical students undertook census enumeration of six small villages with a population ranging between 400 and 1001 by this method. The results obtained for one of the villages, and how these were utilized for practical health planning and administration, are summarized in Appendix I. The Local Government Area was subdivided into three categories as follows:

(1) human settlements with a population under 500;
(2) human settlements with a population under 5,000; and
(3) human settlements with a population over 5,000.

A statistician assisted the physician to obtain by judicious stratified or cluster sampling a representative sample containing the requisite numbers of the populations of the settlements in the three categories. Only the listed settlements need then be enumerated, and the figures obtained can be projected to obtain relatively accurate census figures for the LGA. Thus, if the requisite number of the villages selected from the three categories form ten per cent of LGA, the census figures will be ten times those obtained for the sample. Population pyramids for the area could similarly be drawn from the figures obtained for the representative sample.

It should also be possible to get an average number of inhabitants in the houses in African villages, as most families in rural areas of Africa own their own personal houses, and renting is till largely non-existing.

A fifth improvised method for obtaining a rough census figure for small communities in Africa can thus be obtained as follows: First obtain accurate data on the numbers of small, intermediate, and large sized houses in the villages; then obtain the average number of people residing in a representative sample of the three clusters of size of houses by either *de factor* or *de jure* head count; and lastly project the total census of the village from the percentage cluster sampled. This method is not recommended for drawing the population pyramid or estimating the age and sex breakdown. It is only a very rough guess of the total head count in African villages.

Yet a further method for obtaining a good working census and population pyramid figures for LGAs in Africa consists of randomly selecting *one* out of the usual twelve to nineteen political wards in the LGA, undertaking accurate census enumeration of the entire ward by one of the methods described earlier, and utilizing the obtained figures to estimate the census data for the entire LGA. The population pyramid obtained will yield enough data for formulating a scientifically accurate health plan and undertaking cost effective health administration and management.

Health Manpower Study

An accurate health manpower study should also be conducted. This should involve physically visiting and listing all existing health facilities however sponsored (by government, or by private or other agencies); counting the health manpower working in them, and detailing accurately the results of their achievement. Although records tend to be poor and deficient, yet, as the numbers involved are small, a more accurate idea of the trends of illness and achievements will thus be obtained, as well as a working knowledge of the difficulties encountered by the staff, and the other constraints limiting health development.

Health Survey

As the deplorable poor environmental health situation is now responsible for much of the illness and health problems in Africa, a comprehensive environmental health survey needs to be conducted, so that the existing facilities and resources for effecting town and village planning – water supply, and refuse and sewage disposal; effective drainage and anti-soil erosion measure; food hygiene, and the prevention of soil, water, air, and indoor smoke pollution – can be enumerated. Cultural age-group cohorts, previously utilized for clearing bushes, sweeping streets, and effecting refuse disposal should be kept together, and extended to form sanitary gangs.

A table detailing Messrs Dioxades' provisions for different population groups in the new FESTAC Town in Lagos, Nigeria is attached as Appendix 2. Suitably adapted, similar tables could be provided for every local government area in order to draw up an accurate and comprehensive environmental health plan for the areas. The health administrators or the young community physician could thus make a comprehensive list of diseases and health problems which improvement of the existing poor state of environmental health had helped to control and prevent. Assessments of success achieved are thus relatively the more easily undertaken as they are built into the plan from the start.

National Survey

Poor nutrition contributes a great deal to the prevalence of mortality and morbidity in Africa; hence it is essential that a comprehensive nutritional survey should be conducted. The main objectives will include identifying the sex and age groups chiefly affected; identifying the resources for growing, storing, and distributing nutritious foods to the high risk groups. For example some secondary schools now grow, store, prepare, and serve their own foods; often they have surplus that can be bought by the health administration for distribution to the pregnant, the under-fives, the unemployed, the disabled, and other socially deprived members of the community.

It is possible to establish comprehensive post-primary schools for groups of neighbouring villages, and to make such schools grow enough nutritious food to feed the school children and the high-risk and frequently-malnourished groups in the society. The LGA agricultural department can stimulate the growth, storage, and distribution of such essential food and cash crops; while the state ministry of agriculture can ensure the growth, storage, and distribution of essential foodstuffs which can only be grown in some selected parts of the state and the national government can then take care to ensure the growth, storage, and distribution of foodstuffs which can only be produced in different ecological zones from those which exist in any given state or local government area.

Emphasis should be laid on what individuals and families could also do to promote better nutrition, especially in the way of the development of home gardens, and the prevention of destructive cooking and food-preparation.

Social Survey

Poverty generates diseases and diseases generate poverty, thereby constituting a vicious circle. The great bulk of cases of illness is generated among socially deprived members of the community.

It is thus essential that a comprehensive social survey, to quantify and delineate accurately the socially deprived in the community, should be carried out. This will include quantifying the children under fifteen years of age, as well as the retired and divorced women, the extent of polygamy, especially in towns; the unemployed, the disabled and the chronically ill, the illiterates, and other such groups will also need to be enumerated.

Medical students have been guided to carry out surveys successfully, and to produce registers of such socially deprived persons in villages and towns. Those thus listed then receive priority attention from visiting doctors and the other members of the health team. The spread of communicable diseases from such families is thus prevented or controlled, and the sick receive prompt and early treatment, so that they are made healthier and more productive members of society.

Once the community physician has obtained the confidence of the LGA and the entire community, families will readily reveal those who are socially deprived in all households and houses, and assist the doctor to obtain accurate information on the limits of the assistance for them derivable from their extended families. A register of the socially deprived in all settlements, hamlets, and villages of up to six hundred population might thus be compiled. Trained social or community development or community health aides or assistants could similarly obtain such data, which is what is needed to accurately plan for and provide relief.

Planning Health Record and Accurate Assessment Programmes

Health records and accurate assessment programmes are deplorably deficient in African countries. There is need for a high-powered symposium to abstract the numerous WHO publications on health records, and to recommend feasible and easily adaptable records and assessment procedures for local government areas both in urban and in rural areas of Africa. One such attempt has already been made in this direction in Nigeria, and has been included in the practical handbook written specially for Nigerian Youth Service Corps doctors, who are required to work for a year in a Local Government Area in the country.

The Emerging Health Service

The optimistic aims outlined in the introduction of the chapter will succeed according to the degree to which personnel operating on the periphery, be they medical, paramedical, or traditional doctors, community members, or students and others, are genuinely supported by the local and central government and are soundly trained and supervised. The manpower required is often available, but the training, supervision, and collaboration are often deficient. Sofoluwe and Topley have suggested that the field projects of University Teaching Hospitals are often ideally suited for model action.

Appendix I

Result of a Practical Exercise on Health Planning and Administration in an African Local Government Area, Utilizing Medical Students

A map of the Local Government Area (LGA) was obtained from the LGA's secretariat; a map of the political ward and a detailed map of Idumegan village were drawn by medical students.

A census enumeration for NIFOR community with a total population of about 7,000 was undertaken by 25 medical students, divided into groups to enumerate different sections of the community. Census enumeration of five villages, with a population of between 430 and 700 was undertaken by two medical students each and one village with a population of 1084 was enumerated by 20 medical students.

The detailed results in one of the villages named Idumegan were as follows:

> Total population 634, with 205 males and 229 females. The age and sex breakdown figures were utilized for drawing the population pyramid. Crude birth rate obtained from counting total live births as numerator and total population as denominator was 35 per 1000. Crude death rate obtained was 9 per 1000. Migration figures were obtained as follows:
>
> 52 persons (28 males and 24 females), i.e. 12 per cent of the village, emigrated from the village in 1977. 37 out of the 52, constituting 71.2 per cent of the migrants, were aged 6-25 years; 14, or 27 per cent, of them migrated to attend primary and secondary schools which were not present in the village. The remaining 23, or 44.2 per cent, were aged 16-25 years and had emigrated mainly to look for work or to attend post-primary, trade, technical, or grammar schools. 20, or 4.6 per cent, immigrated into the village. 15, or 60 per cent of the above were aged below 15 years.

Such groups of immigrants vitiate the immunization programme in African villages, since they are not usually immunized when they arrive, and miss immunization in the village, they are usually responsible for introducing or spreading communicable diseases. They tend to be children of married-out daughters of the village. As all in the village are blood relations adolescent girls leave the village, and are replaced by their counterparts from other villages for marital purposes. Population pyramid figures, assisted accurate health planning and administration, as accurate data on numbers in the village requiring BCG, triple antigens, polio, measles and other vaccines were obtained. The numbers requiring antenatal, intranatal and postnatal services were obtained. The numbers requiring other personal preventive and curative health services were similarly obtained. Such a small size of population made it feasible to medically examine all the 434 persons, and to undertake stool, urine, and sputum laboratory investigations. 76 of the 434, or 17.5 per cent of the people, had pathological conditions as follows:

Gastro intestinal–16 had diarrhoea and 6 had worm infestations –	25 or 32.9%
15, all children, had *Tinea Capitis*	15 or 19.5%
13 were diagnosed as having febrile illness, and treated as malaria cases	13 or 17.1%
5 children were diagnosed as cases of malnutrition	5 or 7.9%
3 had tropical ulcers or septic spots	3 or 3.9%
2 old cases of poliomyelitis were found	2 or 2.6%
2 had upper respiratory infections	2 or 2.6%
12, all farmers, complained of aches and pains in all parts of their bodies	12 or 15.8%
3 were found with dental and gum infections	3 or 3.9%
2 old people had a cataract	2 or 2.6%

8 others had the conditions listed below:

snake bite	1
irregular menstrual bleeding	1
inguinal lymphadenitis	1
1 case was queried tuberculosis	1

1 person, constituting 1.5 per cent of those aged 40 years and above in the village had hypertension.

2 cases of burns were seen, constituting 2.6 per cent of the total population.

2 cases of anaemia, constituting 2.6 per cent of the total population, were also seen.

Thus the whole village was screened. It should therefore be possible to undertake complete screening of all villages in Africa of a population of 600 and below.

Environmental health and nutritional assessment of all the villages were also comprehensively undertaken. Assessment of social problems and social assets were also undertaken. Useful results included the finding of an absence of any case of divorce, juvenile delinquency, or children in need of care; and the discovery of the almost complete social security offered to all by all the villagers, who are further assisted by those villagers who have successfully emigrated to the towns.

There was no-one unemployed, as all the villagers, children and adults, males and females, were employed in the farms. The main social problems were the lack of primary or secondary and other schools, and the absence of industries or other intensive labour-employing agencies, which caused a lot of those who attended schools to migrate to towns.

This appendix illustrates that the scientifically accurate health indices hitherto obtained only in the developed countries could also be obtained by improved means in Africa, especially if the continent is divided into small populations of, say, 400 to 600 living in well defined areas, both in the urban and the rural parts of Africa. Thus if all the African countries were divided into districts, wards, sub-wards, and blocks, with well defined borders and small easily enumerated populations of between 600 to 1000, accurate health and demographic data could be obtained.

Appendix 2 culled from a handout from Messrs Dioxades, Architectural Consultants to the University of Benin Medical Students

Hierarchy of Communities and their Functions

The functions given for each community are indicative of their scale. Normally they are not needed for the smaller communities for which they have not been marked in.

		Functions (indicative)								
Order of Community	*Average Population size (Indicative)*	*Education*	*Commerce*	*Business*	*Services*	*Health Facilities*	*Transport and Communication*	*Social and Cultural Facilities*	*Recreational Facilities*	*Industrial Facilities*
Class I	0-80							Small Square		
Class II	300-500	Corner shop						Play area for pre-school-age children		
Class III	1500-2500	Kindergarten, elementary school	Small local market with 5-10 shops		Barber		Bus-stop, Post-office box	Small religious building	Small public garden	
Class IV	6-10 000	Preparatory & secondary school	Small shopping centre	Real estate office, bank branches cobbler, cleaner, photographer, restaurant,	Petrol station plumber, electrician,	Dispensary small post-office, telegraph office	Taxi station, building, local club, child and mother care, youth care centre	Religious field, small park	Playing small industries	Handicrafts
Class V	40-60 000	Technical schools, commercial school	Central market and shopping centre offices	Representative office, bank branches, insurance small hotels	Lawyers, doctors, engineers, restaurants, every two communities of class IV size	General hospitals, private clinics health centre office, rail-way station, port, airport	Local and inter-urban bus station central post-library, cultural centre	Large religious building, meeting, hall,	District park and sports fields estates	Light industries, medium industrial

Order of Community	Average Population size (Indicative)	Functions (indicative)								
		Education	Commerce	Business	Services Facilities	Transport and Health Facilities	Social and Communication Facilities	Cultural Facilities	Recreational	Industrial
Class VI	200-300 000	University centre	Commercial branches of banks, insurance organizations headquarters of local business firms large represen tative offices	Large organizations, restaurant, hotels	Professional hospital	General and inter-urban bus stations, regional port	Large local galleries, small concert hall	Museum art center, parks	Athletic heavy industry industrial estates	Medium and
Class VII	1 000 000 2 500 000	Large University centre,	Large commercial banks, wholesale commerce, warehousing	Central offices of insurance organizations, headquarters of large firms	Restaurants, hotels specialized	Large general hospitals, large airport hospitals	Central rail, bus stations, permanent	National museums, race course, art galleries and exhibition, concert halls	Olympic stadium, special large parks	Heavy industry, industries

51

Detailed Assessment of Health Service Programmes

G.O. Sofoluwe

An Assessment Report

It is often necessary for heads or chiefs to assess the activities of their different departments and units. Sometimes it is necessary to access accurately the quantitative and qualitative aspects of various health services, institutions, and facilities. Here, the essential questions which needs to be answered in order to perform such assessment accurately and comprehensively are listed. For example, it may be necessary to assess the achievement of the existing hospitals, health centres, health clinics, health offices, dispensaries, and maternity centres; or of obstetrical services, orthopaedic services, rehabilitation services, health visiting services, health training schools; or social welfare services for children, for women, for the elderly chronically ill, and so on.

It is often valuable to have a proforma, such as that shown in Appendix 1, which has been utilized for assessing maternity services, orthopaedic services, and health centres; rehabilitation, tuberculosis, leprosy, and industrial health services; welfare services for children and for elderly people, nutrition services, school health services, and other health service programmes throughout Nigeria. Some of the assessments carried out by undergraduate medical students utilizing this proforma have alerted the appropriate health administration to unsatisfactory situations and thus brought about the prompter application to corrective action. For example, in 1964 4,000 out of the 24,000 deliveries accredited to the Lagos Island (Nigeria) Maternity Hospital were found to take place in taxi cabs. This revelation resulted in the immediate decentralization of maternity services, with the provision of 30 maternity beds in the health centres provided in all the eight political wards of Lagos city. The maternity sections of the health centres were placed in charge of a specialist obstetrician and gynaecologist attached to the Lagos Island Maternity Hospital, who worked in each of them in turn on the basis of a rota of three monthly periods.

In addition all the Lagos medical, nursing, and midwifery students were trained to cope with such obstetric emergencies as often tend to occur in the casualty and emergency departments of Lagos hospitals.

A similar assessment of Lagos Royal Orthopaedic Hospital revealed that well over £100,000 worth of equipment had been discarded owing to the breakage of some part or other which could not be replaced from sources within the country.

A Planned Survey

A survey to discover malnutrition undertaken by Benin Medical Students in 1977 in representative census numeration areas of Benin City revealed a low prevalence of clinically visible 'kwashiorkor' cases. The result was attributed to the success of the Nutrition Unit set up and run by the then Bendel State Ministry of Health in Benin City. Similarly, over ninety five per cent of children delivered in the Lagos Island Maternity Hospital since 1960 were found to have been immunized with BCG against tuberculosis. The regulation enacted in 1960 stipulating that all new-born babies in the hospital be immunized with BCG four days after delivery before they were discharged from the hospital had thus been shown to have been effective.

Concluding Remarks

The questionnaire has the added advantage that a quick assessment of health services programmes can be undertaken both before and after introduction of developmental or innovative measures. It also does not involve the use of complicated statistical and computerized calculations. They easily readily report on a survey in which the results can assist in revealing problems that may be partly soluble, and in evaluating the programme.

Appendix I

Suggested Proforma for Accurate Assessment of Health Services

1. Name of the Organization ....

2. Correct Address ....

3. Date of Establishment..

4. Name of Sponsoring Organization(s) ....

   ....

5. Name(s) of Chief Officer(s) ....

   ....

6. Objectives of the Institution:

   (1) ....

   (2) ....

   (3) ....

   (4) ....

   (5) ....

7. Area to be Served (to be stated in details and accurately) ....

   ....

   ....

8. Means for Achieving the Objectives (in a definite estimate year)

   (a) Personnel:

   (i) Senior Category ....

   ....

   ....

   ....

   ....

   (ii) Junior Category..

   ....

   ....

   ....

(iii) Comments on Adequacy or Otherwise..

....

....

....

....

(b) Equipment:

(i) Separate List of Equipment for all the Respective Activities

....

....

....

....

(ii) Comments on Adequacy or Otherwise..

....

....

....

....

(c) Finance:

(i) Income for Capital Expenditure..

....

....

....

....

(ii) Income for Recurrent Expenditure from Different Sources ....

(a) ....

....

....

....

....

(b) ....

....

....

....

(iii) Other Sources of Income or Revenue ....

....

....

....

....

(iv) Statements of Capital Expenditure

....

....

....

....

(v) Statements of Current Expenditure ....

....

....

....

....

(vi) Comments on Adequacy or Otherwise of Financial Situation

....

....

....

....

9. List of Activities Undertaken to Achieve Objectives ....

....

....

....

....

10. Accurate Data on Achievements ....

....

....

....

....

11. List of Constraints Limiting the Achievements of Objectives ....

....

....

....

....

12. List of Future Plans of the Institution ....

....

....

....

....

13. Your Own Assessment of the Achievements of the Institution ....

....

....

....

....

14. Any Other Remarks..

....

....

....

....

Comments on the Questionnaire

Questions 1–5 are absolutely necessary for the accurate and easy identification of the health facility. Question 3 not only enables us to know how long the facilities have been effective, but also assists in research involving cohort studies, and may explain some of the health procedures observed by that establishment.

Question 4 will enable the users to know accurately what payments will be required of them, and also assists health manpower studies, and studies of the extent of the community, private, and public sector involvement in sponsoring health services. The answer to question 5 will enable the users especially to have accurate information on the policy decisions and formulation processes of the establishment.

Many staff in a sizeable proportion of African health facilities are extremely ignorant of the objectives of the health facilities in which they work. This has resulted in wrong or exaggerated information to users, many of whom have had to make expensive wasted journeys only to discover they had come to a wrong facility for their complaints. Accurate answers to question 6 therefore not only prepare the staff adequately for their activities but enable them to undertake a built-in assessment of their achievements and failures. Mission, industrial, and commercial health facilities often have clearly stated objectives, while the majority of governmental health facilities do not.

Leaflets stating accurately the objectives of the institution or facility should therefore be provided and distributed widely, especially during its early years of operation.

Question 7 cannot be answered accurately by the majority of governmental, private, or mission health facilities, as many of them for purely financial reasons, as many of them are not easily accessible to the populace. In fact in many cases the success of health facilities is erroneously measured by the large attendance at out-patient clinics and the large turnover of hospital beds, irrespective of the cost-effectiveness of the services rendered, of whether the diseases seen could have been more cheaply prevented, or of whether those seen survive or die soon after treatment. In Nigeria the 1976 Local Government Edict (which carved out Local Government Areas of manageable sizes of about 100 square miles, and a population of about 150,000) and the National Basic Health Service Programme under the Third National Development Plan (1975 – 1980) have been the first two measures to ensure that health facilities will serve a well defined population living in a well defined area. Recently the national primary health services have further improved on that dramatically.

Nevertheless the answer to question 7 will enable the assessor to delineate the area from where the majority of the users of the health facility are drawn.

Questions 8 and 9 will enable the assessor to know how much effort was undertaken by the providers of the plans, and to build in a health assessment plan to monitor a health programme in terms of the cost-effectiveness of the benefits conferred programme.

Questions 10 and 11 will reveal what pains were taken by the providers for accurate assessment of their activities. As assessment will be a regular and continuous process the data required will improve as years go on.

Question 12 will reveal to the assessor the future lines or plans of development of the health facility, service, or programme, and assist the sponsoring agency to provide a comprehensive health service for the entire nation, state, district, local government area, political ward, or community.

Questions 13 and 14 will enable the assessor to air his unbiased views and, if he or she is a trained health administrator, to offer constructive suggestions on future lines of development.

The questionnaire will thus be found of great value not only to doctors in charge of units, departments, and special health services and offices, but also to the numerous health-team members in charge of the numerous health facilities including for example community health officers or health centre supervisors, community health assistants or health visitors, midwives in charge of health clinics and maternity centres, and those in charge of other such small peripheral health facilities.

Finally, the questionnaire, if methodically completed in this way, will enable an accurate and quick assessment to be made; point out the successes; and not only reveal deficiencies and failure, but readily point out the reasons for all the successes attained and failures sustained. It will thus serve to suggest feasible measures for the correction of deficiencies and the attainment of further development and successes.

52

Rural Public Health Practice in African Countries

F.K. Wurapa

Introduction

At the Alma-Ata Conference (1978), it was agreed that the promotion of the highest possible level of physical, mental and social well being of individuals permitting them to lead socially and economically productive lives should be the key to attaining the goal of Health for All by the year 2000 (HFA 2000). This declaration has since been accepted by all Member States of the African Region of WHO. The universities, health related agencies of other government sectors and non- governmental organizations can contribute to the national primary health care (PHC) effort at the central, intermediate and local levels of the health services. The success of any PHC programme depends on the effective coordination of individual communities, ministries, departments, agencies, organizations – public and private towards the common goal of HFA 2000. In most countries the National Health Council and the Ministry of Health share this responsibility.

The various faculties, of the universities' social, biological and physical sciences have their specific roles to play. The specific ways in which these faculties can co-operate in the national health development is not always clear. The medical faculty's role in training doctors for the national health service is well known. However the new role of the medical faculty in preparing doctors for HFA 2000 activities has not been so clearly defined.

A good department of community health should enable the faculty of medicine to play this crucial role effectively. This chapter describes the activities of a department of community health that can lead the medical faculty to fulfilling its supporting role to the HFA 2000 objectives of the health services.

In the countries of the African Regions, there is a serious time-lag between availability of biomedical technologies and their application for the benefit of the population. It is also true that for any country in the Region, this gap is widest among the rural communities. Some have blamed this time-lag on the inappropriateness of the available biomedical technologies.

Others have felt that the fault lies with the ineffective adaptation of these modern technologies to the variety of existing socio-cultural situations. Whatever the explanation for this progressively widening gap, most medical schools in the African Region, in their institutional as well as their instructional objectives in community health, are determined to produce doctors that can help close this gap.

Preparation for Rural Community Health Practice

In line with the rural development policies of governments of the various African countries, therefore, there have been specific programmes in all African medical schools to teach rural health practice. The following are the type of objectives, both broad and specific, that these rural health practice programmes aim at:

1. Students at the end of the course should be able to:
   (1) Make a diagnosis of the health problems of a community, taking into consideration the major ecological factors which influence health.
   (2) Draw up health programmes relevant to the existing health-care system and the resources and interests of the community.
   (3) Organize and carry out the programmes in collaboration with members of the health team and the community.
   (4) Stimulate the community to modify their behaviour with a view to improving their health status.
   (5) Administer health programmes and personnel, using appropriate management and evaluation techniques.
   (6) Maintain the development of their knowledge and skills in community health.

2. Students should:
   (1) Take part in the programmes being carried out by the health workers in the district.
   (2) Observe closely the roles of the various health workers in the team, considering their background, training, and experience, with a view to a critical examination of their appropriateness for their tasks.
   (3) Evaluate the effectiveness of services, for example, is the service reaching all those at risk? Are the times at which the services are rendered convenient to the community? Are the services technically sound, and are they achieving desired objectives?
   (4) Determine whether the services are making the desired impact on the health consciousness and health status of the community.

There are certain basic assumptions underlying the organization of most of these programmes. First, health is seen as part of a total community development effort. Secondly, the involvement and participation of the communities is deemed to be essential to the programmes. Thirdly, the concept of regionalized health services, with adequately integrated central, intermediate and peripheral services, is considered as a prerequisite.

Rural community health practice can be defined as the type of medical practice that involves the identification of community health needs, organizing appropriate solutions to problems and evaluating the programmes to determine their impact. Rural community health practice therefore is concerned with the definition and solution of health problems. The cycle of activities used in planning any such health service is illustrated in Fig. 52.1. From the foregoing it is clear that the community health practitioner needs to combine health

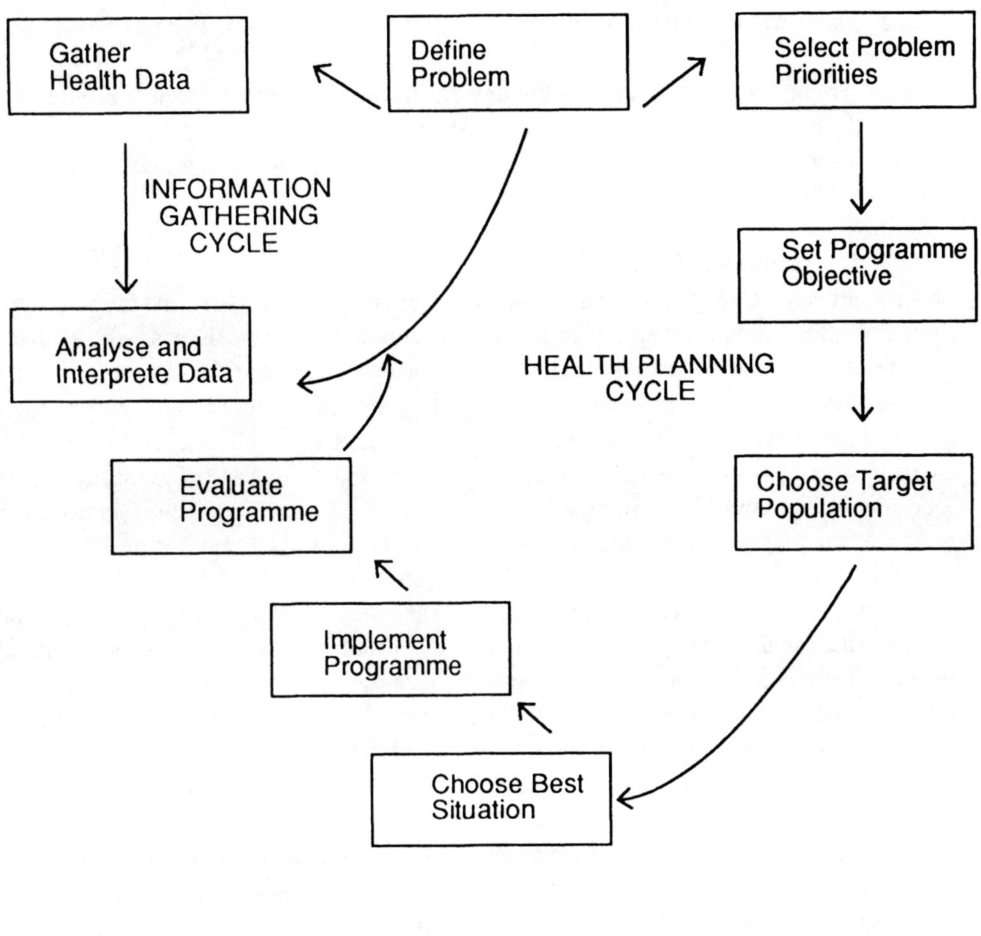

administration and staff development and supervision with the care of patients. The right mix of these activities will vary from one situation to another. The extent of the equipment and other ancillary support at the health facility where the physician finds himself and his own particular interests constitute major determinants. The components of the two cycles indicate the major activities involved in the practice of community health.

Community Diagnosis

The first and most important task in developing a good community health practice is to arrive at a reasonable community diagnosis. Epidemiological methods, coupled with statistical, demographic, and sociological and anthropological methods, are crucial to an accurate community diagnosis. In the following section, an example is given of how the various methods mentioned above can be used to define community health problems through a local health survey. A local health survey can be carried out by reviewing available information sources and supplementing these with a special survey. The type of information that a medical officer would need for planning his programmes can be classified as follows:

(1) general background on population, vital statistics, and environmental sanitation;
(2) the basic information on illness and death; and
(3) information on existing health facilities, health manpower, and the cost of existing health services.

General Background Information

This should include geographic and climatic features, as well as the flora and fauna. There should be information on transport and communications, general cleanliness, and sanitary conditions. The main industries and farming estates, as well as the principal towns and a number of villages, should be identified. A map of the area can be very helpful. Information on the people should cover the number of the total population, as well as other demographic characteristics. The cultural, anthropological, and religious beliefs and customs, as well as food and living habits, are important features to note. Other aspects may include the prevalence of drug and alcohol addiction, the general education level, and the size of families. General social and economic conditions should also be noted. For example, the type and quality of housing, the system of local government and the degree of participation in it by the local people, and the earning capacity of most adults within the population are all important factors affecting health. Accurate demographic data are so basic to effective community health work that a few words should be added concerning them. The enumerated population forms the crucial denominator information needed for all forms of rate calculations. Therefore where accurate national census do not exist or where they are inadequate the census information must be supplemented with a house-to-house survey. The house-to-house survey makes up for the defects of the census with regard to population shifts, whether of agricultural mobility or urban immigration. Most of the previous information can be collected through the census. However, in situations where the census is deficient some of the special instruments need to be developed for the collection of such data.

Information on Illness and Death

For rural health services planning and operation one requires information on the real health problems of the average people in the community. This implies that mere in-patient and out-patient statistics will not be enough. The traditional sources of available health information are: the monthly out-patient and in-patient reports, the number of babies delivered, notifiable communicable diseases and the hospital deaths. Because clinic patient populations tend to be self-selected, and also because several socio-cultural factors affect the use of clinic facilities, data from these sources are unrepresentative. For example, it is known that patient statistics reflect diseases diagnosed in persons who live close to existing health facilities (Belcher et al, 1975). What is more, clinic data are often incomplete and reports are irregular. There is in most countries of the African Region such a long delay in compiling and circulating the data that they are seriously out of date by the time they become available.

It is because of these deficiencies that other supplementary sources of health information must be found. A good alternative would be the surveillance of selected diseases. Surveillance is 'continued watchfulness over the distribution and trend of incidence, through the systematic collection, consolidation, and evaluation of morbidity and mortality reports and other relevant data' (Langmuir, 1963). It is a fact, however, that most countries in the African Region do not have the resources required for successful surveillance (Lucas, 1976). The rural community health practitioner has to look for other forms of supplementary health information. The sample survey, if properly planned and executed, can serve this function. The questionnaire survey can provide a cross-sectional profile of reported illness over a period of a fortnight with an acceptable degree of accuracy (Wurapa et al, 1975). Such interview surveys have the advantage of being relatively inexpensive. However, interviews can seriously under-report significant health problems, including malaria, malnutrition, and diarrhoea (Belcher et al, 1976).

The health examination survey in which a team of health workers goes into a community to examine individuals using a standardized set of diagnostic procedures can be resorted to. Although this approach is more expensive, it provides a more accurate picture of illness and disability. Moreover, if the sampling is well designed, a small number of examined individuals in a community can provide a reasonably representative picture of the whole population. The steps in planning and executing such health examination surveys have been described by several workers (Bucket al, 1970; Belcher, 1975). It has been shown that the instrument for such examination can be modified to suit the level of sophistication of the staff doing the examination. A sample of such a simplified health examination is provided in Appendix 2.

The foregoing activities in data-gathering should naturally culminate in the analysis and interpretation of the data to bring out answers to questions such as: Who is affected by what conditions? Where are the affected individuals, and what temporal considerations are involved? In the following example a multiple data-gathering effort in a small rural community in Ghana was made, and an analysis of the data is given here for illustration (Tables 52.1 to 52.3).

Table 52.1

Characteristics of a Small Rural Health District

District population (1975)	17 931
Population density	245 per square mile
Number of villages	61
Catchment area population	40,000 +
Age distribution	18% below 5; 48.7% below 15; median age 17
Occupation	1/3 of adult population are farmers
Annual rainfall	40 inches peak rains in June
Education	1/3 of adults have never been to school
Transportation	2 major roads; lorries are available only early mornings and late afternoons
Health facilities	One health centre and three weekly satellite clinics
Referral hospital	A district hospital ten miles away

Table 52.2

The Pattern of Diseases Encountered at the Clinics, 1971-1972

Condition	**Percentage Distribution to all Visits to clinics**
Malaria	32.4
Pyrexia of unknown origin (PUO)	3.9
Respiratory infections	14.8
Diarrhoea	7.0
Intestinal parasites	5.0
Skin infections	4.9
Other conditions	32.0
Total	100.00

Table 52.3

Major Health Problems Identified in the Health Examination Survey

1. Preventable communicable diseases:
   (a) Malaria;
   (b) Measles, polio, pertussis, neonatal tetanus;
   (c) Tuberculosis;
   (d) Diarrhoea.
2. Poor environmental sanitation
3. Malnutrition
4. Poor access to health facilities
5. Close birth intervals
6. Inadequate prenatal care

Information from these sources was combined with the community's felt needs, arrived at through careful consultations with the individual village development committees, to produce a list of major health problems. One of these problems was identified as inadequate prenatal care.

Other Crucial Health Information

Data on health facilities, personnel, and costs of services can be assembled from existing records. The poor record system in most health facilities and administrative centres is well known. In any case it helps to start with the available data from the records. The process of updating such data can profitably be built into the regular system of the health service.

It is important for effective planning of community health programmes to have a careful inventory of the health resources – both existing and potential. Infomation on existing health facilities, personnel, and cost of services can be very useful. Usually the quality of record keeping in most central as well as peripheral health facilities is such that one cannot obtain information on these items readily. All the same it is important to start with what information exists in the records. As a means of improving the regular collection of such data, long cumbersome forms can be simplified to make their completion easier. The idea is to encourage a more regular and ongoing collection of these data. For example, the streamlining of the payroll, indenting, and purchasing mechanisms can lead to improved record keeping. Above all, staff at all levels must be encouraged to take accurate recordings of information as a serious responsibility.

Selection of Problem Priorities and Management Alternatives

The most important guides to the proper selection of priority problems are the criteria for the objectives that are to be attained and the political reality of the involved country. The determination of the criteria can be carried out in several ways.

Presently there are no widely accepted approaches to arriving at such criteria. However, consideration such as the number of days lost to the community as a result of a particular disease, based on the degree of the disability caused, have been tried, with rather promising results (Morrow, 1984). This approach has been found very useful in developing countries, where the chief burden of the disease problem consists in debilitating parasitic disease, against which relatively simple measures can produce dramatic results. In using this method, various factors such as the size of the target group affected, the feasibility of preventing the disease or effectively treating it, and the cost of implementing such measures needs to be developed. Such methods, based on a relative objective assessment of the impact of a disease, are to be preferred to the traditional approach derived from more subjective considerations. However, it must be stated that, following an objective determination of the priority rating of a disease or health problem, the result must be subjected to the political reality of the situation if community action is to be effectively organized for its control.

With these considerations in mind, it would appear that improvements in the health of mothers and their children would constitute an adequately high priority in most African countries. Accordingly, the health problems in Table 52.3 could be rearranged to reflect the appropriate priorities. In the process of rearranging the various resources, personnel, facilities, and finance become rather important limiting factors. Also the selection of the management alternative appropriate for a particular problem will depend on the extent of the resources available.

Assuming one decides that inadequate prenatal care is an important health problem, the first task in approaching the solution would be to decide on the group at risk. In this case it would be all child-bearing women. The next step is to identify the contributing factors that give rise to the problem. Present indications of the size of the problem – for example, the incidence of neonatal tetanus, puerperal sepsis, and antenatal as well as postnatal haemorrhage – would be important data to acquire. Also inadequate health facilities, ignorance concerning the proper maintenance of normal pregnancy, and poor midwifery practices need to be identified. The next issue would normally be: how to tackle the problem. Under the circumstances of a rural district, as already described, it would be inappropriate to expect the introduction of modern midwifery services to provide the solution to the problem. A plausible alternative solution might be a programme for the development of the role of traditional birth-attendants.

The rural community health practitioner, therefore, is faced, in this situation, with the problem of the organization of the health workers under him to identify and train the traditional birth attendants. Traditional birth attendants are found in most African countries. Their experience and backgrounds vary considerably. The first task is to identify who the traditional birth attendants are. During this process care should be taken to maintain a good rapport with the community and their traditional birth attendants. The impression must not be created that one is trying to unduly 'criticize' their methods, or to replace them with modern midwives. The next task is to draw up a syllabus whose content emphasizes the simple hygienic routines in midwifery, as well as the elements of prenatal care. The participants can then be involved in a more or less informal dialogue to exchange ideas. Such a course can be completed in six to ten weeks, depending on the frequency with which lessons are given (Ampofo et al., 1976). Following the training and certification stage, the health workers responsible for the programme have the task of supervising the work of the traditional birth attendants. This phase can last for several months to a year or two, during which in-service sessions are provided. Beyond this stage the traditional birth attendant is expected to be integrated into the Maternal and Child Health (MCH) services, and therefore should continue to be supervised by the responsible district public health nurse. There are few health services in Africa in which the traditional birth attendants have been so integrated. The aim of all traditional birth attendants programmes, however, should be to have them integrated into the MCH services.

Assessing Progress

Methods used for such assessment can either be by the use of ongoing service data, or by conducting special surveys. In a community with a fairly good distribution of health facilities, the service data should be adequate for this assessment. This method requires a regular analysis of morbidity and mortality data to determine trends. The importance of accurate baseline data for meaningful evaluation cannot be over-emphasized. Successful programme evaluation depends on the quality of the data upon which the community diagnosis was based. In addition to the documentation of achievable indices of programme objectives, it is important in the assessment of progress to determine the extent to which resources – both human and material – have been effectively utilized. This kind of evaluation can be obtained from a regular periodic assessment of the performance of staff at all levels, as well as from periodic reports on the adequacy of supplies and materials. A programme of improving prenatal care in a community can be assessed in the following way.

What needs to be determined is whether the programme has made an impact on the original status of the complications of pregnancy and delivery. Criteria, for example the incidence of neonatal tetanus and puerperal sepsis and antenatal and postnatal haemorrhage, can be measured to determine any improvement. Maternal mortality rate can also, over a defined period, reflect an improving midwifery service. These are the kinds of problems that the rural community health practitioner has to face in bridging the gap between available biomedical technology and what rural community health care actually receives in most of Africa.

The above procedure can be applied to any of the problems in Table 52.3, and a framework for organizing a solution can be developed. The successful rural community health practitioner operates a cycle of activities starting with a definition of problems and ending up with an assessment of the impact of any programme. It is the extent to which we can increase the influence of such successful community health practitioners that we can hope for a closing of the increasing gap between available medical services and the services that isolated rural communities actually enjoy. In the following section a description of the components of a comprehensive rural health programme is provided. The hope is that by applying the specific method described in the earlier part of the chapter to the components of the comprehensive programme, a functional health delivery scheme can be achieved.

A Comprehensive Health Programme Package in a Rural District

The organization of a comprehensive health care programme can be very complicated and tasking because of the numerous areas that have to be covered, and also because of the large component of community participation which is a *sine qua non* of any community health activity. It is for this reason that we would like to suggest the kinds of activities and programmes that a rural health doctor may have to undertake, and how he might go about organizing some of these activities. Usually the most common component of any health programme in a rural setting is individual patient-care activities. Often this is the best place to begin the contact and association with individuals within the community. Needless to say, the rapport which the health-care providers establish with their patients, as well as the quality of the care of the health facilities, can go a long way in making the community receptive to community-based programmes.

Child Welfare Clinics

There are several activities that can be considered under this conventional category. The management of the minor ailments of children is certainly one of these. The key to an effective clinic in a rural setting, however, is to run a combined well-and-ill-child clinic as many times as possible throughout the week. This implies that the clinic days should be convenient to the mothers. Such an arrangement provides an opportunity for the health provider to attain maximum coverage of the mothers and their children. In most rural clinics over sixty per cent of all patient contacts are with mothers and pre-school children. The clinic is therefore very important.

The immunization of all children should be an activity of high priority. The traditional static clinic approach to immunization coverage, however, has been found to be expensive and inefficient. In its place, a mass immunization campaign organized for a specific target population within the community is recommended. The method of organization and implementation, as well as the evaluation, has been set out in a publication of the Danfa project (Nicholas, et al. 1977). The mass immunization approach can yield up to 60 per cent coverage of the target population, and occasionally even more. This method has the added advantage of freeing the health providers during clinic hours from administering vaccines to a few children only, whose follow-up is often uncertain. The clinic can, however, be used routinely for the administration of booster doses.

Malaria prophylaxis is one activity which can be carried out with very minimal health centre staff involvement, except for the initial stages. The target population is pregnant women. The major hurdle in getting the programme going is how to get the co-operation of the mothers. The best results are obtained by consultations with the chiefs and other community leaders to obtain suitable appointments with the community. Once an audience has been obtained, it is best to outline simply and clearly what the programme entails pointing out particularly what responsibility the individuals will have. From then on it is only necessary to identify a staff member who will co-ordinate and supervise the distribution of tablets and the keeping of records.

The foregoing plan of child health activities should make it possible for health providers to spend more time on their home-visit and follow-up activities. It is the intensification of these activities that can increase the health education input into the health programmes of the district.

Maternal Health

At the district level, it is very convenient to combine the mother and child clinic activities so that the care of sick children and the well ones and their subsequent management causes little inconvenience to the mothers. Again, such an arrangement makes for easy follow-up of hitherto undetected problems that can first be identified in the clinic.

A family planning programme is a necessary component of a maternal health programme. The clinic-centred programme can include the provision of appropriate family planning services. However, it is essential for effective family planning programmes to develop a community-based component. Motivation of mothers, and the provision of family planning methods which do not need to be prescribed by a doctor on a house-to-house visit basis would be a very effective way to promote family planning. The task of motivation, therefore, should be undertaken by health providers at the various places where they make contact with individual men and women.

The traditional birth attendants have been mentioned earlier. The advantages of encouraging and up-grading their skills have been stated. Here it only remains to emphasize that a good maternal health programme in an African rural setting should have an active traditional birth attendant (TBA) scheme. The greatest contribution of a TBA programme is the early identification of maternal problems and their appropriate referral. The TBAs should therefore be considered as partners with other health providers in the district in the task of attempting to lower morbidity and mortality in mothers and their children.

Nutrition and Agricultural Extension

The first place for practical demonstration in nutrition is the clinic. Illustrative talks and demonstrations of the various types of food can also be carried out if facilities are available. Such demonstration becomes easier if a garden for that purpose is provided at the health centre. The nutrition officer or the staff, or else the agricultural extension officer, should be able to discuss the problems of growing the various food items with the farmers. Facilities for demonstrating improved seed and fertilizers can be a great asset to the nutrition education programme. Even greater interest is shown by the farmers if staff from the health centre with an interest in nutrition can visit their farms, and offer on-the-spot advice on their individual crop problems. In the area of nutrition education the health centre staff, particularly the community health nurses, and the midwives, have found organizing nutrition demonstration sessions at the homes of participating mothers a very effective way of achieving not only effective nutrition education but also education of healthful living for the entire family. Small numbers of mothers and young unmarried women are organized into clubs and groups. One or two coordinators are elected by the groups to supervise the details of their various planned activities. The attraction of this approach is that the demonstrations take place at the homes of the members of the group. The ingredients used in all demonstrations must be only the locally available food items. This approach to community health education has proved to be very popular with the few communities where it has been tried. It is recommended because it offers an excellent entry point into the community for badly needed health education. This type of collaboration between health and agricultural workers can be organized to suit the individual situation. There is little doubt that efforts in these directions have been paying handsome dividends in those programmes where these ideas have been tried.

Environmental Sanitation

There has been some debate as to the role of the health centre staff in environmental sanitation. While most health workers in rural communities will agree that improving the environment is as important as treating an acute illness, it is not always clear what role the health centre staff should play in this work. The practical situation is that where the health centre staff have been overburdened with the management of acute conditions, it is not possible to expect such staff to contribute in any significant way to environmental improvement programmes. In the foregoing scheme of a comprehensive rural health programme a deliberate effort has been made to lighten the acute illness management responsibilities of the health centre staff. Under such circumstances it is feasible to involve health centre staff in an environmental sanitation programme. The health inspector (assistant sanitarian) is the obvious leader of the team here. However, other members of the health centre staff in their community- based activities can support and promote family and community-wide activities in environmental sanitation. Communal activities can be organized at the convenience of the people to improve village water sources, improve house refuse disposal systems, build local markets, or cultivate a commercial farm for the support of various community social services. The involvement of the health centre staff in these activities is certainly new. Traditionally, trained health workers have not been accustomed to such activities as part of their responsibility. It is however, in this field among others that rural health workers can increase their impact on the health status of rural populations. We therefore recommend intensive involvement in this area of activity.

Evaluation of the Programme

For the purpose of evaluating the impact of various health programmes it is important that accurate data on the population as well as health activities should be kept. It is the responsibility of the health centre staff to organize this. For the denominator figure, it is helpful to use the latest national census figures for the district. For other ratios concerning population dynamics a simple household registration system can be set up. Several methods have been described (Bennet 1969; Kpedekpo 1972). A simple, low-cost method is to use volunteer school teachers in villages to cover births and deaths in defined clusters of villagers. With regard to patient-encounter record and disease profile, the health centre record should be an adequate source. But there are two factors that tend to render even good systems valueless. The first is over-complicated record forms. These tend to discourage staff from completing them. The second is the human factor of insufficient motivation. The recommendation on these problems are: Design simple short-record forms and pre-coded forms, if possible. Carefully discuss with the health centre staff the importance of carefully completed record forms, and the significance of their responsibility in this regard.

The comprehensive health package, as outlined above, can be very difficult to implement successfully. However, even moderately successful programmes have yielded impressive results, such as lowering the incidence of measles, childhood diarrhoea, noenatal tetanus, and kwashiorkor in the community; achieving wider birth intervals for child-bearing women, reducing the morbidity from puerperal causes, and reducing the infant mortality by at least ten per cent over an eight-year period. The experience from the Danfa project indicates that this level of success is attainable at a district level.

Appendix 1

A list of activities for a rural health team under the direction of a district medical officer:

1. Participate in the organization and the deliberation of village health committees.
2. Participate in the organization of subcommittees for specific activities.
3. Hold combined ill and well baby clinics at an appropriate frequency.
4. Organize adult clinics at an appropriate frequency.
5. Hold mothers' classes at convenient locations throughout the villages.
6. Family planning clinic.
7. Mass immunization programme.
8. Environmental sanitation programme.
9. Problem-oriented visiting –for example, special follow-up of chronic diseases patients on the clinic roll (leprosy, tuberculosis, and other handicapping conditions – for example, orphaned babies).
10. Collection of data and vital events (births, deaths).
11. Malaria prophylaxis programme.
12. Agricultural extension work, with annual farm exhibitions.
13. Annual clean house competition in connection with environmental sanitation programme.
14. Training and supervision of traditional birth attendants.
15. Communal labour campaigns for improved water.
16. Communal labour campaigns for improved latrine construction.
17. Communal labour campaigns for improved house-refuse disposal systems.
18. One-day school for clusters of villages to discuss health topics – for example how to maintain one's health.
19. Training and supervision of village health workers.
20. Periodic staff meetings for review of activities.
21. Joint meetings with community leaders to review programmes in the context of community-based activities.

Appendix 2

Examination Form for a Village Health Survey

Individual Number	Age No.	Age Yr.		Sex M.	Sex F	HH Nr
(1) ....../......./......(7) .../	1	2.	(10)	1	2	(11) ..../.../
Survey number	Village Nr.			Occupation (15 + years only)		Nr. in HH
(16) 9 0 3	(19)			(22)	(24)	

Persons to be queried:

(a) All subjects: Have you made trips or visits to a hospital or clinic for treatment during the past 12 months?
0 = No; 1–7 = 1 to 7 times; 8 = 8 + ; 9 = Don't Know (26) –

(b) 0–4 years-old: Has this child been vaccinated against any of the following diseases?

			Yes	No	Don't know
1.	Measles? (given with a jet gun)	(27)	1	2	9
2.	Tuberculosis? (injection on shoulder leaves scar)	(28)	1	2	9
3.	Whooping cough? (asked to return for 2nd shot)	(29)	1	2	9

What are this child's measurements for:

1.	Weight?	(30) ....kg
2.	Height?	(33).................cm
3.	Arm circumference?	(36) ....cm
4.	Skinfold triceps?	(39) ....mm

(c) For 15–44 year-old women:

1. How many live births have you delivered? (If any, ask;) (41) ....
2. Are they living? (If no, ask;) How many have died? (record if between 0-15 years at death) (43) ....
3. What was the child's age (years) at death?
   (a) .... (44) ....
   (b) .... (46) ....
   (c) .... (48) ....

For all subjects, conduct a medical examination as indicated below. Record whether the condition is present (1 = Yes) or absent (2 = No). If you do not examine a person or feel the examination was unsatisfactory, leave the space blank.

			Yes	No
1.	BCG scar?	(50)	1	2
2.	Yaws (primary or secondary)?	(51)	1	2
3.	Pyoderma?	(52)	1	2
4.	Guinea worm?	(53)	1	2
5.	Pedal oedema?	(54)	1	2
6.	Purulent conjunctivitis?	(55)	1	2
7.	Otitis media (acute)?	(56)	1	2
8.	Palpable spleen (splenomegaly)	(57)	1	2
9.	Poliomyelitis	(58)	1	2
10.	Other conditions (Specify)	(59)	....	....
11.	Other conditions? (Specify)	(62)	....	....

Laboratory test results			Pos.	Neg.
1.	Malaria film	(65)	1	2
2.	Stool hookworm	(66)	1	2
3.	Stool ascaris	(67)	1	2
4.	Urine schistosomiasis	(68)	1	2
5.	Haemoglobin (gramme %)	(69)	....	...

References

Barker, J.P. & Bennett, F.J. (1976) *Practical Epidemiology*. Churchill Livingstone, Edinburgh.

Belcher, D.W. & Wurapa, F.K. (1976). ' A Household Morbidity Survey in Rural Africa' *Int. J. Epidemiol.* 6, 113.

— & Lourie, I.M. (1977). 'Comparison of Morbidity Interviews with Health Examination Survey in Rural Africa' *Am. J. Trop. Med. Hyg.* 25.

—Wurapa, F.K.; Nicholas, D.D.; Kpedekpo, G.M.K.; Ofusu-Amaah, S.; Derban, L.K.A. & Asante, R.O. (1975). Conducting a Rural Health Survey: Experience from the Village Health Survey. –*Danfa Project, Ghana. Danfa Monograph Series*, No. 9.

Buck, A.A.; Anderson, R.I.; Sasaki T.T. & Kwata, K. (1970). *Health and Disease in Chad*. The Johns Hopkins Press, Baltimore.

Helberg, J.H. (1971). *Community Health and the Church*. Christian Medical Commission, World Council of Churches, Geneva.

Lucas, A.O. (1976). *Epidemiology as a Fundamental Science – Its Uses in Health Services Planning and Evaluation* (ed. K.L. White and M.M. Henderson). Oxford University Press, Ibadan.

Kpedekpo, G.M.K. (1972). 'The Planning of Sampling Surveys with Particular Reference to the Epidemiological Survey of the Danfa Project in Ghana,' *Ghana Med. J.* 11, 377–82.

Morrow R.H. Jr. (1984). 'How to Estimate the Relative Importance of Different Diseases: Estimates for Typhoid Fever from Ghana' *Tropical Doctor* 14 (2) 86–89.

Wurapa, F.K. & Belcher, D.W. (1975). 'An Approach to Illness Measurement in a Rural Community – A Questionnaire Sample Survey of Households in the Population of the Project Area in Ghana.' *Ghana Med. J.* 14, 94–105.

The Departmental Objectives and Teaching Programmes. Department of Community Health, University of Ghana Medical School.

53

A Community Laboratory Service as Part of Health Care

Elizabeth Topley

A community laboratory service can help to reduce morbidity and mortality in the community. We are in a period of evolution of laboratory services in many parts of the world. In many areas the work of the laboratory centres on the immediate needs of patients, but increasingly the same community laboratory service can provide the facilities for disease control in the area. The doctor thinking round the illness in his area can help to gear the laboratory to the early diagnosis and effective follow up to recovery which are so difficult to achieve and yet so valuable if preventable mortality and morbidity are to be reduced. Increasingly, concern will be for public health measures as well as patient care.

This chapter is addressed particularly to medical students who learn to order and carry out simple laboratory tests in outstations and in the side rooms of hospitals. In the future a few will have the vision to improve the community laboratory services: many will be leaders collaborating with their laboratory which helps to reduce morbidity and mortality.

The community laboratory service in the Ibarapa Programme of the University of Ibadan, Nigeria, was started in 1971. It will be used as a basis of discussion of the place of the doctor in the community laboratory services trying to improve health care in the developing world. Adadevo (ref. Akinkugbe et al 1973) was emphasizing the concept of overall collaboration from the laboratory angle in this area of Nigeria. Earlier and current reports by the World Health Organisation (1957, 1962, 1972) describe the thinking at the time. Handbooks of the day (Cheesbrough and McArthur 1976) provided simple laboratory teaching on technical methods. Browne's description of the work in the Congo in the 60s should be referred to by all those starting a tropical laboratory (Browne 1979, 1980).

After describing the Ibarapa community laboratory service, we will discuss the role of the medical officer in the community laboratory service of his area today.

Ibarapa Community Laboratory Service

It can be seen from Fig. 53.1 that there were two 'one-man' laboratories in the Ibarapa District of about 150,000 people. One is in Igboora and other in Eruwa. The laboratory service from these simple laboratories is part of the Ibarapa Programme of the University of Ibadan, run in collaboration with the Government departments responsible for the health services of Ibarapa District. University College Hospital, Ibadan, is the specialist reference centre for all types of laboratory support, including the blood bank. More peripherally there are small units, often called maternity and child welfare centres and dispensaries, usually grouped together. For the purpose of Fig. 53.1 all such places are included under the word 'clinic'.

The Nigerian 'Federal Ministry of Health' Plan (1975) envisaged two paramedical personnel serving every 2,000 people in the rural population. These 'health aides' (Ransome-Kuti et al. 1976) go into the community as well as being attached to a health clinic. The 12 villages in the Okolo area and Okolo Health Clinic are shown separately in Fig. 53.1 because it is these villages that were used to learn more about the use of laboratory tests taken by a health aide and about the role of the health aid in referring patients because they need a laboratory test that has to be done at a laboratory (such as very pale mucous membranes indicating that the patient is anaemic and requires a laboratory test to help with treatment).

Table 53.1 compares the population served in rural China (Adey and Smith 1974) with the population served in the Ibarapa Programme as it extends from the Okolo villages through Okolo clinic to Eruwa District Hospital. China concentrates on bare-foot doctors. The Ibarapa Okolo idea concentrates on two whole time paramedical personnel (aides) for 2,000 villagers. Both ideas lay emphasis on collaboration with the community peripherally, and the support of medically qualified doctors and in-service training centrally.

With such a community health service, what are the clinical conditions which a laboratory at this community level can help to diagnose and follow up to recovery?

The Clinical Conditions

Infective Disease or Infestations

Table 53.3, combined with Table 53.4 (Ransome-Kuti et al 1976), covers the common conditions in which the laboratory may help. Table 53.2 lists, perhaps in order of the value of the laboratory in disease control, the diseases commonly diagnosed in the laboratory. It suggests in which instances the laboratory assists in (1) reducing morbidity, (2) mortality, (3) prevalence and (4) improved follow up. The tables do not include diseases such as trypanosomiasis or leishmaniasis important in other areas of the world. But, the microscopist is looking out for rare as well as common diseases.

The laboratory does not rely only on the detection of the organism under the microscope. The laboratory can also help by reporting evidence that there is a host response that could be caused by an infective process, which therefore may need looking for. Such possible clues may include (1) a raised total leucocyte count, or a mononuclear or polymorphonuclear response, or both as judged by a blood film; (2) the presence of a polymorphonuclear cell response (pus cells) or other cellular response in any other specimen such as an exudate or swab; and (3) the presence of albumin or other protein not normally present such as in CSF or urine.

Of immunological test, the Mantoux is the only one listed. This chapter will not discuss the care and control of tuberculosis, apart from emphasizing the importance of the sputum test at this level of health care.

Genetic Disease

The prevalence of SS and SC haemoglobinopathy in Ibarapa varies perhaps from 4% in the first year of life to 1/2% in adults. Screening every new anaemic child by haemoglobin electrophoresis has revealed many previously unsuspected cases, and allows them to be helped at sickle cell clinics (Adeyokunnu and Topley 1977). Such screening was a practical routine because the laboratory worker knew his patients so well. Glucose 6PD deficiency with minimal symptoms is prevalent in Ibarapa. A high index of suspicion is provided by jaundice combined with a severe infection (often detected in the laboratory by the host response) or by haemoglobinuria.

Anaemia

As paramedical personnel get better in detecting pallor of mucous membranes more patients can be referred to the laboratory for testing the degree of anaemia to be measured and followed up. Perhaps in time 10% of the community can be managed effectively for anaemia as part of model primary health care. The degree of anaemia managed will depend on its prevalence and the current health care facilities. In Okolo and in the Gambia (Topley 1968 a,b,c, 1975, 1976 1981, a,b) a study of the most anaemic 10% of the childhood, adult female and adult male population suggested that early diagnosis and careful follow up might result in a reduction of the prevalence of this degree of anaemia from 10% to 2% of the population covered.

The laboratory can help by a precise enough measurement of the degree of anaemia to follow the patient to full recovery. It can also help in suggesting the likely cause of the anaemia. The anaemia is often secondary to malaria and other infective diseases, while iron deficiency may be important especially where hookworm infestation is prevalent or in the presence of menorrhagia or pregnancy. The blood film report can help to suggest the possibility of the anaemia of sickle cell disease, malaria, other infections, severe iron deficiency and folate deficiency.

Other Diseases

The time will come when, for every clinical syndrome, a specialist will be given the opportunity to understand the problem of diagnosis, treatment and referral at every level of health care. Considered opinions will be given on the laboratory support needed at each site of action. This will vary enormously from country to country and area to area and year to year. The limitation often is the skill of the laboratory worker not only to do tests but to maintain equipment. The laboratory has to be cost effective. The laboratory worker should be encouraged to do what it is possible to do well.

Bearing these problems in mind and drawing on the specialists in Ibadan in the 70s it was felt that the side room type tests for anaemia or of urine and stool should predominate. It would be helpful in very rare cases to be able to screen for uraemia diabetes or G6PD deficiency. The doctor at the district hospital may wish to take biopsies especially of lymph nodes. A blood culture may be sent to a reference laboratory without the need to send the patient.

The Survey

The occasional survey, such as one on the prevalence of hookworm infestation in the community, proves valuable in planning the laboratory service and community action. Again, the limit is often the available laboratory workers and field workers.

Public Health

The limitation is the availability of methods of bacterial cultivation. It is highly desirable for the results to be quickly available to local health staff. The method of testing the potability of water, for example by the faecal coliform count, maybe within the range of what the local one-man laboratory could do. If so, it would be easy to add a test for the chlorine content. The time will come when the public health specialist and epidemiologist will apply specialist thinking to how the primary health care laboratories can be much more effective in the control of community health, bearing in mind the local constraints. In public health there is an obvious need for central public health laboratories to be supporting laboratory work relevant to community health as has been developed in the UK (Williams 1985).

The Laboratory Tests

Bearing in mind the diagnosis of the clinical conditions discussed above, Table 53.4 outlines the tests available during the 70s in the Ibarapa Community Laboratory service. It also shows the samples that are taken for those tests more peripherally and the samples that are sent from Igboora or Eruwa laboratories to the reference laboratory in Ibadan.

Of the haematology tests, a precise measurement of the degree of anaemia (Topley 1986, WHO Lab/1984 7) is most important. Table 53.5 shows the details of the blood film report recommended in the light of the experience in Ibarapa (TALC 1986). Table 53.5 includes haemoglobin electrophoresis for the reasons described above. The sodium nitrite reduction test for G6PD deficiency is mainly recommended because of the stability of the reagent. The sedimentation rate has been deliberately omitted, but could be done on request in the rare case where the naturally high fibrinogen levels were not likely to confuse the result.

Added to the pus, smears and swabs should perhaps have been the scrapings for example for ringworm or leprosy (Browne 1980), but such cases were not studied in Ibarapa in the 70s.

Starting a Laboratory from Scratch

The subject is well covered by King (1973), whose book contains a picture of the small room transformed by shelves, a bench, buckets, and the minimal equipment to a good simple laboratory without mains gas, water or electricity. Gas is from a cylinder. Water is in a bucket. A few hour generator electricity is needed for haemoglobin electrophoresis. Otherwise none is essential. Microscopy can be done by daylight.

The appendix to this chapter provides a list of equipment that is more complete in detail than obtainable any where else for the test shown in Table 53.4.

The training of the laboratory staff will not be discussed here. Of importance was the possibility of having a good laboratory technologist to support the laboratory closely, for example by bringing in quality control from the reference centre, doing procedures such as the calibration of a haemoglobinometers and giving in-service training to the laboratory staff.

As the laboratory programme developed, we learned that success depended on close collaboration between laboratory staff and the patients who came for the test and between laboratory staff and doctors. At Igboora the laboratory worker (M.S. Ajagbe) became an excellent collaborator with all who were interested. The supervising technologist was available for expert advice. Emphasis was placed on the need, through the local doctor and visiting experts, for agreement on what tests should be ordered and how follow up could be achieved.

Evaluation of the Ibarapa Community Laboratory Service

Limited data suggests that with the optimum use of the laboratory, the medical and paramedical personnel can treat individual patients better. In particular:-

1. The prevalence of anaemia can be reduced, for example from the degree of anaemia currently affecting 10% of the community to 2% of the community, provided there is no resistance to the antimalarials which would be used as sparingly as possible.
2. Large numbers of patients with sickle cell anaemia can be diagnosed earlier to the clinical benefit of the patient.
3. Weight faltering due to primary tuberculosis and severe anaemia due to hookworm infestation can be picked up earlier and treated.
4. Schistosomiasis producing haemoglobinuria can be detected earlier, and treated, and the appropriate health education to the community slowly introduced.
5. Cases of adult tuberculosis can be detected earlier and treated and the sputum of contacts examined.
6. Infective diarrhoea and urinary pyuria can be spotted by stool or urine microscopy and investigated and followed up as indicated.
7. Cases of possible venereal disease suspected from microscopy and history can be referred for investigation.

The Community Laboratory Service Today

The doctor leading the community laboratory service for health care from the district to the village level is going in the end to improve greatly on the Ibarapa service. But, the Ibarapa type of service will often be the starting point.

There is a certain amount of recent literature to help. Cheesbrough's books *(Medical Laboratory Manual for Tropical Countries* 1987, 1989) help very greatly. The first volume includes in the introduction the general concept of health care at different levels. WHO reports cover the central more than the peripheral laboratories at the moment, but the services at the remote primary health care level are mentioned. WHO/Lab/87.2 discusses the prerequisites, relevance, need for co-ordination, supervision, logistical support, reports and information, collection and despatch of samples, cost effectiveness; Lab/83 11 and Lab/84 4 quality control. Of earlier reports, Lab/83 10 discusses cost effectiveness. Lab/85.7 provides self instruction sheets for users of more complicated 'primary' health care laboratory equipment. Lab/84 7 lists for peripheral laboratories less detailed haematology than used in Ibarapa. Lab/79 1 and WHO 1979 stress strongly the need for continuous support and supervision at all levels.

The doctor responsible for the community laboratory service in his area, including primary health care, must refer to the WHO experiences described above.

To summarize, a community laboratory service helps to reduce mortality and morbidity in the community served. A decision has to be made:

1. What are the local diseases whose morbidity and mortality are likely to be reduced by the availability of a realistic local laboratory? Table 53.2 is basis for thought.
2. What laboratory tests are needed that can be carried out accurately enough to be useful in early diagnosis and careful follow up to recovery of these diseases? Here reference to Tables 53.4 and 53.5 may help, but it is useful to read the WHO literature, Cheesbrough's (1987, 1989) and *Practical Haematology* (Dacie and Lewis 1984) to decide the test to be done bearing in mind the facilities. Should the list in Tables 53.4 and 53.3 be shortened or extended? Can the local pathologist and reference centres help in these decisions?
3. Does the laboratory have to be started from scratch? If so, the list of equipment in the appendix has more minute detail than other published lists. Reference should be made to WHO Lab.87 2.
4. What supervision and quality control is needed from a reference centre (WHO/83 11, WHO/84 4. Cheesbrough 1987, 1989) to maintain the technical efficiency, and accuracy and precision of the results? The reference centre can get advise at the national or international level on how to ask for newly introduced opportunities for quality control such as for testing the degree of anaemia by different methods. The reference centre can send out technical experts to help peripheral laboratories. More often the peripheral laboratory worker has his own contacts when he visits the reference centre.
5. What collaboration and in-service training is needed between patients, laboratory staff and medical and paramedical staff to see that the laboratory service does help

to reduce morbidity and mortality in the community? Staff meetings of all involved may help, together with appropriate visits to the laboratory of non-laboratory staff.

The challenge is a strong one. Laboratories serving the community are in the process of evolution. The dialogue has similarities to the more general dialogue on the future of primary health care. There is perhaps a chance of witnessing to success in model laboratory programmes supported by the universities of developing countries such as the Ibarapa programme.

Acknowledgments

This chapter is possible because of the experts at all levels who have supported the Ibarapa Programme Community Laboratory Service. Particular appreciation is expressed to Mr A. Akintola, AIMLT who is in charge of the laboratory and medical student teaching; and to Mr M.A. Ajagbe, now laboratory chief assistant, at Igboora laboratory. It is they who have been the builders of the laboratory programme.

References

Adey, E.M. & Smith, A.J. (1974) "Medicine in China". *British Medical Journal. ii* 367–379, 429–432, 548–550, 603–605.

Adeyokunnu, A.A. & Topley, E. (1977) Sickle Cell Anaemia, Diagnosis and Care in a Nigerian Health Centre. *Trans. R. Soc. Trop. Med. Hyg. 71*, 416–420.

Akinkugbe, O.O., Olatunbosun, D. & Esan G.J.F. (1973). *Priorities in National Health Planning* Caxton Press, West Africa Ltd., Ibadan.

Browne, S.G. (1979) The Contribution of Medical Missionaries to Tropical Medicine – Service, Training and Research. *Trans. R. Soc. Trop. Med. Hyg. 73*, 357–360.

Browne, S.G. (1980) Discussion in Meeting on Laboratory Support for Rural Health Care *Proc. Roy. Soc. London (Biol.) 209*, 127.

Cheesbrough, M. (1987). *Medical Laboratory Manual for Tropical Countries* Vol. I 2nd Edition. Tropical Health Technology. Butterworth.

Cheesbrough, M. (1989). *Medical Laboratory Manual for Tropical Countries*. Vol. II Revised Reprint. Tropical Health Technology/Butterworth.

Cheesbrough, M. & McArthur, J. (1976). *Laboratory Manual for Rural Tropical Hospitals*. Churchill Livingstone, Edinburgh.

Dacie, J. & Lewis, S.M. (1984). *Practical Haematology*. 6th Edition. Churchill Livingstone, Edinburgh.

Federal Ministry of Health, Lagos (1975). *Challenge of the Basic Health Service Scheme for Change. W July 29–Aug. 4 1975.*

King, M. (1973). *A Medical Laboratory for Developing Countries*. Oxford University Press, Ibadan.

Ransome-Kuti, A.O. et al. (1976). *Community Health Aide: Standing Order*. Institute of Child Health, University of Lagos. Mimeo.

TALC (1986), Topley, E. *Anaemia, Reporting Blood Films*. Teaching Aids at Low Cost. Series Hgy.

Topley, E. (1968) (a) Hookworm Anaemia Among Men, (b) Iron Deficiency Anaemia Among Women, (c) Spontaneously Remitting Anaemia Precipitated by Malaria Parasitaemia. *Trans R. Soc. Trop. Med. Hyg. 62* 579–605.

Topley, E. (1975) Anaemia where Malaria is Endemic. *Trop. Doct. 5* 18–22

Topley, E. (1976) *A Community Laboratory Service as Part of Rural Health Care*. Proc. Annual Conf. Nigerian Medical Association 1975/1976 96–100.

Topley, E (1981a) Common Haematological Problems in the Children of an African Village where Malaria is Endemic *Postgrad. Doctor* 6 209-215.

Topley, E. (1981b) Common Haematological Problems in Adults of an African Village where Malaria is Endemic. *Postgrad. Doctor 6* 296-301.

Topley, E. (1986). *Testing Degree of Anaemia* 16, 3–8.

W.H.O. (1957) The Public Health Laboratory Service. First Report of Expert Committee on Health Laboratory Methods *Tech. Rep. Series* 28.

W.H.O. (1962) Planning, Organization and Administration of a National Health Laboratory Service. Third Report *Tech. Rep. Series 236*.

W.H.O. (1972) Planning and Organization of a Health Laboratory Service. Fifth Report. *Tech. Rep. Series* 491.

W.H.O. Lab/79.1 *Laboratory Services at Primary Health Care Level* 1–21

W.H.O. (1979) *Laboratory Services at the Primary Health Care Level W.H.O. Chronicle* 33 334–337.

W.H.O. *Lab/83 10 Cost Effectiveness.*

W.H.O. Lab/83 11 *Guidelines for the Organization of National Quality Assessment Programmes*. 1–6.

W.H.O. Lab/84 4 *Development and Introduction of the Concept of Reference Value in Health Laboratories.*

W.H.O. Lab/84 7 *Haematology for Peripheral Laboratories.*

W.H.O. Lab/85 7 *Self Instruction Sheets for Users of Primary Health Care Equipment.*

W.H.O. Lab/87 2 *Laboratory Services at Primary Health Care Level.*

Williams, R.E.O. (1985) *Microbiology for the Public Health* Public Health Laboratory Service, London.

Appendix I

Fig. 53.1

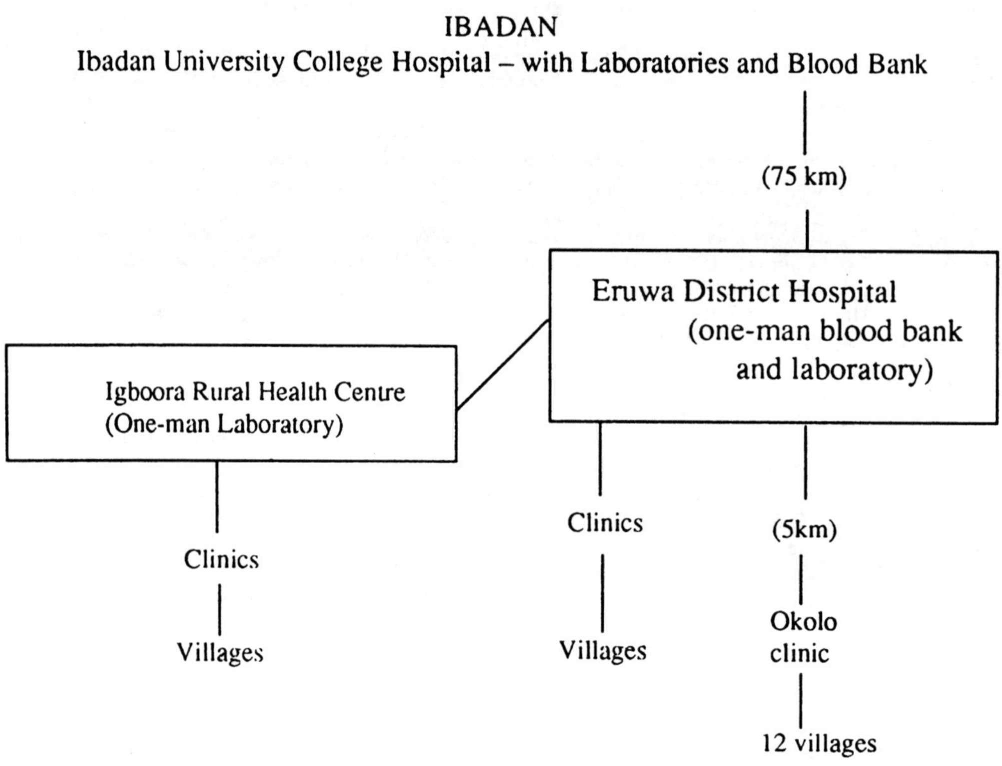

IBARAPA DISTRICT

Table 53.1

Comparison of Health Services in Rural China and the Okolo Area of Ibarapa Programme

China		Ibarapa	
Population Served	**Place of Service**	**Population Served**	**Place of Service**
100,000–200,000	County Hospital	140,000	Eruwa Hospital
2,000–65,000	Community Hospital	50,000	Eruwa Hospital
2,000	Brigade Headquarters	2,000	Okolo Clinic
260–700	Product Hospital Team	50–500	Village

From Adey and Smith 1974

Table 53.2

Infective Diseases or Infestations that Require Laboratory Tests

The laboratory can help to reduce (1) morbidity, (2) mortality, (3) prevalence and (4) improved follow-up in the following bacterial or parasitic conditions:

Tuberculosis	(1), (2), (3), and (4)
Meningitis	(1) and (2)
Gonorrhoea	(1), (3), and (4)
Malaria	(1) and (2)
Urinary infections	(1) and (4)
Amoebic dysentery	(1), (2) and (4)
Bacillary dysentery	(1), (2) and (4)
Onchocerciasis	(1)
Hookworm infestation	(1), (3) and (4)
Schistosomiasis	(1)
Ascariasis	(4)
Septicaemia	(1)

The laboratory helps the health centre staff in:

- Earlier and more precise diagnosis
- Increasing clinical skill in index of suspicion
- Improved follow-up
- Survey and special studies
- Increasing the clinical skill in raising the index of suspicion so as to know when a laboratory test is important, and when it is not necessary.

Table 53.3
List of Main Health Conditions, Health Work and Supportive Tasks in Nigeria

	Health Conditions, Work, Tasks	Laboratory Support
1	Gastro-enteritis (dysenteric diseases)	stool for pus and red cells
2	Malnutrition	stool, urine, blood, mantoux
3	Intestinal parasites	stool
4	Upper respiratory tract infections (acute)	–
5	Tuberculosis	mantoux and sputum
6	Malaria	thick blood film
7	Meningitis (epidemic)	cerebrospinal fluid
8	Measles	total leucocyte (WBC) count to look for added infection
9	Small pox	–
10	Poliomyelitis (prevention)	–
11	Cholera	–
12	Schistosomiasis	urine for red cells and ova
13	Onchocerciasis and filariasis	skin snip or blood test
14	Leprosy	nasal septum scraping
15	Skin infections	scrappings
16	Eye infections and trachoma	smear if? gonorrhoea
17	Veneral disease	cervical or urethral smear
18	Tetanus	–
19	Pregnancy	Screen for anaemia and albuminuria
20	Conditions requiring surgical work	
	Other health work	
21	Immunizations (DPT)	–
22	School health work	blood, urine, stool
23	Health education work	use laboratory results to teach
24	Environmental health work	potability and chlorination of water supplies
25	Community health work	surveys
26	Dental health work	–
27	Laboratory work	–
	Supportive tasks	
28	Patient registration	–
29	Referral of patients	
30	Reporting of statistical information	
31	Training of staff (on-the-job training)	collaboration with
32	Training of TBAs and training of village health workers	all staff on how to use laboratory service
33	Supervision	
34	Logistics of supplies	
35	Mobile team work	

Ransome–Kuti et al, 1976

Table 53.4

Laboratory Tests Carried out in Ibarapa Since 1971

	Tests	*Village clinic sample*	*Test in lab.*	*Sent to reference centre*
Haematology	Packed cell volume	+	+	–
	Haemoglobin	–	+	–
	Total WBC	–	+	–
	Malaria parasites	+	+	–
	Reticulocyte count	–	+	–
	Filaria	–	+	–
	Thin blood film report	+	+	–
	Hb. electrophoresis	+	+	–
	G6PGscreening	–	+	–
Blood quick tests	Urea	–	+	–
	Sugar	–	+	–
Urine	Naked eye	+	+	–
	Albumin	+	+	–
	Glucose	+	+	–
	Urobilonogen	+	+	–
	Bilirubin	+	+	–
	Ketones	+	+	–
	Deposit	+	+	–
Stool	Naked eye	+	+	–
	Microscopy	+	+	–
	Stool count, HW ova	+	+	–
	Occult blood	+	+	–
Sputum	Naked eye	+	+	–
	Tubercle bacilli	+	+	–
Cerebrospinal fluid	Tubercle bacilli	+	+	–
	Naked eye	+	+	–
	WBG and RBC count	+	+	–
	Microscopy	–	+	–
	Albumin	–	+	–
	Sugar	–	+	–
Pus, smear, swabs	Microscopy – cervical, urethral, eye, pus, etc	–	+	–
Tuberculin test (Mantoux)		read result	+	–
Skin snip	Onchocerciasis	–	+	–
Blood culture		–	–	+
Biopsy		–	–	+

Table 53.5

Thin Blood Film Report

Look for the following in every blood film. Report if present:

Hypochromia, hypochromic microcytes –
Macrocytes –
Polychromasia –
Sickle/cells –
Malaria parasites –
Increased or decreased numbers of leucocytes –
Abnormal proportion of different leucocytes –
Cytology suggesting response to infection
  polymorphs –
  mononuclear cells –
Hypersegmented polymorphs –
Malaria pigment –
Nucleated red blood cells –
Increased or decreased numbers of platelets –
Target cells –
Stomatocytes –

Overall comment –

APPENDIX II

Laboratory Equipment
For supply to small 'one-man' laboratories

Igboora Rural Health Centre Laboratory
List of Equipment Needed

Basic – By area of laboratory as it might be planned by a laboratory assistant working alone.

Area	1.	Main working area.
"	2.	Boxes above main working area.
"	3.	Capillary blood testing.
"	4.	Venous blood samples and other samples from patients.
"	5.	Laboratory area of samples (4 above).
"	6.	Staining area.
"	7.	Making up reagents area (including weighing).
"	8.	Chemicals and stains area.
"	9.	Glass and plastic ware area.
"	10.	Record area.
"	11.	Electric centrifuging area.
"	12.	Colorimetry area.
"	13.	Microscopy area.
"	14.	Washing up area.
"	15.	Disinfection area.
"	16.	Disposal area.
"	17.	Heating and sterilizing area.
"	18.	Electrical generating area.
"	19.	Boxes of spares top shelf.

Extra where indicated –

Area	20.	Haemoglobin electrophoresis.
"	21.	Distilled water.
"	22.	G6PD deficiency screening.
"	23.	Blood grouping and cross matching.

Contents of Equipment Kits – 1–20

ML	= Number in Maurice Kings book* (ref.)
New	= Not in Maurice Kings book.

1. Box for main working area – (Opening to make 2 trays)

1	Metal tray – New 25) (supplied outside box)
1	Test tube rack - ML 41) " " "
2	Centrifuge tubes – ML. 46
4	Standard test tubes - ML. 48c
2	Kahn tubes - ML. 48c
2	Graduated centrifuge tubes - ML. 47
1	Filter funnel - ML. 25
1	Box filter paper - ML. 22
2	Pairs forceps - ML. 24
1	Grease pencil - ML. 31
1	Lead pencil - New 1
	Packet razor blades New 2
2	Beakers 500 ml. or plastic cups – New 44 or ML. 58
2	Pasteur pipettes - New 3
2	Rubber teats - ML. 42
1	Piece bent wire for vaseline – New 4
1	Roll of toilet paper – New 5
1	Clean linen cloth – New 6
1	Box glass cover lips – ML. 17
1	Box glass slides – ML. 37
1	Wide mouth bottle for used cover lips – ML. 62
2	Very wide mouth bottle for slides – New 7 (used and unused)
2	Sterile pasteur pipettes – New 3

* *A Medical Laboratory for Developing Countries* by Maurice King.

2. Box for shelf above main working area –

Divide into appropriate compartments.
Make it easy to lift down to bench.

1	Roll cotton wool –New 8
1	Roll toilet paper – New 5
1	Linen cloth – New 6
1	Box filter paper – ML. 22
1	Roll adhesive plaster or 1 box labels – New 22
1	Roll string – New 20
1	Pair scissors– ML 70
2	Boxes litmus paper – ML. 110
2	Boxes universal indicator test paper – ML 109
6	Boxes pH6.8 buffer tablets – New 10
6	Boxes pH7.2 buffer tablets – New 11
12	Spare grease pencils – ML. 31
6	Spare lead pencils – New 1
1	Box glass slides high quality – New 12 (to make spreaders for thin blood films)
4	Boxes glass slides – ML. 37
4	Boxes cover slips – ML 17
1	Glass cutter – New 13
1	Glass cutting marker for slides – ML. 20
6	Rubber teats – ML.42
1	Thermometer – ML. 44
1	Thermometer sheath – ML 45
1	Roll nickel chrome wire for loop holder – ML. 58
1	Spare loop holder – ML. 28
1	Box plasticine – ML. 67
1	Paint brush – ML. 56
1	Spirit pen – ML. 66
1	Spare wick for spirit lamp – ML 54
1	Tin paraffin wax – New 14
1	Tin vaseline – New 15
1	Tin quick drying paint – ML. 64
1	Bottle of ink for spirit pen – New 16
1	Pair pliers – ML. 68
1	Hammer – ML. 61
1	Box swab sticks – New 9

3. Box for capillary blood sample and blood testing

2	Very wide mouthed bottles – New 7 (one for prickers, one for spreaders – see directions)
9	Bijou bottles – ML 14a (for Hb or WBC diluants or EDTA)
2	Universal containers – ML. 14b (for spirit and iodine)
1	Packet plain capillary tubes – New 17
1	Packet heparinized capillary tubes – ML. 123
4	Blood pipettes (0.02 ml) ML. 32, 33, 34
2	Blood pipettes (0.1 ml)
	Neubaurer counting chamber – ML. 15,16.

4. Box for taking other samples from patients

(a) Preparation of syringes and needles
(b) Taking venous blood and blood culture
(c) Pus, smears, scrapes, snips, biopsies
(d) Urine and stool

2	Metal trays – New 25
2	Sterile syringes and needles (see Fig. 4.3 F&G opposite 4.5)* –New 32
1	Sterile needle and rubber tubing (see Fig. 4.3D)* – New 31
1	Length rubber as tourniquet – ML. 50
6	Spare sterile syringes and needles – New 32
1	Oilstone – ML. 62
1	Magnifying glass – New 33
1	Sheet brown paper – New 34 (see Fig. 4.3D)*
12	Polytubes or 6 bijou bottles and 6 universal containers – ML. 14b
1	Roll string – New 20
	Liquid paraffin in one bijou bottle – New 27 in ML. 14a
	Blood culture bottles from reference laboratory
	Heaf test or tuberculin syringe from local reference laboratory
	Packet razor blades – New 2
	Sterile swabs from ward or reference laboratory
1	Box slides – ML 37
1	Box cover slips – ML 17
2	Pairs forceps – ML 27
	Transport medic from reference laboratory
	Urine containers – Universal ML. 14b or disposable
	Stool containers " " "

5. Box for urine, stool, sputum, CSF, pus, smears, swabs, scrapes, snips, and biopsy area

1	Roll cellulose film – ML. 148 (a&b)
3	Urine cylinders – New 21
6	Polypots – ML 14e or other disposal containers
6	Universal containers – ML. 14b
1	Test tube rack – ML. 41
5	Standard test tubes – ML. 48a
4	Kahn tubes – ML. 48c
1	Graduated centrifuge tube – ML. 47
3	Centrifuge tubes – ML. 46
1	Filter funnel – ML. 25
1	Box filter paper – ML. 22
6	1000 ml. reagent bottles – ML. 6
1	100 ml. bottle with cap – New 28
5	Drop bottles – ML. 5
1	Wash bottle – ML. 8
4	Very wide mouthed screw cap bottles – New 7
3	Plastic cups (mortar) – ML. 58
2	Tins – New 29 for paper strips
1	Grease pencil – ML. 31
1	Spatula – ML. 38
	Quick tests occult blood urine – New 23
	Quick tests occult blood stool – New 24
	Quick tests dextrostix sugar stool – ML. 144
2	Pasteur pipettes – New 3
2	Rubber teats – ML. 42
1	Box cover slips – ML. 17
1	Box slides – ML. 37
1	Forceps – ML. 24
	Elastoplast – New 26
1	Metal tray – New 25
1	Hand centrifuge – ML. 12
	Set of proteinometer standards – ML. 36
	Neubauer counting chamber – ML. 15, 16
4	Conical flasks with corks – New 38
	Glass beads – New 39
1	Glass rod – New 40
1	Box large cover slips – New 41
	100 ml cylinder – ML. 18

6. Box for staining area

2	Pieces glass tubing – ML. 51
	Rubber tubing 1–2ft. – ML. 50
1	Bucket – New 35
1	Timer minutes – New 36
1	Slide drying rack – New 37
1	Box filter paper – ML. 22
1	Toilet roll –New 5
8	Dropping bottles – ML. 5
2	Wash bottles – ML. 8
2	Polystop bottles – ML. 7
4	Reagent bottles – ML. 6

A	B	C
Empty reagent bottles labelled ML. 45, and dropping bottle labelled ML. 46	**Empty reagent bottles labelled ML. 45, and wash bottles labelled ML. 47**	**Empty reagent bottles to be labelled**
Giemasa	Saline	10% formol saline
Leishmann	Spirit	Fields stain A
Xylol	20% sulphuric acid	Fields stain B
Dilute carbol fuchsin	Buffer pH6.8	
Conc. carbol fuchsin	Buffer pH7.2	
Crystal violet	Acetone	
Methylene blue		
Grams iodine		
Lugols iodine		

4 very wide mouthed jars Fields stain – New 7.

7. Box for making up reagents (including weighing)

1	Balance (Fig. 5.1) – ML. 1
1	Counterweight – ML. 1
1	Extra weights – ML. 3
1	Watch glass – ML. 52
1	Scoop – ML. 2
1	Spatula – ML. 38
2	Cups – ML. 58
2	Standard test tubes – ML. 48a
1	100 ml measuring cylinder stoppered – ML. 18a
1	1000 ml measuring cylinder – ML. 19a
1	10 ml pipette – ML. 35c,
1	5 ml pipette – ML. 35b,
1	2 ml pipette – ML. 35a
1	Test tube rack – ML. 41
1	Funnel – ML. 25
1	Packet filter paper – ML. 22
1	Wash bottle – ML. 8
1	1000 ml beaker – New 43
1	100 ml – beaker – New 44
2	Glass rods – New 40
1	1000 ml reagent bottles – ML. 6
1	100 ml screw capped bottle – ML. 62

(Collect necessary materials from reagents, chemicals, and stains list; extra glass ware from glass ware area; use burner or spirit lamp for heat).

8. Box for chemicals and stains – New

Stains	**Chemicals**	**Floor or liquid shelf**
Basic fuchsin	Acid suphosalicylic	Acetic acid glacial
Crystal violet	Acid trichloracetic	Acetone
Fields stain A	Ammonium sulphate	Ammonia conc.
Field stain B	Barium chloride	Hydrochloric acid
Methylene blue	Cupric sulphate	
Lieshmann powder	Ferric chloride	Sulphuric acid conc.
Giemas	Iodine crystals	Formaldehyde solution 40%

Lieshmann liquid

Para-dimethyl-amino benzaldehyde
EDTA (sequestrine)
Potassium iodide
Potassium dihydrogen phosphate
Dihydrogen potassium phosphate
Saponin white
Sodium acetate
Sodium carbonate (anhydrous)
Sodium chloride
Trisodium citrate
Sodium hydroxide pellets
Sodium dithionate
Sodium nitroprusside
Oil for immersion lenses
Xylene
1 Bottle parafin – New 18
1 Packet aculute tablets – New 19
1 Bottle trichloracetic acid – New 75

Teepol
Methanol
Spirit (rectified)
Lysol – New 59

9 Box for glass and plastic ware
(quantity is over and above that already listed)

(a) Bottles and cylinders (Put on shelf if shelf is available)
6 Reagent bottles 1000 ml – ML. 6
6 Wide mouthed bottles – ML. 62
6 Very wide mouthed bottles – New 7
Graduated cylinders – 2 1000 ml – ML. 19
4 100 ml – ML. 18
1 10 ml – ML. 47

(b) Smaller bottles and cups (Put in drawer if drawer is available)
112 Bijou bottles – ML. 14a
112 Universal containers – ML. 14b
112 Polypots – ML. 14c
112 Poly tubes – ML. 14d
6 Dropping bottles – ML. 5

6 Polystop bottles – 100 ml – ML. 7
2 Wash bottles 200 ml – ML. 8
6 Plastic cups – ML. 58

(c) Slides, tubes and cover slips (Put in drawer if drawer is available)
12 Boxes glass slides – ML. 37
6 Boxes cover lips – ML. 17
6 Gross heparinized haematocrit tubes – ML. 123
1 Box plain capillary tubes – New 17

(d) Pipettes (Put in drawer if drawer is available)
1 Graduated 2 ml – ML. 35a
2 5 ml – ML. 35b
4 10 ml – ML. 35c
6 Blood pipettes with mouthpiece – ML. 32, 33, 34
6 Pasteur pipettes to be made from glass tubing – ML. 51
2 Graduated centrifuge tubes – ML. 47

(e) Test tubes box (Put in drawer if drawer is available)
112 Standard – ML. 48a
112 Kahn – ML. 48c
1 Centrifuge tube – ML. 46

(f) Glass tubing – ML. 51

10. Box for records and stationery
2 Large stiff backed foolscap size exercise book– New 51
Labels – New 50
Report forms – New 49
1 Pad graph paper for colorimetry – New 52
1 Pad scrap writing paper– New 48

11. Electric centrifuging area
1 Hawksley haematocrit centrifuge – ML. 123
1 Centrifuge reader – New 53
1 MSE minor centrifuge – ML. 122

12. Colorimetry area
1 Grew wedge photometer – ML. 115
1 Grew wedge spare cells – ML. 115
1 Eel colorimeter – ML. 117
1 Page graph paper – New 52

13. Microscopy area
    1 Olympic microscope – ML. 30
    1 Lamp – New 74
    Immersion oil – ML. 96
    1 Bijou bottle – ML. 14a
    1 Plain capillary tube – New 17
    1 Roll toilet paper – soft – New 5
    1 Tally counter – New 54
    1 Neubauer counting chamber and special (spare) cover glasses – ML. 15

14/16. Washing up, disinfection and disposal
    4 Basins – New 55
    6 Very wide mouthed screw cap containers – New 7 for:-
    Needles – in water
    Slides – in water, detergent, lysol
    Cover slips –in water, detergent
    Buckets – water)
    waste)
    disinfect) – 8 buckets – New 35
    wash)
    burn)
    Buckets for actual washing
    1 Jug – New 56
    2 Towels – New 57
    Detergent – See Teepol 8 above
    Soap – New 58
    Bottle brush –ML. 9
    2 Trays – New 25
    Lysol –New 59 (see 8 above)
    Plastic cup for lysol – ML. 58

17. Sterilizing and heating
    1 Box matches – New 45
    1 Spirit lamp – ML. 39
    1 Pressure cooker – hi-dome – ML. 69
    1 Spare gasket
    1 Kerosene (primus) stove – ML. 71
    6 Prickers – New 26
    1 Bunsen burner – ML. 10
    1 Labogas – ML. 150
    2 Gas cylinders – New 46

On and off key – New 47
Rubber tubing – ML. 50
1 Teepol – ML. 42
1 Gauze for burner – ML. 26
1 Loop-holder – ML. 28
(Loop prepared in laboratory)
1 Pan with 2 handles – ML. 65
1 Waterproof metal box volumes more than 600 ml – New 60
1 Hot air oven – New 64

18. Electrical generating
1 Honda generator - New 61
1 Car battery – New 42

19. Boxes of spares top shelf spares
2 Rolls cotton wool – New 8
2kg Glass tubing – ML. 51
20 Feet rubber tubing – ML. 50
2 Rolls toilet paper – New 5
6 Packet filter paper – ML. 22

20. Refrigerator (or use of hospital ward refrigerator)
For tuberculin – from reference laboratory
For grouping and cross matching sera etc. (not listed here)

Extra Items Needed in Nigeria
21. Haemoglobin electrophoresis (extra requirements)
1 Shandon electrophoretic tank – New 62
1 Power control – (Eel) – New 63
1 Rod – New 65
12 Clips – New 66
1 Still – New 67 or other source of distilled water
2 Packets 3mm Whatman Chromatography paper WR Balston Ltd – New 68
Basic/weight – 185/2
Thickness – 0.33 58 x 68
1 Sodium barbitone – New 69
1 Barbituric acid – New 70
1 Tris (Hydroxy methyl) – new 71
1 Diamino-ethane tetracetic acid – new 72
1 Boric acid crystals – New 73

54

Primary Health Care for Countries in Africa

F.J. Bennett

In a textbook on public health, it should hardly be necessary to emphasize the health problems of rural people. However, to interest health personnel in primary health care it is often necessary to jolt them with a realization of these problems, which conventional sickness-oriented services have failed to solve.

In many developing countries, less than 30% of rural people have access to health services, in spite of the fact that often they are mostly exposed to a disease-promoting environment. Furthermore, those who do have ready access often have very expensive services – for example, people in the cities have within their reach a large percentage of a country's hospital beds, medical specialists, and expensive diagnostic equipment. In some countries in Africa health services were modelled on those of the colonizing countries, and were not designed to reach the rural periphery. Mass campaigns were often used as a substitute for health services in the rural areas, but these did not contribute to the establishment of permanent daily services.

Expensive teaching hospitals were put up to train medical practitioners in expensive methods seldom available in a country area, so that this again perpetuated a concentration of the highly skilled and the highly paid in the towns. The real need of the rural poor – immunization, antenatal care, nutritional and other health education, improved water and sanitation, and essential drugs for common tropical diseases such as malaria, worms, respiratory infections and skin diseases – were not met. The bulk of the population who live in rural areas need a readily accessible rural health care that provides solutions for their most common health problems.

The Concept of Primary Health Care (PHC)

It was this realization of the failure of the conventional health services and of the increasing lack of equity in distribution that led Newell (1975) to describe the innovative and indeed revolutional health services in his book *Health by the people*. Similarly, Djukanovic and Mach (1975) produced a joint report for UNICEF and WHO which described alternative approaches to meeting basic health needs in developing countries. Also in 1975, the Director General of the World Health Organisation, in his report to the 28th World Health Assembly, spelt out the seven principles of primary health care. These were:

1. Primary health care should be shaped around the life patterns of the population; it should serve and should meet the needs of the community.
2. Primary health care should be an integral part of the national health system, and other echelons of services should be designed in support of the needs of the peripheral level, especially as this pertains to the technical supply, supervising and referral support.
3. Primary health care activities should be fully integrated with the activities of the other sectors involved in community development (agriculture, education, public works, housing and communication).
4. The local population should be actively involved in the formulation and implementation of health care activities so that health care can be brought into line with local needs and priorities. Decisions upon what are the community needs requiring solution should be based upon a continuing dialogue between the people and the services.
5. Health care offered should place a maximum reliance on available community resources, especially those which have hitherto remain untapped, and should remain within the stringent cost limitations that are present in each country.
6. Primary health care should use an integrated approach of preventive, promotive, curative and rehabilitative services for the individual, family and community. The balance between these services should vary according to community needs and may well change over time.
7. The majority of health intervention should be undertaken at the most peripheral practicable level of the health services by workers most suitably trained for performing these activities.

In a report from the World Health Organization Regional Office in Brazzaville (WHO, 1977a) three further principles derived from the others were more clearly stated for Africa. Primary health care programmes should result from a firm national resolve and decision. An original approach should be adopted in each country, since it is not advisable to adopt a standard model for all, or to act in a uniform way in every case. Primary health care programmes should cooperate with traditional systems of health care, and make positive efforts to ensure integration and/or collaboration.

In September, 1978 the Alma Ata Conference, with 134 nations discussing the subject of primary health care, took place in Russia. It produced in its report (WHO/UNICEF 1978) the now standard definition of primary health care as

> essential health care based on practical, scientifically sound and socially acceptable methods and technology made universally accessible to individuals and families in the community through their full participation and at a cost that the community and country can afford to maintain at every stage of their development in the spirit of self-reliance and self-determination. It forms an integral part both of the country's health system, of which it is the central function and main focus, and of the overall function and economic development of the community. It is the first level of contact of individuals, the family and

the community with the national health system bringing health care as close as possible to where people live and work and constitutes the first element of a continuing health care process.

The Declaration of Alma Ata stated that at least the following eight areas should be included in primary health care. They are: education concerning prevailing health problems the methods of preventing and controlling them; promotion of food supply and proper nutrition; adequate supply of safe water and basic sanitation; maternal and child care including family planning; immunization against the major infectious diseases; prevention and control of locally endemic diseases; appropriate treatment of common diseases and injuries and provision of essential drugs.

The Scope of Primary Health Care

Primary health care embraces all the levels of prevention – from primary prevention (health promotion through good nutrition, housing, and health education, prevention of disease by immunization, prophylaxis, and environmental sanitation), to secondary prevention (early diagnosis and treatment, contact tracing, screening for disease) to tertiary prevention (limitation of disability and rehabilitation). It applies these measures on an individual, family and community basis as necessary.

Life Patterns and Needs of the Community

Most rural communities in Africa are poorly covered by health services, and sometimes the inadequate health services provided are not correctly used. One of the big problems is the distance that people have to cover to seek their first contact with health care; if referred from there to a second, more complex health unit, the distance and problems are magnified. Tertiary health care, in big teaching hospitals equipped for high cost medical care technology, is even more remote and seldom reached. Distance may in fact not be very great, but there may be no roads or adequate means of transport, and no ambulances (Asogwa, 1975). The villagers have their own views about the aetiology of disease and the appropriateness of the medical care provided by institutions, and for many serious conditions for which we have effective treatment or prevention (for example, tuberculosis and measles) they may consider their own traditional management superior. This obviously is a situation requiring both health education and more easily obtained and accessible health services. In many communities in Africa, the common diseases, such as diarrhoea and worm infestations, arise as a result of poor environmental hygiene – again a matter that can only be approached effectively on a local, and almost on a family basis through education, motivation, demonstration, and practical technical disposal of wastes and refuse. Some of the health needs of the communities are related to nutrition, which is bound up with human ecology, food habits, agriculture, and staple crops, etc,; and this obviously implies the need for help from a variety of agencies other than those specifically concerned with health. Agriculture, community development, and veterinary science have an equally great contribution to make.

When considering the needs of a community, there are those that doctors would asses as needs after perhaps a community diagnosis, and there are those which the community deem to be their urgent needs. These two are often different, and the priorities within them are different. It is therefore important to start with the needs as the community sees them.

Primary Health Care and the National Health System

The very term 'primary' presupposes that there is also available subsequent secondary and tertiary care. A continuum of health services is needed, from those available for first contact, for common needs at the village level, to secondary care at a health centre provided by the medical auxiliary, to tertiary care by doctors at district or provincial hospital level. A referral system is necessary to facilitate movement both up and down this spectrum of care. Primary health care also needs supervision, which must provide assistance in monitoring the coverage of the service and its quality, must aim at improving the services by ongoing education of workers, must help in planning of simple health interventions, and must provide inspiration and motivation. This is the medical auxiliary's or doctor's role, and requires careful budgeting of time; and it also requires teamwork from other members of the team, such as public health nurses and sanitarians. Community health workers are the interface between communities and health care system; and Bryant (1978) has given a good description of their allegiance, selection, and training. The interrelationship between community resources and national health services resources needs careful planning and guidance. Both are trying to improve the health of the people; and the balance between initiative from the community and assistance from the health services must be maintained, so that the latter is not imposed from above.

Integration with Other Sectors

Primary health care is one aspect of the development of a community – others are education, agriculture, communication, and water development. In some countries in Africa the decision-making process has been decentralized, and planning is done at the community or district level by a committee – the doctor being merely one technical adviser, who co-ordinates his health planning with other departments. Under these circumstances even transport can be shared.

The primary health care worker has health education duties and these may cover advice on growing foods, feeding children, building houses or protecting water supplies. Obviously there may be other workers also covering some of these aspects and so there is need for a co-ordinated message to be developed, and for all village level workers to work together.

Community Participation

There are many ways in which communities may participate in their primary health care – by providing labour, money and materials, by working along with government personnel, by actual help in organization (for example, of the immunization of children), and by providing selected primary care workers from the community. Examples of active participation are the building of clinics and houses and schools, digging wells or latrines, and making roads that improve communication. These sort of community participation follow on meetings, communities, and other decision-making awareness that may be peculiar to particular communities – for example, in some areas of Africa decisions are made and carried out within lineage groups, and in other areas through church gatherings. UNICEF and WHO have recently analysed nine case studies (UNICEF/WHO 1977), and have listed the factors which appeared to favour successful community participation in primary health care. These indicated that specific government policies to encourage community participation were found to enhance the extent and depth of participation. Another factor was certain existing traditions, which sometimes formed the basis for increased community participation. Non-governmental organizations such as the Church often provided channels for community participation.

A continuing dialogue between the people and the health service is necessary if both felt and unfelt needs are to be met. The people must be allowed to establish their own priorities; and this is best done by discussing and frequent meetings with adequate representation from all sectors of the community. 'Health by the people' or 'Health with the people' are better slogans than 'Health for the people'. The primary health worker (PHW) must be selected by the community, and their duties planned by a local committee. These local communities should also be responsible for some aspects of the supervision of PHWs, and for their remuneration, or for providing other incentives.

Use of Community Resources

If the community doctor sits down with members of the community and discusses existing community resources, it may be quite surprising how many there are. The majority of normal births may be handled quite efficiently in people's own homes, probably by traditional birth attendants. The mentally ill and the mentally retarded are maintained, often with some active function within society. The majority of minor ailments receive placebo or symptomatic treatment with easily obtained herbal remedies. Much of the 'health' education about sexual behaviour, the preparation of foods, breast feeding, care of the aged, and emotional support in times of crisis, is done within the family setting.

There are people with knowledge of the water supplies, people with skill that could be employed in protecting water supplies, and possibly even community mechanisms such as 'Harambee' of the Kenya and 'Ujamaa' of Tanzania that encourage communal work on a project such as water supply.

Resources of manpower and voluntary effort should never be under-estimated – provided the project is a priority in the people's eyes. Even skills are more abundant than was at first imagined – many communities have trained midwives, nurses, health inspectors, and teachers who would be prepared to help their community.

Rural communities are usually poor; and this has given rise to the need for low cost technology. 'Appropriate' or 'intermediate technology' now has many advocates, and journals (such as *Appropriate Technology*) and manuals are available which provide good do-it-yourself instructions for low cost solutions to problems of agriculture, food storage and processing, water supply, etc.

The construction of clinics can often be undertaken by communities on a self-help basis; and they can often employ a more suitable plan than one which comes from a Ministry of Works. The doctors can give guidance in these self-help projects – otherwise sometimes essentials, such as water supply for the clinic, are overlooked.

The use of primary health care workers drawn from the community cuts down costs as special housing is usually not necessary. Some workers may give their services free, some may accept small part time payment, and some may accept payment in kind from patients, but the system of remuneration is for the community to decide.

The Job of the Primary Health Worker (PHW)

The PHW is responsible both to the local community (who selects the PHW for training, arrange remuneration, and provide accommodation) and to the government or voluntary body which organizes the training, supervises the work, helps with the referral of difficult cases, provides other members of the health team, and often provides a source of basic drugs and equipment.

The PHW's job embraces both health care and community development, and in some parts of the world include some demographic duties, such as notifying births and deaths. The health duties almost always include maternal health (advising and providing minimal antenatal care, including education, conduct of a normal delivery, and referral of problems and family planning) and child health and nutrition. There should be an emphasis on the recognition of malnutrition, and the best use of local foods.

Communicable disease control, especially assistance with the community mobilization for Expanded Immunization Programme, is a very important aspect of the PHW's job. Health education will become one of the tools used to promote the improvement of the environment and the construction of latrines and protection of water supplies. In many communities this might well be the starting point for the PHW. First aid and treatment of common complaints will almost certainly be required as part of the PHW's tasks in most communities. The World Health Organization, in a guide for training PHWs (WHO 1977*b*), have suggested the following criteria for establishing in each community which diseases to include: frequency of the disease, demand for treatment by the public, danger to the individual, technical feasibility of action by the PHW, and economic consequences of the problem.

Thus in many parts of Africa, common skin and eye complaints have been included, as well as headaches, malaria fever, diarrhoea, abdominal pains, worms, cough, weakness, mental illness, and sexually transmitted diseases. The emphasis in training is to enable the PHW to know what he can do and what he cannot do – especially when and how to refer patients.

Priorities will however vary – for example, in dry savannah areas health programmes might stress the prevention of blindness by Vitamin A treatment and treatment of families for trachoma. In other areas the diagnosis and follow-up of leprosy and tuberculosis might be considered as fitting in well with the PHW's special advantage of knowing his community.

Many countries do not have the PHW trained in everything, but prefer to have several who have specialized fields of activity for example, a trained traditional midwife to do work with mothers and children, a man to do environmental work, and a third individual to deal with the treatment and referral of illness.

The PHW, according to the World Health Organization (1976) is 'the practical expression of a community's determination to be involved in its own health care and to make up for any deficiencies that might exist in the health service coverage. The PHW should improve the community's involvement in what will be part of an overall service authority with the active contribution of the people'.

Unless however all the senior cadres of the national health services, such as the doctors and public health nurses, accept this philosophy and actively help with the continuing supervision and education of the PHW, such programmes will not be highly successful.

Early Primary Health Programmes in Africa

Some of the pioneering projects in Primary Health Care have been in Africa, and Djukanovic and Mach (1975) described the new strategy in Niger, where previously only 15% of the population had been reached by a curatively oriented health service. The new programme followed on initial sociological research and improved communication with the local population. There were three main elements to the new approach in Niger. The first was the initiation of better health coverage through joint information efforts by the rural development services, the education and literary services, and the health services, supported by the political party. Secondly, there was health protection through the setting up of village health teams (with voluntary participation by village health workers and traditional birth attendants). Thirdly, there was organization of the auxiliary workers towards rural health through the practice of a comprehensive health care.

Another pioneering country in the field of PHC is Tanzania, which provides one of the case studies in *Health by the People* (Newell 1975). For several years Tanzania has been training men and women selected by their 'ujamaa' villages to be their 'Village Medical Helpers'. After a short course in the local district hospital, these workers with only primary school education return to the villages to provide first aid, treat common illnesses, advise on the use of maternal and child health services, help with environmental improvement, referral of serious cases, and notification to the authorities of any unusual outbreaks of disease. Instead of a salary, their work is regarded as a contribution to the communal work of the village. When they run out of drugs, their supplies are replenished by the district health services; and travel expenses are met by the 'ujamaa' village.

Primary Health Care in the Republic of Ghana

Ghana produced a national plan in 1978 titled 'A primary health care strategy for Ghana'. This plan aimed at reaching 80% of the population by 1990; and aimed to prevent and treat the disease problems causing 80% of the unnecessary sickness, disability, and death in the country. Acceptance and initiation of the programme was ensured by a series of workshops, and by retraining the professional staff. In addition, a post was created in the Ministry of Health for the director of the primary health care programme.

Ghana plans to have a three tier system, with the first level for small communities being provided by community health workers selected and paid by the communities, but supervised technically and trained by the Ministry of Health. Three types of workers were envisaged – a retrained traditional birth attendant, a household family health worker, and a local environmental and development worker.

The second level would have broadly trained community health nurse-midwives and environment development officers, who would supervise the primary health level by visits every two weeks, give immunization, and see referred cases. They would also be linked by radio to the District headquarters.

The third level would be the managers, and would consist of the District Health Team (Medical Officer, Public Health Nurse, Health Inspector, and Administrator) and the District Executive Officer, to ensure an integrated approach to village development. This level would need a re-oriented training. Training and logistic support were obviously important areas for consideration in this programme, and were probably the ones which required external aid.

Primary Health Care in the Sudan

The National Health Programmes of the Democratic Republic of the Sudan for the period 1977–84 put special emphasis on a Primary Health Care Programme. This is well set out in various detailed documents – a plan for the Southern Region, one for the rest of the Sudan including the nomadic population, a summary report and a description in the *WHO Chronicle* (Idriss, Lolik, Khan, Benyoussef, 1976). The Sudan aimed at achieving maximum coverage of the population by 1984, and considered that PHC was the only feasible strategy which was socially and politically acceptable.

In rural areas workers would be based at Primary Health Care Units covering a population of 4,000. Five of these units would be supervised by medical auxiliaries in a dispensary, which would also cover 4,000 people. These PHC units would cover a radius of about 16km. In nomadic areas the workers would move with their communities, and would have responsibility for 1,500 people (Benyoussef and Christian, 1977). The need to integrate and co-ordinate the political, administrative and medical machinery for the rural health services was stressed.

In the Southern Region of the Sudan, the new cadre of workers would be called the 'Community Health Worker' (CHW) who was 'an indigenous member of the community selected by that community and paid by the Rural Council to provide primary health care services to a population of approximately 4,000'. These workers were trained for nine months at CHW training centres where the tutors were medical auxiliaries. All auxiliaries in addition received re-orientation training so that they could provide support to the new cadre. The CHW was to be supervised technically by the Medical Assistant at the local dispensary, and administratively and politically by the community through the Village Development Committee, the Village Council, and the Sudanese Socialist Union Basic Unit Committee.

The CHW in Sudan had preventive and promotive activities, and was to provide ambulatory treatment, preventive advice, and referral for a list of twelve common conditions, which included malaria and diarrhoea. He had to keep records and drugs, record births and deaths, and participate in community projects.

Evaluation of Primary Health Care

The methods of evaluating PHC are still being debated, and there is much room for each doctor to try to build in his own evaluation system into each PHC project. Basically, some answers must be obtained for the important aspects of PHC, viz, the degree of accessibility of the basic health services to the community, and the coverage of the population, in terms of meeting their needs, achieved. Participation of the community (as measured by numbers of communities, payment of PHWs, construction of wells, health clinics, etc.) is also an important area to quantify. The doctor should try to evaluate the effectiveness of the referrals between PHW and health units, and the quality of supervision achieved. The actual effects of health measures should also be evaluated – for example, infant mortality rate, nutritional status, and the incidence and prevalence of certain diseases.

For evaluation, certain records will be necessary; and it is wise to have these worked out with the community and the health workers, to decide which of them are absolutely necessary and useful.

Further Development of PHC Programmes in Africa – A Challenge to the Medical and Other Professions

It is likely that almost all countries in Africa will have national programmes of PHC within the next decade. Political and ideological backing are just as essential for successful programmes as are the allocation of funds for the more equitable distribution of basic health services for rural areas. These trends and their implications can be studied by reference to the many official and other publications now appearing, for example, the ones from Ethiopia (Tsegaye Fekade, Solomon Ayalew, Getachew Gizaw, 1978).

Decentralized planning is essential for effective PHC, which depends on finding local answers and methods for a community's problems. The doctor's role in improving the health of his community is thus likely to become even more exacting, as he will have to be responsible for helping the community to determine the most appropriate health technology for their problems. For this, he will have to participate in an exercise of 'community diagnosis'. PHC is likely to demand, excite, and challenge the doctor's ingenuity and social as well as medical skills in the future. It also demands that the doctor adopts a wider view of health, and works together with colleagues from agriculture, education, and other sectors.

It was the Thirtieth World Health Assembly in 1977 which decided on the target of the attainment by all citizens of the world of a level of health that will permit them to lead a socially and economically productive life. This later was interpreted as an acceptable level of Health For All By The Year 2000.

In the address by Dr H. Mahler, Director General of WHO to the conference he addressed crucial questions to the country delegates – the outcome of the conference depending on their response. The questions related to:

- reducing the gap between the haves and have nots;
- proper planning and implementation with other sectors as part of socio-economic development;
- preferential allocation of health resources to the social periphery;
- mobilization and education of individuals, families and communities to ensure involvement;
- relevant trained manpower and appropriate affordable charges in the health system to support PHC technology;
- overcoming political and technical resistance; and
- obtaining political commitment.

In fact these issues have been related to the outcome and success of PHC in almost all countries in the years subsequent to Alma-Ata and they form a good frame work for evaluation.

In 1988, ten years after Alma-Ata, another meeting was held in Riga, USSR which brought together experts from all WHO regions and representatives of UNICEF, UNDP and non-governmental organizations. This meeting surveyed achievements and looked at the future emphasis needed in the period up to the year 2000 and beyond. The Health For All concept had made a very positive contribution to world progress in health as shown by specific indicators (e.g. immunization) and in changes in the organization of services with greater decentralization. Ten actions were described to deal with persisting problems. The first two included maintaining health for all as a permanent goal up to and beyond the year 2000 and renewing and strengthening the strategies. Social and political actions to support health and developing and mobilizing leadership for health for all are also important. Other actions include empowering people by providing information, technical support, and decision making possibilities, and making intersectoral collaboration a force for health. Two of the most important actions for the future are strengthening district health systems based on PHC and planning, preparing and supporting personnel for health for all. The development and rational use of science and appropriate technology is needed. Finally, it was realized that there are persisting problems which have to be overcome.

From this list three topics have been selected to illustrate some of the present approaches in which health workers can play a leading role in Africa. Countries such as Somalia, Sudan, Ethiopia, Mozambique,and Liberia which previously were often quoted as having made progress in PHC and in the training of community health workers are now having to start again from an even lower baseline of poverty, social disruption, low literary levels for women, and deteriorated health and social services. It is in countries such as these that the process of empowerment is really needed now to produce an upsurge of self help activities for health and to enable communities to participate in the management of local health care.

Equity

One of the principles of Primary Health Care is equity. This means equal distribution of resources based on need. It also means equal access of all to essential health services. One of the glaring examples of lack of equity is the adequate resources for health in towns (trained staff, building, expenditure per capital) as compared to the poor resources going to rural areas. Government employees often contribute to state health insurance schemes which enable them to use expensive private hospitals at a cost far above what the average citizen could afford. Equity is related to improving services to underserved areas and also making sure that the more vulnerable who require services more, have them readily accessible and of equal quality. Children and women are more vulnerable and their needs for immunization, antenatal care, and growth monitoring constitute essential health care. Even if it costs more to bring these services to a remote village every child or pregnant mother should have access to them. The 'All' in health for all is a very important word and it should be prominent in every district health plan. A target of 100% coverage of BCG immunization might be unrealistic but a target of 80% implies that 20% cannot be reached or monitored and these might be the most vulnerable and most neglected. Health workers can identify disparities in the use of services if there is a good health information system. This system will show utilization rates for different services, e.g. family planning, immunization, skilled delivery – these will possibly show differentials by education and distance from the facility. Some of the differences in utilization will be due to differences in physical accessibility, or lack of attractivity of a health unit because of poor staffing or equipment. Reasons for disparities within a district must be sought as there is an implied lack of equity. Within urban areas there will similarly be squatter areas or slum or deprived parts where some aspects of health services are lacking and yet where need is greatest.

A big problem lies at the national level where the curative urban based services always take the big share of the health budget. Few countries have been able to show a very significant and sustained shift of resources to the rural periphery, although some such as Tanzania, Zimbabwe and Botswana have made major strides to bring services within the reach of the majority of their population.

District Health Systems Based on PHC

One of the important features of Primary Health Care is decentralization to lower levels so that planning, decision making and integration of sectors is done closer to, or within, communities. The district level has thus come into focus as the level most important for development and health management. In the African region a 3–phase scenario for Primary Health care has been developed in which the national level is responsible for policy formulation and the regional level provides technical support to the district level where implementation takes place.

The district health system includes all those services and agencies which contribute to health and which thus need to be co-ordinated – these usually include government health services, non-governmental health services such as mission hospitals, private medical practitioners, industrial health services, municipal health services, traditional healers and other sectors contributing to health and community-based activities.

The services which however need special effort at co-ordination are those provided by the district hospital and the communities. The clinical curative services need to be linked with promotive, preventive and rehabilitation activities as PHC embraces the whole spectrum of care.

The aspects of a district health system that are crucial for PHC are a good health information system and epidemiological analysis, good leadership and management, logistics and teamwork. With these elements in place high risk groups, lack of equity in resource distribution, and health problems are easily identified and disparities can be reduced. If all parts of the system are co-ordinated then planning is easier, communication between actors is improved and resources are fully used. Information, education and communication can use all resources and channels, and thus individuals and communities can be more readily mobilized for health.

Some countries such as Kenya and Zimbabwe have already made great progress in developing the district focus and have many good district health managers. Other countries such as Namibia are just beginning to decentralize to district level and still have a variety of components (government, local authority, church based health services) which are not yet integrated into one system with a common set of goals and objectives.

Co-ordinating mechanisms such as District Development Committee, perhaps with a PHC sub-committee, can bring all agencies and sectors together to plan and set targets and develop suitable indicators for monitoring. Where church-based hospitals have preceded the government in training community health workers it is necessary that some co-ordination with government be established and that some guidelines for PHC and community based health care be set up. Otherwise some areas might provide community health workers with drugs or with different instructions about activities such as oral rehydration, or there might be differences in payment whereas government might focus on volunteerism.

Empowering the People

Empowering has many connotations – for some it is a process by which individual families or communities take steps themselves to control their own development through mobilizing their own resources and management skills. For others it implies some outside agency, service, or ministry providing information and support and facilitating decentralized decision making through political reform.

It is a process which comes about through many approaches, the important ones being information, education and communication (IEC). Many ministries of health now have divisions or units which started as health education units and which have evolved to a broader IEC approach which undertakes social mobilization and multi-sectoral approach. Ministries of health, education, information and broadcasting, community development, and local government are co-ordinated in an effort to use all social groups and leadership in the effort to involve people in action for their own health and development.

Education of women has been identified as one of the important factors in enabling poor countries to achieve better reduction of indicators such as infant mortality. Education empowers women to take on leadership roles and to make decisions about their own families, development and welfare. In many African countries the status and education of women has been restricted but with increasing urbanization and with men migrating to towns women are increasingly left in charge of farming activities and rearing the family.

Important approaches to women's education have been made through functional literacy classes, women's groups for church or cultural activities, farming, income generating or co-operatives. Special efforts to prevent girls dropping out from school, to prevent teenage pregnancy, and to involve girls not in school are needed. Family planning allows women to make decisions about family size and also gives them time to take more active part in community meetings which augurs well for Primary Health Care. Associated with improved education and high status of women goes better use of health services and so immunization coverages improves and indicators of maternal health and survival also improve. Although there have been improvements in MCH indicators in most African countries there is still room for improvement especially in those countries which are least developed.

Some of the steps in empowerment are the same steps as undertaken in the managerial cycle. First stimulation, motivation or facilitation of the community to assess its own problems – to make a community diagnosis or situation assessment. Then to analyse what the priorities are and what actions are needed and finally to implement these actions with local resources in a spirit of self reliance. When communities undertake these steps they are making decisions and become responsible for the outcome. This is the basis of community involvement – empowering alters mere participation in someone else's decisions and activities into one of real management. This triple A (Assessment/Analysis/Action) has been used very successfully in PHC activities in Iringa region of Tanzania.

Empowering also has an individual meaning – it is a strengthening of an individual's ability to achieve the inherent potential for developing socially, mentally and physically and achieving health in a holistic sense. This occurs with a communication dialogue when information leads to education and when behavioural and lifestyle changes occur. Primary health care aims to facilitate and provide motivation for these changes but it is a slow process requiring a balance between health inputs and development stimuli – something best achieved by a co-ordinated multi-sectoral approach.

Supporting Health Workers for Health For All

Support for health workers in primary health care and community based health activities must start with their basic training. In many countries medical students and nurses in training receive only a small proportion of their training in communities or situations outside the teaching hospital walls. Subjects such as communication, group work in communities, management, and community assessment, receive little attention. This is partly due to the curriculum but other factors such as lack of funds and transport prevent students from going out into communities to learn how to work with people in their own environment. Some of the newer schools, e.g: Moi University in Kenya have attempted to have innovative curricula but many schools face problems of lack of teaching staff motivated to work in communities. The student training needs to be done in communities which have community based activities managed by the communities and supported by various different sectors and NGOs.

Even if the basic training is community orientated and gives insight into the management skills needed for promoting community involvement and intersectoral co-ordination as well as indicating a desire to reach all and ensure equity, there is still a need for continuing support of workers. This support is in continuing education or refresher courses or more specific training as facilitators and trainers for community based health care (CBHC). Some communities will require some of their members to be trained as community health workers or be given particular skills, e.g. as community based distributors of contraceptives. In these districts some PHC facilitators will require training and these then train trainers for CBHC. The latter are usually health staff working in more local facilities such as health centres or clinics which are within communities. An initial role of the facilitators and trainers is arousing awareness and sensitizing families and communities to their own latent ability so that they become motivated to take their own initiatives in health and development.

Besides these inputs of training of staff other support measures are needed – transport, equipment, and means of communication for referral purposes to the next higher level of care.

Regular supportive supervision which provides a stimulus and improves morale rather than undermining it is important. Maintaining morale of staff in peripheral health units is very important – in many countries in Africa at present there is poor maintenance of buildings, no continuing education, erratic supply of drugs, no feedback of health information and little attempt to improve staff housing or benefits. Doctors and nurses in charge of a district must take a very active part in supporting health staff concerned with primary health care and its peripheral component of community-based health activities. It is these more peripheral components which increase access and coverage and help to reach the underserved.

The three most numerous and important types of community based health workers in Africa are community health workers (CHW), Traditional Birth Attendants (TBA) and community based distributors of contraceptives (CBD). These workers are selected by the communities of which they are members and are trained as near to or in the communities. The duration of training and its content is determined by the community and trainees and is related to the local problems and culture. Rewards and incentives are provided by the community but in many countries CHW are voluntary workers who have a small workload, e.g. 20-40 families, so that they are part time workers. Support for them is also necessary in the form of continuing education, possibly supplies and 'supervision' which can be monthly meetings with their co-workers and trainers. Support often comes both from the health and other sectors as well as from the community group or committee which initiated the community based health care activities. Communities will support their community health workers if they find them useful and effective in their work. They are more likely to be effective if their training has made them good motivators and communicators with the correct information and skills to deal with relevant local health problems as prioritized by the communities. The type of training commonly used in eastern Africa is the 'psycho-social method' which is learner-centred, problem-based and problem-solving, promotes self discovery and is action-oriented.

Community Based Health Care

In many countries small projects often run by aid agencies or church based organizations were started which aimed at stimulating a partnership between the communities and the health services. As these projects aim at arousing awareness of the communities' own ability to deal with their problems they work towards communities taking a greater part in management especially the planning and leadership. The name of community based health care (CBHC) is now given to these activities as they are rooted in the community and not in the health service or donor. The methods of community development are used and the emphasis is on health care rather than medical care.

This peripheral element of PHC requires the training of facilitators who then arouse awareness in the community using adult approaches to education about health and social development. Communities might then wish the facilitators to train committees or groups (e.g. women's groups) in specific knowledge and skills to deal with problems they identify. They might also wish to have community health workers, traditional birth attendants or other community resources people trained.

All of this training has cost implications especially if on a wider district or national scale – as one CHW may only be able to serve adequately one small community or segment of a community. If the resources are coming from government national, regional, or district funds then it might be quite difficult to train and sustain a significant number: only some selected communities are then included. The national programmes which are successful in achieving greater coverage have also had to spend considerable funds on reorientation of the hospital and clinic staff to be able to support CBHC. This requires very dedicated staff and a very successful community sensitization and training process if it is to be sustained without any additional input of outside funds or expertise. CBHC has proved of greatest benefit in environmental improvement, in MCH and family planning and has great potential in control of vector-borne diseases and AIDS. In getting down to the causes of these problems, e.g. social disruption, poverty, poor education system and lack of democratic government, the achievements have been slower and less dramatic. However, there is every hope that CBHC could help to vitalize and bring communities up from the depths into which war or disaster has plunged them, and that it can be the start of a true dynamic partnership between the people and the government (or mission) health services.

Community-based health care however requires the backup of a good referral system to deal with the inevitable medical problems – the obstructed labour, the fractures, the diabetes and the severe infections. The liaison between the CBHC and the government district services is essential and requires good district health leadership.

References

Appropriate Technology Journal – Intermediate Technology Publications Development Group, London, England. (1975)

Asogwa S.E. (1975). 'The Problems in the Delivery of Primary Health Care at Rural Health Centres. *Proceedings of Conference on Research and the Delivery of Health Care*, Nairobi.

Benyoussef A. & Christian B. (1977). 'Health Care in Developing Countries.' *Social Science and Medicine*, Vol. II pp. 399–408.

Bryant J.H. (1978). 'Community Health Workers. The Interface Between Community and Health Care Systems' *WHO Chron.* 32, 144–8.

Democratic Republic of Sudan (1975). *National Health Programme 1977–8 – 1983–4, Khartoum.*

—(1976). *Primary Health Care: Eastern, Northern, Central and Western Regions, 1977–8 – 1983–4*

—(1976). *Primary Health Care Programmes, Southern Region* 1977–8 – 1983–4, Juba.

Djukanovic, V. & Mach, E.P. (1975). *Alternative Approaches to Meeting Basic Health Needs in Developing Countries.* A Joint UNICEF/WHO Study, WHO Geneva.

Idriss, A.A., Lolik P., Khan R.A., & Benyoussef A. (1976). "The Primary Health Care Programme in Sudan", *WHO Chron.* 30, 370–4.

Newell, K.W. (1975). *Health by the People* , WHO, Geneva.

Republic of Ghana(1978). *A Primary Health Care for Ghana.* National Planning Unit, Accra.

Tsegaye Fakade, Solomon Ayalew, Getachew Gizaw (1978). *Primary Health Care Status in Revolutionary Ethiopia.* Ministry of Health, Addis Ababa.

UNICEF/WHO (1977). Paper No. JC21 (UNICEF/WHO 77.2 Con 1). *Community Involvement in Primary Health Care. A Study of the Process of Community Motivation and Continued Participation.*

WHO (1975). *Promotion of National Health Services* A 28/9 18 April, WHO, Geneva.

—(1977). *Primary Health Care.* Africa Technical Report Series No. 3. WHO Brazzaville.

—(1977). *The Primary Health Worker — Working Guide.* Guidelines for Training, Guidelines for adaptation. Working document WHO Geneva.

WHO/UNICEF (1978). *Report of the International Conference on Primary Health Care*, Alma-Atala, 6–12 September, 1978. ICPHC/ALA/78.10. WHO, Geneva.

WHO (1988) *From Alma-Ata to the Year 2000 Reflections at the Midpoint* Geneva: WHO

55

Health Legislation in Africa: the Example of Nigeria

O.O. Sosan

The practice of public health administration in both the developed and developing countries of the world requires both legislation controlling the movements of the personnel involved in such administration, and unwritten code of ethics for such administering personnel. Health legislation can thus be described in terms of the statutory duties of the medical officers made legally responsible for enforcing them, who is called the medical officer of health, usually for a well-defined population living in a well-defined area.

The duties of a medical officer of health are many and varied, and include the following:

1. to be aware of some environmental factors injuriously affecting the public health;
2. to investigate the causes, origin, and distribution of infectious diseases;
3. keeping himself informed by inspection of conditions injurious to health;
4. advising his council or government on all matters affecting health in his area of jurisdiction;
5. on the outbreak of an epidemic, visiting the place and inquiring into the causes and circumstances, and taking measures to prevent the spread of the disease;
6. directing the work of public health inspectors;
7. where necessary dealing with unsound food;
8. performing all duties laid on him by by-laws and regulations of his council or government;
9. dealing with offensive trades;
10. making periodical reports;
11. making weekly notification of communicable diseases, especially as directed by the World Health Organization for scheduled disease, and by the state or national health authorities for others; and

12. making annual reports on
    (i) influences affecting health in the area:
    (ii) all general and special inquiries instituted in the year;
    (iii) the work of the public health inspectors;
    (iv) conditions affecting the wholesomeness of food;
    (v) the condition of the water supply;
    (vi) the pollution of rivers and streams;
    (vii) drainage and sewage disposal;
    (viii) the removal of house refuse;
    (ix) housing accommodation; and
    (x) vital statistics.

The first stage in the evolution of the health activities of the medical officer of health as enumerated above was concerned with the environment of the individual. The efforts of the health officers were directed to obtaining healthy surroundings, freedom from nuisances, the provision of a satisfactory water supply, and the protection of food.

The successful administration of these essentials involves the mobility of the officers and a measure of encroachment on the privacy and access into the dwelling places of the members of a community which, more often than not, are viewed unkindly, and sometimes thoroughly detested. It is in support of this aspect of the health officers' duties that the Public Health Laws are primarily enacted to grant a *right of entry* to statutorily entitled officers of health, affording them an uninterrupted approach to the discharge of the above duties.

For the sake of setting out an objective appraisal of public health laws reference will be made to those which in fact represent the model for almost all Anglophone countries in Africa. When the practice of sanitation was permanently introduced into Nigeria in 1917 a chapter in the Laws of Nigeria was designated *The Public Health Ordinance* — Cap. 56 Vol. 1 — which was reproduced in book form, as the *Sanitary Manual*— which is still obtainable today at the National Archives. The Laws were revised in 1923, and the chapter then retained its form and designation, thus:— Cap. 56, Vol. I Laws of Nigeria, 1923. With subsequent revisions in later years up to the regionalization of the country in 1957, these laws finally emerged as Public Health Laws, No. 25 of 1957 (Western region), becoming operative in August, 1959. Subsequent legislation from the period 1966 to 1974 is listed in Appendix I.

An aspect of the revisions worthy of note is the continuous use of the original terminology in much of the wording, which is still subsisting. This gives an added advantage to scholars of the laws in many parts of the Republic to keep abreast with the theme, aims, and objectives of the original laws, without many difficulties other than those occasioned by local amendments.

The meaning of the term 'health officer' in this context includes:

> a medical officer of health, superintendent or inspector or other person acting under the authority, whether general or special, of the medical officer of health, and whether such superintendent, inspector or other person is serving in the medical or sanitary departments of the government of the region or of a competent council.

As the effective performance of the duties of a health officer demands a very high degree of knowledge of the pathology of communicable diseases, a list of Notifiable Infectious Diseases in relation to human beings is given, which term is to be taken to mean:

> plagues, cholera, yellow fever, smallpox, typhus, relapsing fever, puerperal fever, whooping cough, measles, scarlet fever, cerebrospinal meningitis, chicken pox, diphtheria, rabies, typhoid, dysentery, poliomyelitis, tuberculosis, yaws and trypanosomiasis, (and includes) any disease of any infectious or contagious nature which the ministry may by public notice declare to be a notifiable infectious disease within the meaning of this law.

With the above definition, a health officer possessing a good knowledge of the pathology and the epidemiology of these diseases stands a good chance of locating the causes of these diseases and their appropriate control measures, which is the sum total of his professional assignment.

The medical officer of health is first and foremost a registered medical doctor, with a post graduate qualification in Public Health. But section 3 subsection (1) of the law imposes on a medical practitioner in certain circumstances the designation of medical officer of health, even though he has not acquired a post-graduate qualification; and it reads:

> Section 3(1). The Governor may appoint a qualified medical practitioner to be government medical officer of health for the purposes of this law in any specified area or generally for the regions, and in the absence of any such appointment for any area the medical officer in charge of the area shall be the medical officer of health for the area.

A competent council (such as Lagos or Nairobi or Lusaka City Council or Okpebho Local Government Authority) may appoint a qualified medical practitioner to be medical officer of health of the council for the purposes of this law in the area of authority of the council. The duties of a medical officer of health and, for that matter, of a health officer, are given in a concise form as 'to inspect the area . . . to abate nuisance'. Section 5(1) reads:

> It shall be the duty of every medical officer of health to inspect the areas to which he is appointed to abate nuisance and otherwise to enforce the powers vested in him under this law.
>
> It shall be the duty of every competent council in an area in respect of which no medical officer of health is appointed to ensure that the provisions of this law are enforced.
>
> The Public Health Law is then divided into parts:

Part I

Section
1. gives the Short Title, commencement, and application;
2. gives the interpretation of the various terminology;
3. gives a definition of the Officers of Health;
4. give the powers of Senior Health Officers to direct; and
5. gives the duties of Medical Officer of Health and Council.

Part II

Section 6 deals with *nuisances* which may be abated summarily:

any premises in such a condition as to be injurious to health; any premises which are so dark or so ill-ventilated or so damp or in such a condition of dilapidation, as to be dangerous or prejudicial to the health of the persons living or employed therein;
any premises which contain rat holes or rat runs or other similar holes or which are infested with rats or in which the ventilating openings are not protected by gratings in such manner as to exclude rats therefrom; any pool, ditch, gutter, watercourse, cesspool, drain, ashpit, refuse pit, latrine, dustbin, washing place, well, water tank, barrel, sink, collection of village water, receptacle containing stagnant water, or other thing in such a state or condition as to be injurious to health; any animal or bird so kept as to be injurious to the health of man or molesting to neighbours and any animal or bird suffering from a noxious or contagious disease; any hole or excavation, well, pond, or quarry in or near any street which is or is likely to become dangerous to the public;
any stable, cowhouse, pigsty, or other premises for the use of animals or birds which are in such a condition to be injurious to the health of man or of such animals or birds;
any noxious matter or water flowing or discharged from any premises into any public street or into any gutter or side channel of any street;
any accumulation or deposit of rubbish of any kind whatever, or any decaying animal or vegetable matter, whether in the form of refuse, manure, decayed or tainted food, or in any form whatever;
any growth of weeds, cactus, long grass, reeds, or wild bush of any kind which may be injurious to health and any vegetable that of itself is dangerous to children or others either by its effluvia or through eating its leaves, seeds, fruits or flowers;
any premises certified by the health officer to be so overcrowded as to be injurious or dangerous to the health of the inmates;
any premises on which servants or workmen are employed and suitable and adequate sanitary conveniences are not provided;
any act, omission, place or thing which is or may be dangerous to life, or injurious to health or property;
any plant or tree which may be specified by the Minister by a notice published in the Regional Gazette as being favourable to the breeding of mosquitoes, found in any area which may be specified in the said notice.

Section 7 directs the action to be taken on the abatement of nuisances, and provides the penalty for non-compliance, conferring power to sell premises:

A health officer shall, if satisfied of the existence of a nuisance, serve a notice, hereinafter called an abatement notice, on the person by those acts, default or sufferance the nuisance arises or the premises on which the nuisance arises requiring him to abate the same within the time specified in the notice, and to execute such works, and to do such things as may be necessary for that purpose, and, if the health officer thinks it desirable (but not otherwise), specifying any works to be executed.

The officer may also by the same or another notice served on such person, occupier or owner require him to do what is necessary for preventing the recurrence of the nuisance, and, if he thinks it desirable, specify any works to be executed for that purpose, and may serve that notice notwithstanding that the nuisance may for the time being have been abated if the health officer considers that it is likely to recur on the same premises.

Where the nuisance arises from any want or defect of a structural character, or where the premises are unoccupied, the notice shall be served on the owner.

Where a notice has been served on any person (including an occupier or owner) under this section and either – the nuisance arose from the wilful act or default of such person; or such person fails to comply with any of the requisitions of the notice within the time specified, he shall be liable to a fine of fifty pounds or six months imprisonment.

Section 8 deals with court action in making a Nuisance Order for non-compliance with an abatement notice:

If either – a person (including the occupier or owner) on whom an abatement notice has been served as aforesaid makes default in complying with any of the requisitions thereof within the time specified; or the nuisance, although abated since the service of notice is, in the opinion of the health officer, likely to recur on the same premises, the health officer shall make a complaint and the court hearing the complaint may make on such persons a summary order, in this Law referred to as a nuisance order.

A nuisance order may be an abatement order, a prohibition order, or a closing order, or a combination of such orders.

An abatement order may require a person to comply with any of the requisitions of the notice, or otherwise to abate the nuisance within a time specified in such order.

A prohibition order may prohibit the recurrence of a nuisance.

An abatement order or prohibition order shall, if the person on whom the order is made so requires, or the court considers it desirable, specify the work to be executed by such person for the purposes of abating or preventing the recurrence of the nuisance.

A closing order may prohibit any premises from being used for human habitation.

A closing order shall only be made where it is proved to the satisfaction of the court that, by reason of a nuisance, premises are unfit for human habitation, and, if such proof is given, the court shall make a *closing order, and may impose a fine of fifty pounds or six month imprisonment.*

The court when satisfied that the premises have been rendered fit for human habitation, may declare that it is so satisfied and cancel the closing order.

If a person fails to comply with the provisions of a nuisance order with respect to the abatement of a nuisance he shall, unless he has satisfied the court that he has used all due diligence to carry out such order, be liable to a fine of one pound a day during his default; and if a person knowingly and wilfully acts contrary to a prohibition or closing order he shall be liable to a fine of two pounds a day during such contrary action; moreover the health officer may enter the premises to which a nuisance order relates, and abate or remove the nuisance, and do whatever may be necessary in execution of such order.

If an order of the court or notice of the health officer for the abatement of a nuisance by the occupier or owner is not complied with because the occupier or owner cannot be found or because the occupier or owner is imprisoned, the health officer may apply to the court for an order to have the nuisance abated, and all costs of and expenses incurred in connection therewith shall be paid to the health officer by the occupier or owner, and may be recovered as a debt.

If no owner or occupier can be found or if the expenses are not paid within six months after the completion or the abatement of such nuisance, the court may order the premises upon which the work shall have been done, or any part thereof, or any movable property found thereon belonging to such occupier or owner to be sold to defray the said cost and expenses.

The rules of court relating to sales in execution of decrees shall *mutatis mutandis* apply to such sales.

As the successful prosecution of public health duties involves incursion into people's apartments and private settlements by the health officer, he is given a legal backing under Section 10. Sub-sections (1) (a), (b), 2 and 3 in the form of his *right of entry*.

Section 10 (1)

(a) It shall be lawful for the health officer to enter any premises at any time between the hours of six in the morning and six in the evening for the purpose of examining as to the existence thereon of any nuisance, or until a nuisance found to exist has been abated or the works order to be done are completed or the closing order has not been complied with or has been infringed, to enter premises at all reasonable hours for the purpose of securing the execution of the order.

(b) If the admission to premises is refused, the court may require the person having the custody of the premises to admit the health officer into the premises during the prescribed hours and if the person having the custody of the premises is found the court may authorize the health officer forcibly to enter on such premises.

(2) Any such order shall continue in force until the work for which the entry was necessary has been done.

(3) Any person who refuses to obey such order or in any way hinders, prevents or obstructs the execution of the order shall be liable to a fine of fifty pounds or six months imprisonment.

Section 11 deals with the Cost of Execution relating to Nuisance.

All reasonable costs and expenses incurred in serving the notice, making a complaint or obtaining an order or in carrying the order into effect shall be deemed to be money paid at the request of the person on whom the order is made, or, if no order is made, but the nuisance is proved to have existed when a notice was served or the complaint made, then the persons by whose act default or sufferance the nuisance was caused; and in the case of nuisances caused by the act or default of the owner of the premises such cost and expenses may be recovered from any person who is for the time being owner of such premises.

Part III Notifiable Infectious Diseases

Under Section 12 of the Law, the Medical Officer of Health becomes the 'appropriate Medical Officer of Health' and the significance of his duties is reflected by the qualifying epithet 'appropriate', which singles him out as the collating officer to whom all information relating to the occurrence of a notifiable infectious disease should be made during an epidemic in his area of jurisdiction.

Under this qualification he has exclusive powers to deal with containing an epidemic. Section 13(1) (a) and (b) make it obligatory for:

1. the head of family of an inmate suffering from notifiable disease, and in his default;
2. the nearest relatives present in the building or in attendance on the patient, and in default of such relatives;
3. every person in charge of or in attendance of the patient, and in default;
4. the occupier of the building, as soon as he becomes aware that the patient is suffering from a notifiable infectious disease, to send notice thereof to the appropriate medical officer of health.
5. Also every medical practitioner attending on, or called to visit the patient shall, as soon as he becomes aware that the patient is suffering from a notifiable infectious disease, send to the appropriate medical officer of health, a certificate stating the name of the patient, the situation of the building and the disease from which, in his opinion, the patient is suffering.

A penalty for default in notifying the appropriate medical officer of health is imprisonment on such a person, consisting of a fine of up to fifty pounds or six months imprisonment.

This is a clear indication of the determination of the authorities to deal with the outbreak of notifiable infectious diseases. Under notification, it is also mandatory upon all medical officers of health to issue a *Weekly Bill of Health* according to the specifications of the *World Health Organization*, through which the organization is able to publish the *World Health Bulletin*. It will therefore be observed how correct and regular collation of reports on notifiable infectious diseases are of great importance in relation to world health. Still under the terms of this important part, the appropriate medical officer of health is empowered to:

1. order post-mortem examination;
2. mark premises where infectious disease has occurred or is suspected;
3. order disinfection of such building;
4. order the destruction of building and formites;
5. order destruction of animals carrying or suspected to carry notifiable infectious disease;
6. remove and detain persons and suspects; and
7. isolate contacts.

In going through the Notifiable Infectious Disease Ordinance one is apt to feel that both the health officer and the appropriate medical officer of health are given very wide powers, such as could be misused by the unwary. Again, one will easily arrive, from the scope of these powers, at an awareness of the determination to contain outbreaks of notifiable infectious diseases by the appropriate authorities.

There is usually a Compensation Board appointed by the Minister to deal with cases of claims on buildings, animals, or articles destroyed in the interest of public health. Such Boards usually consist of two persons, 'one of whom shall be unconnected with the Government Service', and who 'shall have all the powers of a High Court of the Region'. Section 33 of the Law empowers the Minister to make regulations:

(a) for isolating all persons suffering or suspected to be suffering from a notifiable infectious disease, or brought into contact with any person so suffering, or suspected;
(b) for inspecting and granting permits to persons travelling by sea or land from a place where a notified infectious disease has occurred, and for disinfecting their clothes and effects;
(c) for closing, destroying, disinfecting, cleaning or otherwise rendering harmless, houses, building, latrines, wells, dust-bins, dumping grounds and any place that by reason of the existence of infectious disease it may be deemed advisable so to deal with;
(d) for prohibiting the removal of property from an infected house;
(e) for prescribing the mode of burial or disposal of the bodies of persons dying from a notifiable infectious disease;
(f) for the removal of persons from an infected area the evacuation of which has been ordered by the Minister;
(g) for establishing a cordon around any place where a notifiable infectious disease has occurred or otherwise preventing persons departing from or going to any such place;

(h) for prescribing the reporting of cases of sickness and death;
(i) for the disposal or destruction of refuse and sewage;
(j) for the erection of temporary huts, mortuaries and similar buildings by the chiefs or headmen of towns or villages;
(k) for prescribing the acts of things, done under any rule, in respect of which compensation may be paid;
(l) for declaring whether compensation shall be paid out of general revenue of the Region, or out of the funds of a local government council;
(m) for the publication within the area affected of any notice under section 28 or regulation made under this section;
(n) for prescribing the procedure to be adopted by a compensation board; and
(o) generally for the better carrying into effect of any of the provisions of this Law relating to infectious diseases.

Part IV Sale of Food

From early recorded history civilized countries have recognized the importance of safe food, and the obligation to produce sanitary and safe food rests upon the producer, processor, or manufacturer. Regulatory control is generally the responsibility of the health staff. Sanitation in food handling establishments is of prime importance in the prevention of food contamination. A sanitation control programme includes such items as:

1. location of premises;
2. exterior environmental appearance;
3. good construction with easily cleaned interiors;
4. cleanliness of equipment;
5. good house-keeping;
6. education of personnel in the use of hygiene and sanitation procedures; and
7. sanitary methods for the disposal of all wastes.

Under Section 34 of the law:

A health officer is empowered at all reasonable hours to examine any food intended for human consumption, which has been (i) sold or (ii) is offered or (iii) exposed for sale or (iv) is in possession of or (v) has been deposited with or (vi) consigned to any person for the purpose of sale or of preparation for sale, and if it appears to him to be unfit for human consumption or diseased or unwholesome, may condemn the same and order it to be destroyed or so disposed of as to prevent it from being used for human consumption.

2. Any person to whom food condemned under this section belongs or in whose possession or premises it was found shall be guilty of an offence and liable on conviction to a fine of ten pounds for each article condemned and for every subsequent conviction to a fine of fifty pounds or imprisonment for six months.

The health officer is also empowered to apply and effect a search warrant where he believes there is an article of food for human consumption in any building, carriage, receptacle or place which is diseased or unwholesome or unfit for human consumption. For regulatory control of food preparing premises, Section 36 empowers the Minister to make by-laws as regards the slaughter of animals and regulated premises as follows:

36. Subject to the provisions of this Law, a competent council may, with the approval of the Minister, make by-laws for all or any of the following purposes:
   (a) licensing slaughter-houses and regulating the slaughter of animals intended for the food of man, and the management and use of slaughter houses;
   (b) providing for the inspection of such animals;
   (c) regulating the preparation and sale of meat;
   (d) prescribing the charges for the use of slaughter houses, and fees for inspection and licences;
   (e) the prevention of unnecessary pain or suffering before or in the process of slaughtering animals, and prescribing the methods of slaughtering;
   (f) regulating the sale, preparation, storing and exposure for sale of food;
   (g) preventing the sale, preparation, manufacture, conveying or exposure for sale of food which is unwholesome or diseased;
   (h) licensing and regulating corn-mills, rice-mills, bakeries, aerated water manufactures and other establishments for the preparation of food and drink; and
   (i) regulating and prescribing the cleanliness, water supply, drainage and sanitary conveniences of any premises in which food is sold, prepared, manufactured, kept or exposed for sale;

Part V Vaccination Ordinance

This contains details about the Vaccination Ordinance, which has been omitted here because smallpox has been successfully eradicated in most countries in Africa, and from the whole world.

Part VI Yellow Fever Ordinance

Yellow fever, an internationally quarantinable disease, is mosquito-borne, and immunization against it is an essential health requirement in immigration. Section 53 interprets inoculating to include re-inoculation, and a 'temporary visit' to mean a stay of seven days. Sections 54-65 emphasizes and defines:

1. the liability for inoculation;
2. the inoculation of adults;
3. the inoculation of children;
4. the power to make rules;
5. record-keeping by health officers;
6. the supply of inoculation certificates; and
7. penalties.

Under the section of penalties, one can gather the authorities' determination to effect a check on defaults from the heaviness of the penalties imposed; for example, Section 61 reads:

Any person who, without reasonable cause, the burden of proving which shall be upon him, contravenes or fails to comply with the provisions of Sections 55 and 56 of this part or of any rule made under Section

62 shall be liable on a first offence to a fine of fifty pounds or to imprisonment for six months or to both such fine and imprisonment, and on conviction for a second or subsequent offence to a fine of one hundred pounds or to imprisonment for one year or to both such fine and imprisonment.

Section 62 empowers the Minister to make rules:–

The minister in relation to any order of the Governor-in-Council made under Section 54 or Section 63 may make rules generally for the carrying out of the provisions of this part, and in particular for:

(a) prescribing the forms to be used for any purpose under this Part;
(b) the duties to be performed and the procedure to be adopted by a town council, or local government council either generally or in respect of any prescribed area;
(c) the duties and power of any person engaged or employed in the administration of this Part;
(d) the keeping and examination of books and other records in connection with the administration of this law;
(e) exempting from the provisions of this Part any person or class or classes of persons;
(f) prescribing the standard of any serum or virus to be used for the purposes of inoculation;
(g) prescribing the period on the expiration of which re-inoculation may be required;
(h) specifying penalties for breaches of any rule made under the provision of this section and providing for different penalties in the case of successive breaches.

Part VII: Sanitation and Housing Ordinance

Apart from the details in all the foregoing, it should be realized that the government provides ample measures for the maintenance of public health, and using the proper administrative machinery, it delegates its powers to competent councils to make by-laws to each ordinance, approvable at ministerial level. A competent council, in the context of the Public Health Law, is one which is viable enough to employ the full time services of a medical officer of health.

In its entirety, therefore, the administrative machinery to practise Environmental Health Control is not a monopoly of the government; but in general this responsibility is in part delegated to the local government councils, within a framework of the enacting of by-laws and regulations not dissimilar in aims and objectives to those of the parent public health law.

It is in this context that the present ordinance, sanitation and housing, operates; for Section 64 covers the majority of the environmental aspects of sanitation and housing, and imposes a responsibility for:

(a) the maintenance of public latrines, urinals, dustbins and manure and night-soil depots in sanitary conditions;
(b) surface scavenging, and the removal and disposal of night-soil and other refuse;
(c) the cleansing of streets;
(d) the provision and proper construction of rubbish receptacles on private premises;
(e) the prevention of overcrowding in premises or rooms either in respect of human beings or animals, including the designation of an officer to fix the maximum number of human beings or animals which may occupy any particular premises or room;

(f) the destruction of rats, mice and other kinds of vermin, and of fleas, bugs, or any other such parasites as it may be deemed advisable to destroy and for rendering houses rat-proof;
(g) the sanitary maintenance of workshops, breweries and places of public instruction, recreation or assembly;
(h) the regulation of laundries and wash-houses;
(i) the admission into any urban area of animals;
(j) the construction, position and proper sanitary maintenance of all places where animals are kept;
(k) the methods to be adopted in cleansing and disinfecting places which have been occupied by any animal suffering from a contagious or infectious disease;
(l) requiring the owner or occupier of any land or tenements to clear and keep free from vegetation the road, streets, or paths adjoining their land or tenements;
(m) prohibiting or regulating the making of borrow pits or excavations;
(n) prohibiting or regulating the sinking of wells and providing for the closing of wells.

Section 65 deals with buildings and their construction. The competent council is empowered to make by-laws dealing with:

1. the construction of buildings and the materials used;
2. free air space, lighting and ventilation, and the dimension of rooms for human habitation;
3. height of buildings; the height above the roof or the rest of the building of chimneys within buildings;
4. the provision of sanitary conveniences, drainage, and means for conveying refuse water;
5. the refuse collection service;
6. wells, tanks and cisterns in buildings; for water storage for human consumption;
7. stoves and cooking appliances (not being electricity supplied) for the purpose of preventing fire accidents; and
8. septic tanks and sewage.

Section 67 deals with measures to be taken on the fouling of water in any well, stream, tank, reservior, aqueduct, or pond used or intended to be used for human consumption with any deleterious substance, and imposes a fine of ten pounds for the first offence and two pounds for everyday during which the offence continues.

Part VIII General Provisions

The Public Health Law takes care of every aspect of maintaining environmental health in the country, and throughout the law efforts have been made to safeguard this principle, both in terms of preventing the perpetrating of actions inimical to the public welfare, and in preserving the authority of the administering officials. Further, under the above Part, Sections 68 to 75 deal generally with likely environmental encounters and relate them to penalties to be imposed. Section 68 imposes penalties for obstructing execution of the law. Section 69 imposes penalties for the obstruction of the owner of premises from complying with health requirements by their occupiers. Section 70 prescribes further the mode of service of abatement notices, which includes (a) fixing the notice on some conspicuous part of the premises; (b) delivering the notice to the person to be served; and (c) delivering the notice at the usual or last known place of abode of such person to some adult member or servant of his family.

Section 71(1) compels the occupier of any premises to give his name and the address of the owner of the premises (2) penalizes to the extent of a fine of five pounds any occupier declining to give or wilfully mis-stating the name or address either of himself or of the owner.

Section 72 gives the powers and privileges of a police officer to a health officer for the purpose of enforcing the provisions of this law, including (a) detaining or arresting any person who has or is reasonably suspected of having committed an offence against this law and (b) appearing for the prosecution of such an offence in a magistrate's court or a customary court. Section 75, the all important section, absolves the health officer of any liability for his actions done *bona fide* in the execution of the Public Health Law. It reads:

> A health officer or other person shall not be liable to any action, liability or demand or account of anything done by him *bona fide* for the purpose of executing this Law.

By the foregoing enactments environmental health control is thus effectively taken care of.

The concern of the authorities may be assessed by the severity of the penalty clauses appearing in the law. When it is realized that the economy of the nation is reflected in the buoyancy of the health of its manpower, and that the main scourge that saps this energy is *malaria*, one will not then be surprised at the introduction of the Mosquitoes Destruction Law as Cap. 103 of the Laws of Nigeria, 1948.

Mosquitoes Destruction Law, 1948

This law gives an interpretation of 'house' to include a dwelling house, etc.; 'mosquitoes' as the insect including its eggs, larvae, and pupae; and 'owner' as the person for the time being receiving the rents of any premises, whether on his own account, as agent or trustee or as receiver, or who would receive the same if such land or house were let to a tenant – which includes the Crown and any local government council.

'Sanitary authority' is the terminology used under this Law for the medical officer of health or any other person appointed by the Governor by notice in the Regional Gazette.

The law empowers the sanitary authority to do the following:-

1. to effect entry to premises and inspect them;
2. to order action;
3. to prohibit the clearing of undergrowth;
4. to order the covering of tanks and receptacles;
5. to take preventive measures;
6. to comply with orders in default, and recover costs;
7. to be subjected to appeals against orders; and
8. to pay no compensation for any expense or damage incurred in pursuance of the law without reasonable cause.

In effect, the object of the Mosquito Destruction Law is to emphasize the dire need to eliminate the propagation of mosquitoes by means of the imposition of heavy fines for acts favourable to their breeding. Penalties enacted under the law may amount to a fine of as much as one hundred pounds, or one year's imprisonment, or both such fine and imprisonment. This is far in excess of the maximum penalty under the Public Health Law; and it also enables more specific work against mosquito propagation by the public or by the sanitary authority to be carried out.

International Health Regulation

This is the Regulation under which health officers operate at Immigration Centres, at both sea and air ports. When properly organized and operated, it serves as an effective check against the transmission of Quarantinable Notifiable Infectious Diseases.

The International Health Regulation is published in annotated editions of reports adopted by World Health Assemblies; and it is usually issued at ten year's intervals by the World Health Organization.

It is a directive which gives uniformity to the control of diseases through agencies concerned with travel, and it streamlines its universal action by international patent authority.

Because of its peculiar terminology it is essential that operators should be practically involved in port health duties, so that routine duties as required by the regulations can be continued correctly and without hitches.

The regulation makes provisions relating to each of the quarantinable diseases. It defines '*Aedes aegypti* index', 'aircraft', and 'airport', and (a) 'arrival in the case of a seagoing vessel'; (b) 'in the case of an aircraft'; (c)'in the case of inland navigation vessel, either at a port or a frontier post'; and (d) 'in the crew of a train or road vehicle, at a frontier post'. It also defines: 'baggage', 'crew', 'day', 'direct transit area', 'epidemic', 'health administration', 'health authority', 'imported case', 'imported local area', 'infected person', 'international voyage', 'isolation', 'local area', 'medical examination', 'port', 'ship', 'suspect', 'valid certificate' and 'yellow fever receptive area'.

It also describes measures and procedures permitted by the regulation as the maximum measures applicable to international traffic required by a state for the protection of its territory against the quarantinable diseases.

In one of the articles it is stated that: 'sanitary measures and health formalities shall be initiated forthwith, completed without delay, and applied without discrimination'.

Factory Law

The definition of a factory may be classified as follows:

1. all places in which mechanical power is used in the aid of manufacturing process; and
2. all places, whether mechanical power is used or not, in which certain specified industries are carried on.

The use of water, steam, or any other form of mechanical power for manufacture in any workshop or workplace converts it into a factory. The Ministry of Labour enforces the Factory Law through Factory Inspectors; and among their main duties are:

1. to see that every factory is provided with means of escape in case of fire;

2. to see to the provision of suitable and sufficient sanitary conveniences; and
3. to see that every building used as a workshop or factory, or where persons are employed in any trade or business is provided with suitable and sufficient sanitary conveniences.

The Public Health Officers ensure that:

1. premises are kept in a healthy and clean state;
2. are ventilated in such a manner as to render harmless as far as practicable any gases, vapours, etc; and
3. they are not overcrowded.

Domestic factories or workshops include private houses, rooms, or places which, though used as a dwelling, are by reason of the work done there a factory or workshop, and in which the only persons employed are members of the same family dwelling there. Premises in which offensive trade is carried on also come within the inspection of the health officers. These trades include:

(1) bone boiling; (2) blood boiling or drying; (3) gut scraping; (4) fat and tallow melting; (5) skin or leather tannery; (6) paper making; (7) oil mills; and (8) rice mills and similar dusty trades.

The Factory Inspectors are concerned with the occupational hazards likely, i.e. possible risks of accidents; while the health officers are concerned with the concomitant environmental health control, properly carried out under thorough knowledge and routine as specified under the Public Health Law.

General

The Public Health Law, as health education teaches, is to be applied as a 'last resort' after all efforts at persuasion have failed.

In the actual administration of environmental health control it is more often than not a question of encountering recalcitrant defaulters whose attitudes in public towards environmental health control have been highly unco-operative, and whose influence in the community may constitute a serious deterrent to effective control. After all genuine approaches through health education have failed to make an impact, the law invariably becomes the last resort.

Unfortunately health legislation takes years to enact in many African countries. For example, the drafting of the Food and Drugs Act in Nigeria commenced in 1962 and was only completed in 1975. Other major constraints rendering health legislation in African countries ineffective include the lack of law enforcement personnel and public health laboratories, and a tremendous shortage of legal manpower and courts. Nevertheless, newer legislation is slowly being added on mental health, Indian hemp, narcotic drug abuse, industrial safety, occupational health in general, and many other health topics. Laboratories for enforcing the Food and Drugs Act are now being developed not only in the Federal and State capitals, but in other major cities and settlements as wel[1].

Appendix I

Supplementary Federal Gazette Publications from 1966 Containing Enactments

1.	Medical Practitioners (Temp. Regu.) Decree 1966	page A 303
2.	Midwives Decree 1966	page A 325
3.	Nigerian Council for Medical Research	page A 293

Acts and Decrees not in force at 31/12/66
Cap. 209 Venereal Disease Act
1952 No. 16 Medical Auxiliaries Registration Act 1952
1965 No. IX Food and Drugs (Lagos) Amendment Act 1965
Decree No. 72 of 1966 Nigerian Council for Medical Research Decree 1966 (Except S.10)
Decree No. 79 of 1966 Midwives Decree 966

Subsidiary Legislation (Jan. – Dec. 1966)
Medical and Dental Practitioners Act 1963 No. 9 – Legal Notice 65 page B337

Subsidiary Legislation applicable to city of Lagos only Jan-July 1967
Public Health Rules (Cap. 165)
Lagos Public Health Rules (Pigs) Amendment Notice 1967
Legal Notice No. 12 page B15 – Amendment of Public Notice 99 of 1943 (1958 Laws Vol. IX p. 1997)

Decree No. 2 of 1970 Establishing the Nursing Council of Nigeria
Decree No. 42 of 1st April, 1971 – Nigerian Livestock and Meat Authority.

Legal Notice 45 of 1971
Immigration Act 1963. Immigration Act (Visa abolition) Order 197 of 1st June, 1971.
Immigration (Amendment) Decree 1972 No. 8 of 10th April, 1972

Decree No. 35 – Food, Drugs, Cosmetics and Devices of 1974

Legal Notice 6 of 1974. Merchant Shipping Act 1962 Decree No. 30 of 1962
Merchant Shipping (Collision) Rules 1974 of 1st January, 1966

Local Government Edict No. 5 of 1976 for Oyo State, 1 September 1976 section 64b – Sanitary inspection, sewerage, refuse and night soil disposal comes under direct control of Local Government.

Ibadan Wastes Disposal Edict, 1973, establishing the Ibadan Wastes Disposal Board.

56

Health Services and the Quality of Life

John R. Goldsmith

A. Variation in the Attitude Towards Quality of Life

Once risks to survival have been reduced to a certain level, concern about diseases gives way to concern about the capabilities of a person or community to participate in and enjoy life. These concerns have been focussed on the quality of life.

Quality of life is a highly subjective matter, and each of us may have a different operative definition which is part of our culture, philosophy or religious convictions. For one person,quality involves beauty, happiness and freedom from responsibilities; for another it involves being part of a family or tribe or people; for a third it involves absorbing knowledge of the world around one and using the knowledge in constructive ways; for a fourth it involves dedication to right the injustice and unfairness of the world; for a fifth it involves accumulation of goods, money, power and/or privileges. Some of these desiderata are in terms of positive accomplishments and actions, and others are in terms of freedom from risk, constraint or impoverishment of mind, spirit or body.

Health services, involving both publicly provided services as well as those affected by market conditions, can be seen with little reflection, to affect any of these possible attributes of the quality of life. Health services can also be dissected into those intended primarily for treatment of established disorders and those primarily intended for prevention of a disease, impairment or disablement. Both sectors involve quality of life considerations.

Rather than attempting to treat the relationship of health services to quality of life in a systematic or didactic fashion, it is well to recount three samples which seem to reflect health problems associated with the quality of life.

B. The Rise and Fall of Cigarette Smoking

Certainly the American Indians, to the best of our knowledge, the first tobacco smokers, found the practice of smoking tobacco satisfying or they would not have taken it up. It must have contributed to the quality of their life. And when European explorers were introduced to it, the attractiveness of the habit was found to be cross-cultural. Different forms of tobacco consumption did tend to disseminate in different cultures; the person who savoured a fine Havana cigar tended to be different from the person who chewed snuff and from the pipe smoker. The ritual of snuff inhalation had its own adherents. Cigarette smoking was a relatively minor mode of tobacco consumption until the first World War, when cigarettes were widely given to soldiers as a way of boosting their morale (or distracting them from their fear and misery). In the 1920s, the number of cigarette addicts was in the millions, and the advertising industry promoted the habit by identification of it with prominent figures in the social and sporting worlds, among other things.

The encouragement of cigarette smoking continued during World War II with promotion of smoking among the recruited soldiers, sailors and airmen, even in areas of food shortage and among starving refugees, distribution of cigarettes was encouraged. But within a decade the connection with lung cancer was recognized, and medical recognition of the role of smoking cigarettes in other chronic diseases, such as heart disease, doudenal ulcer, peripheral arteriosclerosis, other forms of cancer and in unfavourable reproductive outcomes led to professional and governmental efforts to halt the practice or at least to modify it in a favourable direction. Offering a visitor a cigarette was no longer considered a precious gesture in the United States, and the casual assumption that the smoker could light up when and where it pleased him, began to be replaced by the notion that non-smokers had a right to smoke-free air.

By this time, governments had learned how lucrative it was to raise money by taxing cigarettes, but many smokers, especially young persons, had to come to terms with the fact that they had become addicts. Survey after survey showed that a high proportion of smokers wanted to quit. It was learned that the advice of one's physician was the most influential approach for many who were able to terminate their smoking practice voluntarily.

The evidence of health risk to the 'bystanders' exposed has been documented and the quitter makes a contribution as well to the quality of life of his family and co-workers.

In the 1990s, the treatment of cigarette addiction was one of the most useful contributions a physician could made to preventive medicine. For most of the serious health effects, the uptake of the smoking habit is earlier by years or decades than the first manifestations of unfavourable health effect. Impairment of the quality of life of both smokers and non-smokers becomes an important consideration, motivating the smokers to quit. In the latter case, regulations restricting smoking in public places and in worksites have been found useful in the U.S. and in Europe and now in Nigeria.

The tobacco industry has, however, increased its promotion of smoking among developing countries, for whom the prospects of governmental revenue from taxation of tobacco products is very attractive. To wait in each country for the development of the serious health problems associated with smoking before taking preventive action would be to doom the residents of such countries to hundreds of premature deaths per thousand in the population. It may prove to be more effective to emphasize the smoking-related impairment of quality of life, such as the malodour in the house and of the breath, the rubbish from cigarette packaging and filters, and the need for larger air conditioning units and better fire protection if smoking becomes more widespread.

Thus health risk recognition has catalyzed a change in the quality of life associated with smoking from recognition of a gratifying habit to the awareness of the advantages of a smoke-free world.

C. Urban Housing Standards and the Quality of Life

Historically, there is no doubt that urbanization in Europe, Asia, and the Americas was associated with substantial risks of bubonic plague, cholera, dysentery, rheumatic fever, and tuberculosis, both of the latter of which have long term health consequences. One approach to avoiding the health risks from poor housing, widely used in Europe and North America, was to develop housing standards, including minimal space per resident, stipulating the acceptable type of construction materials, and requiring running water and water-borne waste facilities, among other attributes. Such provisions are often excessively costly for poorer individuals and populations, who make up most of the urbanizing wave of the last generation.

This dilemma was put before an Expert Committee on Epidemiological Aspect of Housing in the World Health Organization. The committee noted that in some urban slums, mortality and morbidity did not seem to be elevated, despite the obvious fact that housing was substandard. Furthermore, in several programmes to improve substandard housing to meet the standards, the cost of the improvements was so great that housing costs had to be increased; in some locations this led to lowered levels of health because family budgets were no longer adequate for food and clothing. Thus it was clear that the engineering approach to urban housing quality was not a sufficient one.

The committee then emphasized certain functions which urban housing needs to fulfill, such as shelter, adequacy of water and waste disposal, reasonable freedom from insects and vermin, physical safety, and conformity with the cultural and social values of the community which uses the housing. The committee was impressed by evidence that with a strong family structure and community support, health can be sustained under a great variety of physical conditions.

Its report encouraged local authorities to help urban slum dwellers to improve the defects in their physical environment by providing construction materials, cement slabs, sanitary ware or approved types of pipes for water supply and waste disposal. Such experience as has accumulated with this approach has been favourable, not least because the people who built the houses were more likely to take good care of them than those for whom the building was done by someone else's labour. Their quality of life was enhanced because they had participated in improving their own environment. Of course disease prevention and treatment remain important requirements, but the quality of urban life in many crowded centres is improving not only because of specific disease prevention activities, but because matters of human dignity, as well as power and prestige within a community have been shown to be useful concepts for the improvement of urban housing and the resultant health of urban residents.

D. Technical Means for Adaptation to Chronic Illness and Prolonging Life

Among the major ethical problems facing physicians in Western countries and their health service system are:

1. maintenance of patients with end-stage renal disease through transplantation or renal dialysis;
2. the choice of which patients are to have coronary bypass surgery, a procedure for which the supply of surgical and hospital services is either scarce or expensive;
3. how long to provide life support for patients with no chance for independent living; and
4. when and how to use toxic and often costly anti-cancer drugs, radiation, etc.

In facing such decisions, although the technical factors loom large, to an increasing extent, quality of life considerations are becoming prominent. It is well recognized that the successful treatment of end-stage-renal failure by transplantation leads to a better quality of life than is the case for treatment by renal dialysis. Such criteria as an ability to hold a steady job, have freedom of movement by bus, train or on foot, to undertake moderate physical activity and normal sexual activities have been shown to be important criteria of quality of life.

Conversely, as increasing numbers of older persons or those with chronic diseases at all ages survive with or without these technical aids, their active involvement in the life of their community is also a factor in the quality of their lives. While many are no longer able to earn a regular wage, to assume that they will thrive without income, social contact and the dignity that can be realized from constructive activities is not realistic. A person, with or without health problems, who is forced to retire from useful work at age 65 (if male) or at 60 (if female) has lost an important qualitative dimension of his or her life.

These illustrate some of the problems which beset us when we face the real world of providing 'Health for All'. A few generalizations seem justified.

1. Among any group of persons, different variables will be seen as relevant to quality of life. Health services should be responsive to these differences. This is another way of saying that health services should be responsive to the value systems of the individuals receiving services.
2. Although it is natural to assume that, as a nurse or physician, your patients should be treated as you would like to be treated if you were in the same situation, this 'golden rule fallacy' should be resisted, at least until you learn whether the patients share the same values as you do. When they do not, your well-intentioned intervention (or lack of same) is likely to cause hostility, resentment, and impair

other aspects of health management, and even have a negative impact on the quality of your patients' lives.

3. The dignity of the patients and their families is precious and needs to be reckoned with in any health services decision.
4. Innovative health services, as well as new procedures and their use and efficacy are a large source of potential disagreement among communities, patients and health care providers. They deserve deliberate and careful planning and discussion prior to being used on an individual or community basis.
5. Because some intervention or procedure is technically feasible, it does not necessarily follow that it is acceptable to all members of the community.
6. Some contributions that physicians and nurses can make to the quality of life are based not on the care of individual patients, but on community resources, understanding, and policies.

References

Health Principles of Housing W.H.O.,Geneva, 1989, and "Uses of Epidemiology in Housing Programmes and in Planning Human Settlement" Report of a WHO Expert Committee, *WHO Technical Report Series No 544*, Geneva, 19874.

PART EIGHT

Health Care Services in Economically Developed Countries: Lessons for Africa

57

Health Care Systems in Israel

Vital Barell and Pnina Zadka

In the 30-year period prior to the founding of the State of Israel, its health services developed in a pattern that persists to this day. The mandatory government initiated some basic public health services, while personal preventive and some hospital and outpatient services were developed by voluntary charitable agencies such as the Hadassah Medical Organization. Personal care services (including hospitalization and drugs) were developed through the voluntary health insurance funds that were largely organized through the labour movement. The existence of the Sick Fund goes back to the early 1920s, when it was founded by the Confederation of Labour, whose aim was to assure the state of health and well being of its members and their families. Direct care services were provided through their own facilities, including hospitals and drugs.

With the creation of the State of Israel in 1948, the Ministry of Health together with its district offices took responsibility for the basic public health services. Many of the services initiated by voluntary agencies, especially in the field of child care, geriatrics, and psychiatry, were also taken over by the ministry. Present trends are toward the transfer of direct services from the Ministry to other care giving agencies, such as the Sick Funds, with the Ministry focusing on setting standards and supervising the health services.

The insurance and services initiated by the Labour and Trade Union Movement, developed into the General Sick Fund, which covers 80 per cent of the population. This provides prepaid comprehensive health insurance and has its own facilities for providing direct primary, secondary, tertiary, convalescent, and rehabilitation services.

Organization

The current organizational framework of the health services in Israel is given in Figure 57.1. The Ministry of Health is responsible for priority setting and allocation; planning and supervising of health care services; and licensing and standard setting for the health professions. In addition, it provides a significant share of preventive, curative, and rehabilitative services. The ministry operates twelve general hospitals which provide 48 per cent of all acute care beds, as well as more than half of the psychiatric services. 69 per cent of all mother and child health stations are also provided by the ministry, while 25 per cent are provided by the Sick Funds and about 6 per cent by municipalities.

The four voluntary Sick Funds active in the country cover 95 per cent of the population for prepaid medical, hospital, drug, convalescent, and other services. These Funds employ close to 60 per cent of the country's physicians and operate 1,300 health clinics. These include more than 200 MCH centres, providing ambulatory, primary and speciality care.

Preventive and ambulatory primary health care services are present in nearly every village, and neighbourhood, town, and city in the country. They are readily accessible, including secondary referral access to speciality clinics and outpatient hospital services. Three-quarters of the community clinics serve populations of under 5,000 individuals, with half of these in small agricultural settlements with a single doctor. Fifteen per cent of the clinics, all in urban areas serve between 5,000 and 10,000 members, and the remaining 10 per cent have larger populations. In urban areas the average list size of the family doctor is 1,500 insured population, while primary paediatricians have a smaller load of about 1,000 children. The rural doctor generally has a list of 1,200 individuals, and serves a small village or a number of agricultural settlements.

The ambulatory services provide secondary referral access to specialty clinics and hospital services. A survey of health services showed Israelis to be relatively high users of ambulatory care services, both preventive and curative, with over twelve visits to a physician per person per year.

The Sick Fund runs eight general hospitals, providing about 30 per cent of acute case beds, and many laboratory, convalescent, rehabilitation, and other facilities. No additional fees for services are required from members, except for very low co-payment for prescriptions and the cost expenditure for dental care.

Health Manpower

The health industry, large by Israeli standards, directly employs 60,000 people (about 6 per cent of the civilian labour force) in medical, paramedical, administrative, and support services. Israel currently has more than 8,000 registered physicians (21/10,000 population). The vast majority of Israeli physicians work primarily as employees either of the Ministry or of the Sick Funds. Very few are primarily self-employed in free-for-service practice; however, a large percentage carry on some free-for-service, self-employed practice; in addition to their primary employment. Of the 19,000 nurses employed (46/10,000 population) 55 per cent are practical nurses and 45 per cent are registered nurses. There is a relatively high dentist-to-population ratio in Israel (5.4/10,000) but a large proportion of dentists work only part-time.

Population Characteristics

Israel has about 21,000 square kilometres. Topographically, it is constituted by four general areas: the coastal plain – fertile, humid, and thickly populated – stretches along the Mediterranean; the central hills include the Hills of Galilee and Golan Heights in the north and the Negev Hills in the south; the Jordan Rift Valley with the lowest point at the Dead Sea; and the Negev Desert, which accounts for about half the country's area. Israel is a country with a rapid population growth–1.37 million persons in 1950 to 2.15 million in 1960, 3.02 million in 1970, 3.84 million in 1980 and it reached 4,063, 700 by the end of 1982. It is heterogeneous with regard to ethnic origin and sociocultural characteristics, with successive waves of Jewish immigration from 108 countries. There are considerable differences in population characteristics in the two national groups (Jewish and Arab). The Jewish population is composed of four major ethnic groups – European, North African, Mid-Eastern and Yemenite. The non-Jewish groups are composed of Moslem and Christian Arabs, as well as à sizable Druze population.

There are 95,000 births per year – 25 per cent of which are non-Jewish. The crude birth rate among the Jews is 23/1,000 population and 35/1,000 population among the non-Jewish. The total fertility rate among Jews is 2.91/females, and among non-Jewish 4.7/female.

Israel is an industrialized nation, but atypical. The number of immigrants and the fact that many of them have come from developing societies have had their effect. Side by side with the diseases and problems of industrialization and relative affluence in some groups are other problems related to lack of hygiene awareness and poor enforcement of public health regulations.

Mortality rates and life expectancy in Israel reflect the patterns prevalent in Western countries.

Table 57.1

Life Expectancy at Birth, 1983

Sex	Jews	Non-Jews
Males	73.0	70.8
Females	76.3	73.3

Among Jews acute myocardial infraction is the leading cause of death: 132.8/100,000 in 1980 down from 213/100,000 in 1970–74. For the non-Jewish population, mortality rates reflected a younger population–ischemic heart disease death rates were 72/100,000 in 1969–72, 76.4/100,000 in 1973-76, and 120/100,000 in 1980. The increase can be attributed to rapid industrialization and urbanization processes.

Cerebrovascular disease declined slightly as a cause of death among the Jewish population during the same periods and increased slightly among the non-Jewish population.

Morbidity from the major infectious diseases has declined dramatically over the years, although infectious diseases such as hepatitis and gastrointestinal disorders still constitute a public health problem.

Service Utilization

Israel's patterns of health care use are quite different from those in the United States. Americans spend almost one and a half times as many days in acute care hospitals as Israelis do; Israelis make three times as many doctor visits as Americans do. These differences are unexpected, for the two countries are similar in their patterns of disease and death and in the percentage of their aged population (Table 57.2).

National Expenditure on Health (NEH) by Service, 1978

Hospitals in Israel consume 44 per cent of all health expenditure, even under a policy of restraints. Ambulatory and preventive health services consume about 32 per cent.

The central government is the source of about 40 per cent of the national expenditure on health (Ministry of Health 35.7 per cent, and other central government sources about 4.3 per cent). The National Institute for Social Security provides about 3.5 per cent of the NEH. This includes collection and distribution of the employer's contributions to health insurance schemes and financing hospitalization of maternity cases and newborns.

Voluntary Health Insurance schemes provide about one-third of the NEH and the private sector provides another 15 per cent. Local authorities, voluntary associations, universities, and donations account for the residual 8.5 per cent of the NEH.

Obstetric and Neonatal Services

Following are a number of tables which summarize the obstetric and neonatal special care services in Israel. As can be seen from Table 57.3, the government sponsors almost one-third of the obstetric beds in the country, the Sick Funds sponsor another 28 per cent, and the private sector sponsors less than 4 per cent. The overall bed occupancy rate is 96 per cent with an average length of stay of 4.1 days. The occupancy rates in Government and Sick Fund obstetric services are over 100 per cent. The occupancy rates differ considerably by geographic area (Table 57.4).

There are 300 neonatal special care beds in Israel; 36 per cent of these (120 beds) are authorized neonatal intensive care beds. Because of reporting artifacts, it is not possible to separately identify admissions for prematurity, special care and intensive care.

Government and Sick Fund hospitals provide more than 75 per cent of the neonatal special care wards in the country, and there are no wards of this type in private hospitals. The average occupancy rate in these wards is 108 per cent with an average length of stay of almost 16 days.

Overall, there is one neonatal special care admission for every 13.5 maternity admissions, though the ratio varies throughout the country, as do the occupancy rates.

Sixty per cent of the hospitals with obstetric services also have special neonatal care units. All of the services have 5,000 or more births yearly, as well as ten of the eleven services with 3,000-4,999 annual births. One hospital with less than 2,000 births has a special care ward as well.

Problems in MCH Services

Fragmentation of services and care is one of the major problems in maternal and child services in Israel. From the beginning of pregnancy through to the end of one year of infant life, care is given in multiple sites. This, of course, puts considerable strain on the flow of relevant information from one site to another and the consequent continuity of care. Even within the same facility, there is often discontinuity in medical records and in care-giving policy.

Health service policy in Israel today is directed toward the provision of continuity of care and adequate flow of relevant information over multiple sites, as well as maintaining the generally high quality of services.

In addition, emphasis is being put on the following:

- Appropriate use of high-technology.
- Equitable and efficient distribution of scarce resources.
- Reorganization of services and proper routine of high-risk maternity cases and infants.
- Targeting high-risk populations and designing appropriate interventions to reduce infant mortality and morbidity.
- Maintaining a high level of preventive services and increasing the capabilities of heterogeneous populations to comply with health directive.

Table 57.2

General Utilization Data

Acute care beds (27,247)	2.92/1,000 population
Bed days	966/1,000
Average length of stay	6.1 days
Bed occupancy	91.8 per cent
Total bed ratio	6.7/1,000 population
Ambulatory visits	12/person/year
• infants born in hospital	less than 99 per cent
• infants fully immunized	84 per cent
• receiving care by trained personnel	mothers – 90 per cent
	children – 90 per cent

Table 57.3

Obstetric Services in Israel: 1982

Ownership	Hospitals	Beds	Admissions	Occupancy rate	Average length of stay
Total					
Number	35	1266	104,857	96.0	4.1
Per cent		100.0	100.0		
Government	11	33.4	36.4	103.4	4.0
Municipal	2	9.2	8.0	87.7	5.3
Sick Fund	8	28.2	33.0	112.6	4.3
Hadassah	2	3.9	4.8	106.4	3.7
Mission	4	10.1	6.0	52.3	3.8
Voluntary	6	11.4	9.1	89.4	4.0
Private	2	3.8	2.5	45.9	2.9

Table 57.4
Obstetric Services by Regions: 1982

Region	Number of hospitals	Beds	Admissions	Occupancy rate	Average length of stay	Number of Beds	
						Range	Average
Total							
Number	35	1266	104,857	96.0	4.1		
Per cent		100.0	100.0				
North	11	32.6	28.8	84.2	3.9	15-58	35.5
Sharon	6	18.4	18.4	105.3	4.4	25-55	38.8
Central	4	15.2	18.3	107.0	3.9	36-60	49.0
Tel Aviv	2	9.5	8.0	75.2	4.9	40-80	60.0
Jerusalem	9	14.8	13.3	88.0	3.7	8-30	20.8
South	3	11.3	13.2	124.0	4.7	7-90	47.7

Fig. 57.1
Organizational Framework of Health Services in Israel

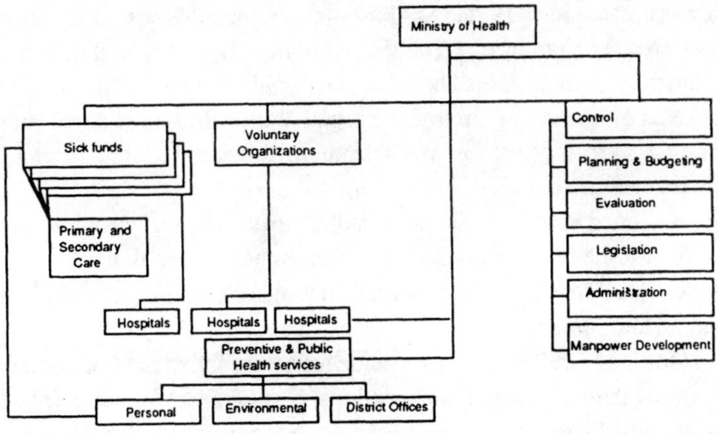

Figure 1: *Organizational framework of health services in Israel*

58

*The Main Goals of the National Health Service in the United Kingdom**

G.T. Pollock

The Origins

An organization on the scale of the United Kingdom National Health Service (NHS) clearly can come into being only after many years of consideration of tentative ideas emanating from a wide range of individuals and groups, motivated by a broad spectrum of aspirations. Furthermore, in attempting to take a historical perspective of a major public sector initiative of this kind, one finds genuine difficulty in knowing exactly where to begin as apparently formative activities frequently are found, on closer study, to have their origins in even earlier events.

Perhaps it was the rich variety of voluntary, religious and philanthropic activity in the 19th and early 20th century England which pointed the way to some kind of rationalization of medical care being necessary and requiring, in all probability, a national co-ordinating focus. However, although a Ministry of Health was created in 1919, the establishment of the NHS was still thirty years off.

Nevertheless, the existence of a relevant Central Government Department did, in fact, provide a framework with which the idea of a national health service could receive an encouraging hearing. Although, in the ten years or so leading up to the Second World War, traditional public health administrative legislation took precedence in Parliament, focusing on the need to improve unsatisfactory environmental conditions.

The six years of war stiffened the country's determination to have better conditions in the future. This included the shifting of the main focus from the environment to the individual, leading to a post-war package of social welfare legislation designed, amongst other things, to eliminate poverty and to promote, maintain and protect health.

The overall goal of the NHS Act 1946 was to provide for the establishment of a comprehensive health service available to all and, with minor exceptions, free of charge at the point of delivery. (It is, perhaps, necessary to stress this point as, of course, no service of this kind can be 'free'; the NHS was at its inception, and is now, funded mainly out of taxation). The duty was placed on the

Foot note

*A number of minor administrative differences distinguish the way in which health services are provided in the constituent countries of the United Kingdom; the details given in this chapter relate to England.

Minister of Health to promote the establishment of such a service 'designed to secure the improvement in the physical and mental health of the people and the prevention, diagnosis and treatment of illness'.

The question of the service being 'available to all' meant, of course, a great deal more than simply being free of charge to the consumer, although this was probably the benefit most immediately perceived. For example, it ended the anomaly by which an employed, insured man could receive free treatment from his General Practitioner whereas his wife and children could not. It clearly also had to mean, for example, equal access to hospital medical care. This required quite a major organizational initiative in order to attempt to spread hospital resources as evenly as possible in terms of both quantity and standards throughout the country. Fourteen Regional Hospital Boards were set up to cover the whole of England and, within each Region, Hospital Management Committees were set up to administer local hospitals on a day-to-day basis. Because the Central Government was to determine the national strategy, the hospital service could be said to be centrally directed, regionally organized and locally administered.

All hospitals, whether voluntary (mainly acute services) or municipal (mainly long stay – elderly, mental illness, tuberculosis etc) were transferred to and vested in the Minister of Health on the appointed day. The senior medical staff of both types of hospital were able to be considered for appointment as Consultants or Senior Hospital Medical Officers (a specialist but Sub-Consultant grade) in their designated specialities. The deliberate creation of Consultant vacancies in the various provincial regions did much to ensure an even distribution of specialist skills throughout the country, although this took some little time in those Regions covering the industrial North and Midlands.

Similar arrangements were made in order to ensure the availability of General Practitioner services throughout the country. Local Executive Councils were set up to administer the contracts of doctors and dentists providing services in their areas. However, a national committee took on the task of overseeing the even distribution of these services throughout the country by declaring which ratios of practitioners to population were acceptable and which localities could, or could not, support further practice development.

The local authority health departments, those of City and County Councils, still under the direction of their Medical Officers of Health, although losing their municipal hospitals to the new Hospital Management Committees, were assigned a set of functions broadly concerned with community care and prevention. The provision of a community nursing service and the control of communicable diseases were clearly essential public health functions which could not reasonably be provided by hospitals or General Practitioners by the continuation, under the local authority umbrella, or pre-school child health clinics and the school health service was perhaps, in retrospect, more difficult to justify in an era in which each individual was to have free access to the services of both General Practitioner and hospital.

The 1974 Reorganization

It was unthinkable that a new organization of this national scale, brought into being one day – which would no doubt these days be referred to as a 'big bang' – could possibly be perfect in all respects;

indeed controversy not only on its detailed arrangements but also on its very first principles continued for at least fifteen years. Furthermore, although the overall goal to provide a comprehensive health service for all had been clear from the start, that goal was manifestly going to require support from a number of subsidiary objectives related to the effective and efficient planning and delivery of the service.

It was these very terms 'effectiveness' and 'efficiency' which dominated discussions on public sector management in the 1960s. As part of the glossary of the management theory of that decade, these terms, along with a variety of so-called management techniques, were imported from the United States, initially into British industry and commerce and subsequently into the British public sector, perhaps into local government a little before the health service. The various forms of management theory were not, however, wholly technical. The concept of consensus management was also being brought into the discussions so that the behavioural sciences were brought to bear alongside the quantitative methods and systems analysis which were bringing new and exciting ideas into project management and resource allocation.

At the same time the objective of integrating the three separate parts of the NHS was finding favour in all quarters, both professional and political. What were, in effect, three discrete services could survive only by virtue of a multiplicity of liaison committees and arrangements for cross-representation and the idea of an integrated service began to appeal greatly. (An illustration of the practical difficulties, often quoted in the discussions of the period, was that of a mother in labour. The normal confinement of a mother in labour at home, supervised by the local authority domiciliary midwife, could develop complications requiring the attendance of the professionally independent General Practitioner. This might, in turn, require the admission of the mother to the local maternity hospital for specialist care within a service planned and managed quite separately from the other two.)

Furthermore, the need to seek and take into account the views of those providing and receiving the service was becoming an objective in its own right. These views in the run-up to the now inevitable major reorganization plans were made to secure both professional advice and the voice of the consumer in the new management arrangements.

The 1974 reorganization attempted to achieve these various objectives and did so with a fair measure of success, although not without reservations from some quarters – from the local authorities because of their loss of control of the community health services to the new, all-embracing Area Health Authorities; from health care professionals, suspicious of the new managerial jargon; and from Medical Officers of Health, whose posts had ceased to exist in the new set-up and who were not necessarily comfortable with their new speciality of Community Medicine, let alone the fact that they had to compete for these new posts in the reorganized service.

More seriously, it was perhaps unfortunate that the introduction of the reorganized service coincided with economic difficulties and subsequent industrial recession, precipitated by events remote from the United Kingdom, which brought a new concern over the resourcing of the service.

The 1982 Restructuring

Two additional structural issues soon called for attention. In order to try to reconcile planning functions with those of operational management, two separate levels had been introduced in each locality – the Area, coterminous with the matching local authority and the District, covering the catchment population of each general hospital. The District was not managerially accountable to the Area but was to be 'monitored' and 'co-ordinated' by it. This relationship caused much perplexity and frustration. Similarly, there was a growing dissatisfaction that dialogues between Area and District were overlooking the key importance of management at the operational level. The 1982 restructuring took care of both of these anomalies by simply eliminating the Area level and by strengthening the management function at Unit level. A 'Unit' was being defined as a general hospital, a group of related hospitals or the community health services of a District. This restructuring greatly simplified the organization by giving us the District Health Authorities which we have today and by emphasizing the value of good management within the Units.

The Introduction of General Management

Since 1982, a great deal has happened in a comparatively short time. Following the settling of the main structural issues, a further objective became overt to provide the best possible service to patients within available resources. This may seem self-evident but, following the NHS Management Inquiry carried out in 1983, the government came to the conclusion that in order to secure this particular objective, it would be necessary to introduce the general management function into the service – to have, at each level in the organization a general manager who would have the individual responsibility for planning, implementation and control of performance. On the face of it, this appeared to be the end of the consensus approach within the service. However, it may well have re-emerged in a different form – in the sense in which the word can be said to mean 'general support for a proposal'. Certainly the most successful general managers are those who have been persuasive rather than authoritarian, who have used their clinical and other colleagues as 'sounding boards' and who have worked hard at attempting to carry people with them before taking policy decisions.

The Public Health Function

Two unexpected events occurring within a few months of each other led to the health service having to bring a sharp focus to bear on its public health responsibilities. In August 1984, an outbreak of over 400 cases of food poisoning took place at a hospital in the North of England and in April 1985, a large outbreak of Legionnaire's disease occurred at a hospital in the Midlands. Both outbreaks were the subject of public inquiries which subsequently identified deficiencies in the organization of surveillance, preventing and control of communicable diseases. In response, the government established an 'Inquiry into the Further Development of the Public Health Function' under the chairmanship of its Chief Medical Officer, the report of which was published in January 1988. The government accepted its main recommendations and both Regional and District Health Authorities are now required to accept the additional objective of ascertaining the health status of their respective populations and taking such steps as are necessary to secure improvements in that health status.

What began, in effect, as a positive response to a concern over the possible vulnerability of the population to outbreaks of communicable diseases quickly developed into a much wider review of the public health function in England – the first, incredibly enough, since the Report of the Royal

Sanitary Commission in 1871. At a time when a review of the NHS was being carried out, it was clearly sensible to re-examine the public health responsibilities of Regional and District Health Authorities alongside their responsibilities for the delivery of medical care.

As a means of taking these issues forward, each Regional and District Health Authority is now required to appoint a Director of Public Health (usually the existing Regional or District Medical Officer) who is to be responsible for the provision of public health advice, including the provision of an annual report on the health of the population. Initially it was felt that such an annual report would essentially identify key local health problems as a basis for health promotion and disease prevention but, as it is mentioned later, more recent discussions have identified wider uses of such a local public health information base.

The Government's White Paper 'Working for Patients' 1989

Throughout the 1980s, the Government has presided over a very considerable expansion of the NHS but it has become increasingly clear that more needs to be done because of rising demand and an ever-widening range of treatments made possible by advances in medical technology. At the same time there is clear evidence of a wide variation in performance up and down the country. Following the review of the NHS carried out in 1988, the Government's White Paper presents a programme of action with the intention of giving patients better health care and greater choice of the services available and providing greater satisfaction and rewards for those working in the NHS who successfully respond to local needs and preferences.

The detailed proposals include a number of key changes including the ability of individual hospitals to apply for 'self-governing' status within the NHS and improved arrangements for money required to treat patients to be able to cross administrative boundaries. Furthermore, in order to improve the effectiveness of NHS management, Regional and District management bodies are to be reduced in size and reformed on business lines, with executive and non-executive directors. Lastly, to ensure that all concerned with delivery services to the patient make the best use of the resources available to them, quality of service and value for money are to be more rigorously audited.

The short time-scale within which the public health and review reports have been produced has suggested a degree of cross-fertilization. The establishment of a public health information base within each District Health Authority is clearly going to have value beyond simply identifying targets for health promotion and disease prevention. The same information base will do much to guide the new District Authorities in deciding what are their priorities for the development of medical care delivery.

At the time of writing (December 1989), these proposals are the subject of much detailed discussion.

Conclusion

Present intentions are that the original goals of the NHS are to be preserved, that the service will continue to be available to all, regardless of income, and to be financed mainly out of general taxation. However, the White Paper makes it clear that the major task is now to bring all parts of the NHS up to the very high standard of the best, while preparing for the needs of the future.

59

United States of America International Health Agencies with Interest in Africa

Timothy D. Baker

Professor Timothy Baker, Head of the Division of International Health in the School of Health in the world famous Johns Hopkins University in Baltimore has kindly supplied us a Computer Matrix Locator – a list of some of the United States of America (USA) International Health Agencies with interests in Africa classified under (A) Disaster Relief, (B) Environmental Services, (C) Health Education, (D) Health Planning/Management to training, and for countries of Africa listed alphabetically from Angola to Guinea Bissau.

The second edition of our book therefore has in Table 59.1, the names of such agencies listed alphabetically starting with 'A' from the 'African Development Foundation' to the 'American Leprosy Missions Inc.

Table 59.2 contains the key for listing the agencies by the services they render specifically: (A) Disaster Relief; (B) Environmental Service; (C) Health Education; (D) Health Planning/ Management; (E) Hospitals/Health Centres; (F) Material and Child Service; (G) Equipment and Supplies; (H) Nutrition Services; (I) Population and Family; (J) Primary Care; (K) Research; (L) Disease Initiatives; and (M) Training.

Table 59.3 details the international health agencies operating in specific African countries from Angola to Guinea Bissau.

Prof. Timothy Baker will gladly supply either part or the full listing of USA international health agencies for all or just particular African countries especially alphabetically after G. Guinea Bissau.

The Editors and the University Press PLC, Ibadan, Nigeria, are very grateful to the Professor for such valuable data from a great country which extends her great wealth of knowledge and experience not only to the developing countries of Africa but also to much richer countries.

Table 59.1
Some of United States of America International Health Agencies with Interests in Africa, Listed Alphabetically — "A" Only

African Development Foundation 1625 Massachusetts Ave. NW Washington, D.C. 20036 Category: Govt. Agency Activities: A,B,C,D,E,F,G,H,K	ABT Associates Inc. 4250 Connecticut Ave., NW, S 500; Washington, D.C. 200 Category: Small business/consulting Activities: D,C,E,H,I,J,K	American Baptist Churches International Ministries P.O. Box 851, Valley Forge, PA 19482–0851; Category: Religious Activities: A,E,F,H,J,M
African Medical and Research Foundation 420 Lexington Ave., New York, NY 10170; Category: PVO Activities: A,B,C,D,E,F,G,H,I,J,K,L,M	Academy for Educational Development (Clearing house Development Communications) 1255 23rd St., NW, Suite 40 Washington, D.C., 20037 Category: Private, non-profit Activities: C,D,F,H,I,J,M	American College of Nurse-Midwives 1522 K Street, NW, Suite 1120 Washington, D.C. 20005 Category: PVO Activities: F,I,J,M
Africare 440 R Street NW, Washington, D.C. 20001 Category PVO; Activities: A,B,C,D,E,F,G,H,I,J,K,L,M	Action for Corporate Accountability 3255 Hennepin Ave, South, Suite 230; Minneapolis MN 55408 Category: PVO Activities: C,D,E,I,J,M	American College of Surgeons 55 E. Erie Street Chicago, IL 60546; Category: Professional/Trade Assoc. Activities: D,M
Aga Khan Foundation USA 1800 K Street, NW Suite 920 Washington, D.C. 20006 Category: PVO Activities: C,D,E,F,G,H,J,M		American Foundation for AIDS Research 5900 Wilshire Blvd., 2nd Floor, East Satellite LosAngeles, CA 90036 Category: Private Foundation Activities: C,K,L
Agency for International Development State Department, Washington, D.C. 20523; Category: Govt. Agency; Activities: A,B,C,D,E,F,G,H,I,J,K,L,M	Adventist Development and Relief Agency 6840 Eastern Ave., NW Washington, D.C. 20012 Category: PVO; Activities: A,B,C,D,E,F,G,H,I,J,K,L,M	American Friends Service Committee 1501 Cherry Street Philadelphia, PA 19102 Category: PVO Activities: A,C,E,F,G,J,M
Albert Schweitzer Fellowship 4520 NW 36th Street, Oklahoma City, OK 73122 Category: PVO; Activities: A,B,C,D,E,F,G,H,I,J,K,L	Africa Evangelical Fellowship 702 State Farm Road, Boone, 28607; Category: Religious Activities: A,B,C,D,E,F,G,H,I,J,K,L,M	American Jewish World Service 729 Boylston St. Boston, MA 02116; Category: PVO Activities: A,G,J
Amanda Wash & Associates International 22 S. Figueroa #216 Los Angeles, CA 90012 Category: Small business		American Leprosy Missions, Inc. 1 Broadway Elmwood Park, NJ 07407 Category: PVO; Activities: A,C,D,E,I,J,K,L,M

Table 59.2

Key for Listing Agencies

A:	Disaster Relief
B:	Environmental Services
C:	Health Education
D:	Health Planning/Management
E:	Hospitals/Health Centres
F:	Maternal and Child Services
G:	Equipment and Supplies
H:	Nutrition Services
I:	Population and Family
J:	Primary Care
K:	Research
L:	Disease Initiatives
M:	Training

Table 59.3

Matrix Locator

Countries	A Disaster Relief	B Environ-mental Services	C Health Education	D Health Planning	E Hospitals	F Maternal and Child Services	G Equipment and Supplies	H Nutrition Services	I Population and Family	J Primary Care	K Research	L Disease Initiatives	M Training
Angola	8	8	31, 246		8, 36, 246	31, 246				8,31,246		36	8, 31, 36, 246
Benin	235	235, 244, 297, 333,	235, 244, 297, 333, 347	235, 244, 297	36, 235, 244, 333	235, 244, 297	235, 244	235, 244, 297, 333	244, 297	235, 244, 297, 333, 347		36, 244, 297	36, 235, 244, 297, 347
Botswana	7, 8, 235	7, 8, 235, 426	7, 65, 208, 235, 364, 426	7, 65, 208. 235, 247, 364	7, 8, 10, 235, 364, 426	7, 10, 208, 235, 247, 364, 426	7, 181, 235	7, 235, 426	364, 426	8, 10, 235, 247, 364, 426	124, 364	124	8, 10, 65, 208, 235, 247, 364, 426
Burkina Faso	7, 13, 235, 316	7, 13, 235, 244, 297, 316, 333, 418	7, 13, 172, 235, 244, 297, 316, 244, 297, 316, 333, 207, 347, 418	7, 13, 172, 235, 244, 297, 308, 207, 293	7, 10, 13, 172, 235, 244, 308, 333	7, 10, 13, 97, 172, 235, 244, 297, 308, 316, 293	7, 13, 172, 181, 235, 244	7, 13, 172, 235, 297, 316, 333	13, 97, 196, 297, 316, 293, 418	10, 13, 172, 235, 244, 297, 308, 316, 333, 207, 347, 418	13, 97, 244, 308, 293	13, 172, 297	10, 13, 97, 172, 235, 244, 297, 316, 207, 347, 418
Burundi			102	53	36		53	102	53		53	36	36, 53
Cameroon	7, 35, 235, 316	7, 74, 235, 299, 316, 398	7, 115, 172, 231, 235, 242, 270, 299, 316	1, 7, 84, 172, 231, 235, 242, 299, 293	7, 36, 115, 172, 235, 242, 270, 299	7, 74, 115, 172, 234, 235, 242, 299, 316, 293	7, 181, 172, 235, 242	7, 74, 172, 234, 235, 242, 316, 398	196, 234, 242, 299, 316, 293	74, 84, 172, 231, 235, 242, 270, 299, 316	242, 293, 398	36, 172, 242	36, 74, 84, 172, 235, 242, 270, 299, 316
Cape Verde	13	13, 244	13, 70, 208, 244, 347	13, 208, 244, 393	13, 244	13, 70, 208, 244, 393	13, 244	13, 70	13, 393	13, 244, 347	70, 244, 393	13, 70, 244	13, 70, 208, 244, 347, 372
Central African Republic	13, 235	13, 235	13, 235	1, 13, 235, 293	13, 36, 235	13, 235, 293	13, 235	13, 235	13, 196, 293	13, 235	13, 293	13, 36	13, 36, 235

Chad	7, 13, 137, 235, 410	7, 13, 74, 137, 206, 235, 410, 418	7, 13, 137, 172, 206, 231, 235, 410, 418	7, 13, 137, 163, 172, 206, 231, 235, 410	7, 13, 137, 172, 235, 410	7, 13, 74, 163, 172, 206, 235, 410, 418	7, 13, 137, 172, 206, 235, 410	7, 13, 74, 137, 172, 235	13, 206, 418	13, 74, 137, 163, 172, 231, 235, 410, 418	13	13, 172, 410	13, 74, 137, 163, 172, 206, 235, 410, 418
Comoros	235	74, 235, 426	235, 426	53, 235	36, 235, 426	74, 235, 426	53, 235	74, 235, 426	53, 426	74, 235, 426	53	36	36, 53, 74, 235, 426
Congo		74			36	74		74		74		36	36, 74
Djibouti				163		163				163	369	369	163
Ethiopia	7, 13, 20, 34, 35, 59, 95, 114, 118, 137, 161, 235, 316, 410	7, 13, 74, 137, 235, 299, 316, 329, 233, 410	7, 13, 31, 107, 114, 118, 137, 161, 172, 235, 242, 245, 246, 299, 316, 233, 347, 410	7, 13, 53, 137, 172, 235, 242, 299, 329, 410	7, 13, 20, 34, 36, 95, 107, 114, 118, 137, 172, 235, 242, 245, 246, 299, 329, 233, 410	7, 13, 31, 34, 74, 90, 95, 114, 172, 235, 242, 245, 246, 294, 299, 316, 329, 410	7, 13, 20, 53, 95, 107, 118, 137, 161, 172, 181, 235, 242, 245, 329, 410	7, 13, 20, 34, 74, 90, 114, 172, 235, 242, 245, 316, 233	13, 53, 242, 294, 299, 316	13, 31, 34, 74, 90, 95, 107, 118, 137, 172, 235, 242, 245, 246, 299, 316, 329, 233, 347, 410	53, 76, 242	13, 36, 172, 242, 410	13, 31, 34, 36, 53, 59, 74, 76, 137, 171, 172, 235, 242, 245, 246, 299, 316, 347, 410
Gabon	8	8			8					8			8
Gambia	13, 235, 316	13, 235, 316	13, 235, 316	1, 13, 235, 293	13, 235	13, 90, 235, 316, 293	13, 181, 235	13, 90, 235, 316	13, 316, 293	13, 90, 235, 316	293	13	13, 235,316
Ghana	7, 114, 118, 137, 235	7, 137, 148, 197, 235, 299, 418	7, 114, 118, 137, 197, 235, 242, 245, 299, 314, 418	7, 53, 137, 148, 235, 242, 299	7, 114, 118, 120, 137, 235, 242, 245, 299, 314	7, 24, 97, 114, 148, 197, 234, 235, 242, 245, 299, 314, 418	7, 53, 118, 137, 181, 235, 242, 245	7, 114, 137, 148, 197, 234, 235, 242, 314	24, 53, 97, 197, 234, 242, 299, 418	24, 97, 118, 120, 137, 197, 235, 242, 245, 299, 314, 418	53, 97, 120, 197, 242	242	24, 40, 53. 97, 137, 148, 197, 235, 242, 245, 299, 314, 418
Guinea	13	13	13, 93, 170	1, 13, 93, 170, 195	13	13, 93, 170	13	13	13	13, 93, 170		13, 170, 195	13, 170, 195
Guinea-Bissau	13	13	13, 31, 131	1, 13, 293	13	13, 31, 131, 293	13	13	13	13, 31, 131	293	13	13, 31, 131

60

The Impact of Environmental Sanitation Upon Health and Economic Development in Singapore

Wai-On Phoon

Introduction

Singapore is a small island republic located just north of the equator in South-East Asia. It used to be the headquarters and bastion of British might in that part of the world in the colonial era. A population of 2.6 million lives in an area of 602 square kilometres, making Singapore one of the most densely-populated countries in the world. At the same time, the gross national product per capita has reached the standard of developed countries. Self-government was achieved in 1959 and independence in 1963 as part of Malaysia. In 1965, Singapore separated from Malaysia and became an independent country.

Infectious diseases have declined markedly in recent years. Tuberculosis, the leading cause of death less than a generation ago, is virtually extinct. Cardiovascular diseases and cancer are now the leading causes of death. The average life expectancy has increased to approximately 70 years for males and 73 years for females.

Organization of Environmental Health Services

Several years ago, the Ministry of Health was responsible for all health matters, including environmental health. Under the Director of Health Services were two Deputy Directors, one for public health and the other for hospital services. Nowadays, the Ministry of Environment is in charge of environmental matters, such as pollution and vector control, and the Ministry of Health looks after preventive and primary health care programmes.

Agencies Responsible for Education in Environmental Sanitation

There is only one university in Singapore, the National University. Very soon a second university, the Nanyang Technical University, will be established. Within the National University of Singapore (and its predecessors) public health has been taught at the postgraduate level since 1973 and occupational health in the same year. In the Faculty of Medicine, medical students undergo training in both subjects, mostly over the third and fourth years of their five-year course. Aspects of the environment are also taught in the Faculties of Engineering and Architecture.

Training for public health inspectors is conducted by the Ministry of Environment. Public health inspectors have a wide range of functions, such as the inspection of food establishments, and the enforcement of measures against the breeding of insect vectors.

There used to be a special course of training for Public Health Nursing, but this is subsumed in a post-basic nursing course which includes other subjects as well as Public Health Nursing.

In the schools, 'Human and Social Biology' can be taken as a subject for the School Certificate Examination. The syllabus was originally based on that for the Cambridge School Certificate, but since 1983, it has been more adapted to local needs, and the textbooks used tend to reflect the same trend.

The Population Issue

Although the population is not strictly environmental in nature, a rapid growth of population and overcrowding could have a significant impact upon the environment, both in terms of available natural resources, demands upon sanitary facilities, and a greater likelihood of pollution from the increased consumption of energy and production of garbage.

In the early post-World War II years, the population of Singapore grew by leaps and bounds. In the 1950s, the average growth rate was 4.8 per cent. Part of the growth was due to natural increase and part due to transmigration from Malaya, which was under British rule and was virtually part of the same country as Singapore. A vigorous family planning programme began in the 1980s through the National Family Planning and Population Board.

By 1975, the average growth rate declined to 1.6 per cent only. The success in population growth reduction was probably also contributed to by many other factors, among the most important being:

(a) Reduction in infant mortality rates (measured per 1,000 of infants) from around 60 or more in the 1940s, 30 in the 1960s, to presently 9-11. This meant that most parents could reasonably expect that all their children would reach adulthood.

(b) The increasing proportion of women in the reproductive age group taking up paid employment. At present more than 50 per cent of such women have joined the labour market.

(c) A mixture of incentives and disincentives instituted by the government. From the 1970s to the mid 1980s, abortions were permitted virtually on demand. Tubal ligation for mothers with three children or more was encouraged and also rewarded under certain conditions with a cash bonus. Conversely, disincentives were imposed upon families with more than three children (and later on even on those with more than two children). Such disincentives include the withholding of paid maternity leave, the subsidy of accouchement fees in government hospitals, and the withdrawal of preferential admission of children into schools where their older siblings were already studying.

The national population policies had to take a round-about turn, as Singapore currently has a tight labour situation. There are approximately 150,000 migrant workers from overseas. Nowadays, mothers, especially those with graduate qualifications, are encouraged to have four or more children, and generous tax rebates are given as incentives for their so doing.

Pollution by Inorganic Wastes

Pollution from industries has been minimized by the proper joining of different types of enterprises.

'Dirty industries' are located away from residential areas. Singapore is a major manufacturer and exporter of petroleum products. All the refineries and petrochemical plants (except one) are located in the small islands around Singapore (which are gazetted as industrial areas) rather than in Singapore itself.

Pollution from road traffic is less in Singapore than in many other cities because stringent curbs are imposed on the growth of the car population. There is a very heavy import tax on cars, and all cars are imported. Since 1990, there is a kind of government-run auction for the privilege of owing a car.

The banning of cigarette smoking in public places and a similar prohibition in many private buildings has also reduced the amount of tobacco pollution in indoor buildings.

Pollution by Organic Wastes

Pollution by human wastes has been considerably lessened by the implementation of the water carriage system throughout the country. About 10 years ago, the bucket system of night soil removal was still used in certain remote areas.

Until very recently, septic tanks were used in many housing estates, but they are rapidly being phased out in favour of centralized sewage treatment plants, which makes the control of sewage effluents easier.

Pollution by animal wastes has been largely eliminated by the phasing out of most of animal husbandry. Pig farming used to pose formidable problems in waste disposal, especially since the shortage of living space in Singapore rendered the heavy concentration of the animals necessary. Pig farming is now being phased out altogether.

Housing

The residential environment in Singapore has changed radically since a generation ago, when most of the population lived in low-rise buildings, such as shop-houses, detached bungalows and atap huts. High-rise apartments are now the normal housing milieu for most Singaporeans. Most of such apartments have been built by the Housing and Development Board (HDB), which began in 1960. By 1970, the HDB had built 120,000 housing units. By 1980, there were about 370,000 such units, housing 6-70 per cent of the population. Phoon *et al* (1976) studied 438 households who moved into such apartments. In the majority, there was an improvement in hygienic conditions from the previous accommodation. Thirty-five per cent of the sample reported that they were in better health after moving into the flats while six per cent said that their health worsened. The remainder reported no change.

Control of Vector-borne Diseases

Malaria of endogenous origin has not existed for several decades. Imported cases from endemic countries in the region do occur. Cases of dengue haemorrhagic fever (DHF), both as endemic cases and epidemic, have occurred since the late 1950s. The vector, *Aedes aegypti*, has been found breeding in water containers in construction sites and domestic establishments. Stricter laws to prevent this have been passed, including the levy of sizeable fines on offenders. The Vector Control Unit was established in 1968. An integrated system of *Aedes* control, using health education, law enforcement and source reduction was implemented. House-to-house inspections, publicity through mass media, and strict imposition of fines on offenders breeding mosquitoes proved successful. The DHF morbidity rate for 100,000 population fell from 32-42 during the period 1966-8 to 9.2 in 1969, 3.4 in 1970, 5.5 in 1971 and only 3.0 in 1972.

Control of Food-borne Diseases

The re-siting of itinerant hawkers in modern, hygienic hawker centres has reduced the hazard of food-borne diseases. All food handlers are subject to registration. All food premises are subject to inspection. In the 1960s the Minister of Health established the Food Establishments Licensing Board which set up a large number of guidelines and standards for this purpose. Moreover, sanitary disposal of faecal and solid waste, direct access to piped water supply, fly control and better housing conditions have markedly reduced the transmission of most diarrhoea diseases, including those caused by parasitic infections.

Control of Occupational Diseases

Workers exposed to specific occupational hazards are required by law to undergo statutory medical examinations. These can be undertaken only by medical practitioners who have undergone a course of approximately eighty five hours of teaching in occupational health and who have passed the requisite examination. This course provides instruction on the prevention, diagnosis and treatment of occupational diseases. It is generally thought that the services of such trained practitioners must have contributed significantly to the reduction of occupational-related disorders.

A Multi-Disciplinary Approach Towards Solving Environmental Problems

It has long been realized in Singapore that environmental issues can be exceedingly complex and a multi-disciplinary and inter-disciplinary approach is usually required. In 1971, the Singapore Professional Centre was established with the support of both the Singapore Government and Commonwealth Foundation. The centre has a membership of twenty six professional associations. One of its main purposes is to provide a forum for professionals to meet together and address issues of national importance, including those relating to the environment.

A National Approach towards Solving Environmental Problems

Special campaigns are organized by the government with the help of community and professional organizations to focus on national issues, many of which are environmental in importance. For example, the series of 'Keep Clean' campaigns have probably contributed much towards the 'clean and green' conditions in Singapore. Throughout the country, there are competitions, exhibitions, poster, radio and television broadcasts on chosen themes for the duration of each campaign.

Conclusion

It is extremely difficult to assess how much impact the improvements of environmental sanitation had on the health and economic development of Singapore. However, there is little doubt that the indicators of health and economic prosperity have improved steadily in recent years. Environmental problems, such as pollution and water-borne and vector-borne diseases, have been well-controlled. Nevertheless, continued vigilance is always needed, especially since Singapore is so geographically vulnerable to the importation of environmental problems from abroad.

References

Chan, K.L. (1985). 'Singapore's Dengue Haemorrhagic Fever Control Programme'. Tokyo: Southeast Asian Medical Information Center, pp. 73-75.

Goh, K.T. 'Diarrhoeal Diseases Surveillance in Singapore.' In *Epidemiological Surveillance of Communicable Diseases in Singapore*. Tokyo: Southeast Asian Medical Information Center, pp. 89-130.

Phoon, W. O. (1980). 'Department of Social Medicine and Public Health.' In '*75 Years of Medical Education in Singapore*', pp. 46-47.

Phoon, W. O., Chew, P. K. and Goh, E. H. (1986). *Comprehensive Human and Social Biology* (3rd ed). Singapore, Kuala Lumpur, Hong Kong.

Phoon, W. O. (1989). 'Epidemiological Transition in Asian Countries and Related Health Policy Issues'. *Asia-Pacific Journal of Public Health*, 3, 139-144.

Phoon, W. O., Quah, S. R., Tye, C. Y. and Leong, H. K. (1976). 'A Preliminary Study of the Health of a Population Staying in Apartments of Varying Size in Singapore'. *Annals of Tropical Medicine and Parasitology*, 70, 232-246.

Phoon, W. O. (1985). 'The Designated Factory Doctors' Course in Singapore'. In *Proceedings of XI Asian Conference on Occupational Health*, Manila, pp. 97-100.

Phoon, W. O. (1973). 'The Mobilization of Human and other Ecological Resources in Singapore.' In *Human Ecology in the Commonwealth*. H. Bowen-Jones (ed). London: Charles Knight, pp. 164-5.

Singapore Professional Centre (1990). *The Singapore Professionals*, 13, 10.

PART NINE

Medical Sociology, Nutrition, Health Education and Training in Public Health in Africa

61

The Role of Private and Voluntary Organizations and Communities in the Promotion of Health

G.O. Sofoluwe

Introduction

A productive and successful public and community health practice aims to achieve the best level of health for everyone in the community, by their own efforts and by judiciously utilizing the resources of the community.

Innovations in community health care services in developed countries now include community health councils, which decide the people's health needs and assess the type of care given them by the health professionals and the government. The councils also harness community resources for solving the prevalent health problems.

In Africa the communities, the missionaries, and commercial and voluntary organizations have contributed a sizeable proportion of the existing health (and indeed also educational) facilities; they have blazed the trail for the development of all welfare services, including, for example, homes for the motherless, centres for the poor and needy, and youth organizations, before the government eventually took over some of the services. In fact in 1965, a Nigerian National Health Manpower Survey revealed that the missionaries built and ran 50 per cent of all Nigerian health facilities, including hospitals, maternity centres, dispensaries, etc., and almost 100 per cent of the leprosy welfare services, clinics, and hospitals, especially in the then Northern and Eastern Nigeria; and that they excelled in improvization and in running cost-effective health establishments.

The World Health Organization, especially since 1973, have based their innovations in increasing basic and primary health services coverage throughout the world on the harnessing of communities' own resources and on self-help activities. It has thus been possible to catalogue a long list of successful projects sponsored by community efforts, private general practitioners, and voluntary organizations, where remarkable basic health services coverage has been achieved at low cost or at a cost which most of the people served could afford.

Classified lists of such voluntary organizations in Nigeria have been compiled through the Society of Health in Nigeria and the University of Ibadan by Sofoluwe and Professor J. Owen of

NISER. These and similar studies reveal that a good number of voluntary organizations exist, and undertake among others the following health activities.

1. Care for the handicapped, and deprived children and adults. Hitherto, in Africa, extended families took care of such groups in the villages; but with the hetero-ethnicity in the African towns, the phenomenal increase in the cost of living, and the breakdown of extended families in towns, and with the lack of funds supplied by governments, voluntary organizations, sponsored mostly by women's organizations, have been formed to provide such welfare services in some African towns. Such organizations include the Child Care Services of the Nigerian Women's Voluntary Organizations; the Nigerian Societies for the Blind and for the Deaf; the Leprosy Relief Association; Cheshire Homes; and similar bodies in Nigeria, Ghana and Kenya.
2. Voluntary organizations, such as the Citizen and Leadership Training Centre; Marriage Guidance Councils; the Red Cross Society; the Discharged Prisoners Aid Society; Rotary Clubs and similar bodies help to provide social services in African countries.
3. Youth organizations, such as the Boys' and Girls' Brigades; Boy Scouts; Girl Guides; African Lads and Lassies Brigades; Religious Youth organizations; Young Men's and Women's Christian Association (YMCA and YWCA); Nigeria Youth Councils; Students' Union, etc., cater for the needs of youth.
4. Women's organizations: These include the Women's Voluntary Organization; the Nigerian Business and Professional Women's Association; the National Council of Women's Organizations; the Nigerian Child Welfare Mother's Union; the Women's Corona Society, etc., help to run normal and special schools and promote comprehensive health services.
5. Professional organizations: for example, the Hotel and Catering Association; Chambers of Commerce; Medical, Engineers', Lawyers', and Accountants' organizations, etc., help to improve nutrition, food hygiene, provide employment opportunities, produce health promotive articles and promote health in many other ways.
6. Co-ordinating voluntary organizations: These include the Christian Churches' Councils; the Council of Parents/Teachers Associations; National Youth Councils; the National Advisory Councils for the Blind, Deaf, etc.; the Society of Health, Nigeria, and many others, help to promote health as their names imply.
7. Missionaries and church organizations: for example, Anglican, Methodist, Catholic, Baptist, Presbyterian, Salvation Army, Ahmadiya and other Muslim organizations, etc. Most of these build and run hospitals, health centres and maternity centres, and are now also developing primary health care services to assist African countries to provide basic health services, especially for rural dwellers.
8. Sports and recreational organizations: There is, in many African countries, an organization for almost every sport and recreative activity. There are now Sports Councils in each of the thirty states, and several Sport Committees on zonal or local government basis, in every state of Nigeria. Many African countries have similar sports organizations; and the Supreme Council for Sports in Africa co-ordinates sports activities and development in the continent.
9. Miscellaneous organizations, such as the Society for Prevention of Cruelty to Animals and

the League of Bribery and Corruption Scorners and others help promote zoonotic health services and improve human moral health.

10. There are also many community and ethnic or tribal voluntary organizations. Owen (1967) and his research assistants (medical students) were able to list well over three hundred such bodies in one state of Nigeria alone.

Although he says precise classification of such indigenous welfare organizations was not possible, yet he discusses the following main groups, based on their activities: family unions, lineage groups, townspeople's unions, credit societies, OSUSO (Urhobo), and self-help groups, trade associations of rubber growers, farmers, herbalists, motor vehicle owners, youth organizations based on age cohorts, social clubs, for example, football associations, special traditional, ritualistic, and cultural organizations such as circumcision societies and healing groups (Ukoko).

All the above-named groups of voluntary organizations have sponsored the following health promotion activities:

1. Curative services: by building hospitals, health centres, maternity centres, or dispensaries, or just financing a wing of a hospital, or providing some essential equipment or the payment of certain salaries, or by donating staff to man such facilities;
2. Curative, preventive, and welfare services for the blind, deaf, and paralysed, and for mental, tuberculous, leprous, and other diverse physical and mental diseases;
3. Orphanages, motherless babies homes and homes for deprived children including those in need of care;
4. Welfare activities for well children; for example, day nurseries and working mothers' children play centres.
5. Marriage guidance and family health activities.
6. Preventing boredom and crime among children through directed activities among the youth, as provided by Boy Scouts, Guides, etc.
7. Assisting women to fulfil their role successfully as wives, hostesses and mothers; and also in harnessing women's great empathic potentials.
8. The professional organizations help to promote health by gearing their professional knowledge to solving communities' urgent health problems. As, for example, engineers arrange conferences and congresses to tackle the problems of urgent water supply, sewage disposal and other environmental problems in urban and rural areas; while hoteliers organize schemes for improving nutrition, food hygiene, etc.
9. Some special organizations seek mainly to improve nutrition: for example, OXFAM (Oxford based voluntary organization for actively improving nutrition in the developing countries) and a Farmer's Rural Training Centre sponsored by the Nigerian Christian Council.
10. General welfare services for adults, seamen and prisoners.
11. Disaster relief in Africa has hitherto been almost entirely provided in the villages by the family and ethnic groups, and in the towns by voluntary organizations. The governments in Africa are only just beginning to form Disaster Relief Agencies. The Red Cross Societies have constituted and still constitute the backbone for providing such relief, even though the various governments now subsidize them by some sizeable annual grants.

12. Rehabilitation in almost all its forms has hitherto in Africa been provided by voluntary organizations in the towns and the extended family system in the villages. Internationally and nationally government sponsored medical and vocational rehabilitation projects are now being developed, however.
13. Some voluntary organizations, such as the Council of Parents and Teachers Associations, the Society of Health in Nigeria, and many others concentrate their activities on assisting the governmental agencies to promulgate health policies based on scientifically accurate data.
14. Sports and recreative activities have not only offered youths good vents for their energies but have generated lots of employment. (Many prominent Nigerians and Africans have now attained fame through sports, e.g. Keino of Kenya, Fibayi of Tanzania, and numerous other examples in all African countries.)
15. Drama groups have helped moral development and eased physical and mental stresses.
16. The numerous indigenous, ethnic, community and self-help groups have been responsible for building schools, health facilities, water supplies, rural electrification, road construction, and for meeting many other basic socio-economic and health needs of their villages and areas. The Iludun Oro Community in Kwara State in Nigeria have exemplified this by the electrification of their town, the erection of a community hospital, staffed and managed successfully by community resources; the erection of day nurseries primary and secondary school buildings, the building of roads and the provision of scholarships. They will soon build a dam for providing water to a community of about 30,000 people. *Contact* – (a magazine) has also recorded a case in Northern Nigeria where a community sponsored and provided a comprehensive health service in the local government area by their own (not government) efforts.

The doctor is therefore advised to make an exhaustive and comprehensive local health study to provide a comprehensive list of such organizations in his area of practice. Such study has the additional benefit of introducing the doctor to those in the community who have demonstrated by their activities, deep interest and involvement in health promotion. Everybody should be involved in providing a comprehensive community health service in Africa.

References

Directory of Voluntary Organizations in Lagos, Published by the London Organization for Advancement of Africans, London on Behalf of the Society of Health, Nigeria, and Printed by the Daily Times of Nigeria 1966.

Directory of Voluntary Organizations in Western Nigeria, Compiled by Professor J. Owen and Published Jointly by NISER (Nigerian Institute of Social and Economic Research) and the Department of Preventive and Social Medicine (both of the University of Ibadan, Nigeria) by the Baptist Press (Nigeria) Limited, Ibadan, in 1967.

Directory of Voluntary Organizations in Midwestern Nigeria, Compiled by Professor J. Owen and Published Jointly for NISER (Nigerian Institute for Social and Economic Research) and the Department of Preventive and Social Medicine (both of the University of Ibadan, Nigeria) by the Baptist Press (Nigeria) Limited, Ibadan in 1967.

62

International Health Agencies and the Promotion of Health

J.W. Kwaimina Duncan

The International Health Organization

The history of international co-operation for health protection dates back to the ancient times. The great epidemics of the middle ages were thought to have been introduced into Europe from the East. Local and national quarantine was established in an effort to prevent the spread of plagues or cholera. The city of Venice established what seems to be the first formal quarantine organization in 1328, and was followed by many other city states. Co-ordination was lacking until 1831 when the Egyptian Quarantine Board was formed to advise the local government on matters of plague. Also the repeated appearance of cholera in moslem pilgrims to Mecca was recognized as a serious threat to Europe. A Superior Health Council was created in Turkey in 1938 consisting of four Turkish representatives and one representative of each of the major European powers.

However, the first and formal International Health Co-operation came from the conference held in Paris in 1851 in which twelve nations participated and the first treaty dealing with sanitary conventions was drawn up and signed by the representatives attending. This first conference was followed by a series of similar conferences all having the primary purposes of drafting international quarantine regulations.

During the intervening years, there was growing recognition of a need for a more formal and more permanent international health organization. At the conference in Rome in 1907, the representatives approved the establishment of a permanent International Health Organization with offices in Paris and a permanent committee of senior public health officers of member governments. This organization was to receive and transmit to member nations notification of such diseases as cholera, plague, smallpox, typhus and yellow fever. A further purpose was the study of the development of sanitary conventions and quarantine regulations on shipping and train travels. In 1909 I' Office International d'Hygiene Publique was established in Paris to carry out the above functions, and it remained in existence until it was absorbed by the World Health Organization in 1948.

Running parallel to activities of international health co-operation in Europe were activities also initiated in the Americas. The first of such regional sanitary conventions was held in Rio de Janeiro in 1887. In 1889-90, the first International Conference of American States was held in Washington DC which approved the provision of the Rio de Janeiro convention for general application to the American states. The second conference of American States held in Mexico City in 1901-1902 approved the establishment of an International Health Organization called the International Sanitary Bureau with offices in Washington DC and with functions similar to those of l' Office International d'Hygiene Publique. In 1924 it became the Pan American Sanitary Bureau and was designated the regional office of the Health Section of the League of Nations. In 1949, it became the Pan American Health Organization and the regional office of WHO for the Americas.

Health Organization of the League of Nations

One of the tasks of the League of Nations, formed after the First World War, was to take steps in the matter of international concern for the prevention and control of diseases. At the League Assembly in 1923, the plan for the Health Organization of the League of Nations was approved, and this Health Section co-existed with l'Office International d'Hygiene Publique in Europe during the period between the two world wars. On the other side of the Atlantic, the third international organization, the Pan American Sanitary Bureau continued to function. Consultative and co-operative arrangements existed among all three organizations.

World War II caused extensive destruction of property, loss of human lives and displacement of people. International health work was almost completely destroyed. Recognizing the need for early action on health, the United States of America suggested in 1943 the development of an international relief organization. Forty-four nations met and set up the United Nations Relief and Rehabilitation Administration with the main functions of supplying relief to the suffering in devastated countries; rehabilitation of medical and health services; and provision of medical supplies and facilities for epidemic control. The UNRWA was responsible for the conference held in New York in July 1946 which approved the constitution of the World Health Organization.

The World Health Organization

When the Charter of the United Nations was drawn at the San Francisco Conference in 1945, it was recognized that there should be an international health organization. The following year, an international conference held in New York set up an Interim Commission and approved the constitution of the World Health Organization (WHO). This came into force on 7 April, 1948 when the twenty-six governments (out of the sixty-one who signed it) formally ratified it in their national parliaments. The scope of WHO's work in health was vastly greater than that of any previous health organization but it is pertinent to note that the establishment of WHO is the culmination of efforts at international health co-operation that had started almost a century before in Europe and America.

The World Health Organization is one of the specialized agencies of the United Nations family. Its aim as defined in the constitution is 'the attainment by all people of the highest possible level of health'. A new dimension was added in 1981 when the World Health Assembly (the policy organ composed of delegates representing 166 member states) unanimously adopted a global strategy for Health for All by the year 2000 which embodied the eight essential elements of primary health care set forth earlier by the International Conference on Primary Health Care at Alma-Ata in 1978.

The eight elements of primary health care are:

(i) education concerning prevailing health problems and the methods of identifying, preventing and controlling them;
(ii) promotion of food supply and proper nutrition;
(iii) an adequate supply of safe water, and basic sanitation;
(iv) maternal and child health care, including family planning;
(v) immunization against the major infectious diseases;
(vi) prevention and control of locally endemic diseases;
(vii) appropriate treatment of common diseases and injuries; and
(viii) provision of essential drugs.

The World Health Organization consists of three constituent bodies: the World Health Assembly, the Executive Board and the Secretariat. Sessions of the Assembly are attended by delegations from all 166 member states. Its main tasks are to approve the biennial programme and budget, and to decide upon major questions of policy. The Executive Board consists of 31 persons technically qualified in the field of health, each appointed by designated member states elected by the Assembly. The Executive Board functions as the executive organ of the Assembly. The Secretariat is the staff of WHO with the Director-General as its technical and administrative head.

A characteristic feature of WHO is its decentralization. It has six 'regional organizations' each consisting of a Regional Committee and a Regional Office. The head of each regional office is a Regional Director. The regional offices are located in Alexandria, Egypt (Eastern Mediterranean Region); Brazzaville, Congo (African Region); Copenhagen, Denmark (European Region); Manila, Philippines (Western Pacific Region); New Delhi, India (South-East Asia Region); and Washington D.C., United States (Regions of the Americas).

The WHO Regional Office for Africa

The regional office for Africa has a staff of some 760 people made up of 280 professional staff and 480 general services staff, most of which are assigned to countries of the region. In addition there is a regional Onchocerciasis Programme with headquarters in Ouagadogou, Burkina Faso with compliment staff of 60 professionals and 490 general service staff. The regional office operates under the authority of the Regional Director elected by the Regional Committee and appointed by the Executive Board. The staff of the regional office are appointed by agreement between the Director-General of WHO and the Regional Director. Their make-up includes six programme directors/managers responsible for general programme development, management, co-ordination and support services; and regional officers who carry out the technical health activities in the region with the support of field teams headed by WHO representatives located in the various countries of nearly forty-five authentically African member states. There are also three Sub-regional Health Development offices based in Bamako, Mali for Sub-region I countries, Bujumbura, Burundi for Sub-region II countries and Harare, Zimbabwe for Sub-region III countries. The implementation of health programmes in the African region is continuing despite the prejudicial effects of the world economic recession, and the world pandemic of an unprecedented challenge to mankind, the acquired immune deficiency syndrome (A.I.D.S). The new orientation in accelerating the achievement of health for all Africans (defined in 1985) was to concentrate on community-based health and related activities – which are the foundation for economic and social development. They would have to be sustained by appropriate operational, technical and strategic support at the local (district), intermediate (province/region), and central levels respectively. This is the three phase health development scenario which makes the district the corner stone of the organizational framework for implementing the primary health care approach. Community participation, intersectoral collaboration, and affordable technologies constitute the key strategies.

Health services alone do not ensure the well-being of individuals, family and community. Health activities must therefore be well co-ordinated with the social, educational, economic and cultural policies of countries. To this end, WHO AFRO collaborates very closely with others inside the UN system and outside of it; in particular with the United Nations Development Programme (UNDP), the United Nations Children's Emergency Fund (UNICEF), The United Nations Environment Programme (UNEP), the Food and Agriculture Organization (FAO), the International Labour Organization (ILO), the United Nations Educational, Scientific and Cultural Organization (UNESCO), Organization of African Unity (OAU), the Economic Commission for Africa (ECA), the African Development Bank (ADB), the League of Arab States (LAS), non-governmental organizations (NGOs) and others.

The United Nations Development Programme

The United Nations Development Programme (UNDP) is the largest organization for economic development and co-operation within the United Nations System. It came into being on 1 January 1966 as a result of the merger of the United Nations Technical Assistance Board and the United Nations Special Fund. The key to the accomplishment of the UNDP's task is the mobilization of voluntary financial support from governments world-wide, and the conversion of that funding into effective development services. As the world's largest channel for international technical co-operation, UNDP serves as a vital catalyst for collaboration between the industrialized and the developing nations and among the developing countries themselves. At the national and regional levels, UNDP supports activities in education and training, inventory of latent natural resources, enlargement of technological capabilities and planning the most effective use of all potentials for progress.

UNDP assistance is incorporated into national or regional development efforts, and provided to all developing countries according to a formula which is periodically revised and which takes into account many factors including the overall economic status of a country and the population. These Indicative Planning Figures (IPFs) allow the government and the UNDP representative to estimate the share of UNDP resources the country might expect to receive. UNDP funds are expended entirely in the form of project grants executed in certain instances by UNDP itself, but more commonly by the specialized agencies of the UN system.

A UNDP-supported national project for health is in most cases a tri-partite venture, with the recipient government, UNDP and one or more of the UN specialized agencies as partners. Collaborations with WHO in particular has progressed in the area of basic sanitary measures. Approximately 50 projects relating to the International Drinking Water Supply and Sanitation Decade received support from UNDP in the African region amounting to some US$53 million. WHO continues to be the executing agency for UNDP supported projects in health, environmental pollution, environmental planning and management, and occupational health resources from UNDP have thus substantially augmented the resources available from the regular budget of WHO.

The United Nations Children's Fund

The United Nations International Children's Emergency Fund (UNICEF) was created in December 1946 by the General Assembly of the United Nations, with its headquarters in New York, to provide assistance to the children of those countries most seriously affected by World War II. In 1950, when the emergency needs of these countries declined, the organization extended its field of operation to other countries, and to programmes of long-range benefit to children in the developing countries. To reflect the new orientation, the organization's name was shortened to 'United Nations Children's Fund' in 1953. Through mutual agreement, the World Health Organization gives technical advice to the medical and environmental health programmes being supported by UNICEF in the countries.

UNICEF co-operates with governments to carry out vital programmes in such fields as health, nutrition, education, provision of safe and sufficient water supply, personal hygiene and sanitation and social welfare for the benefit of mothers and children. Its assistance includes supplies of medical equipment and drugs, training grants for the in-service training of medical personnel, supplies of vehicles and tools for rural projects, and where necessary, the provision of fellowships and experts. UNICEF also maintains regional and field offices in many African countries, headed by Regional and Country Representatives to whom much of the responsibility for the programme activities of UNICEF has been delegated.

The United Nations Environment Programme

Since its creation in 1972, the United Nations Environment Programme (UNEP) has been active in the promotion of environmental protection and improvement within the framework of the Stockholm Plan of Action for Human Environment. In 1973 the Governing Council of UNEP met for the first time Geneva, and adopted areas of concentration of interest. From the activities of UNEP have emerged major United Nations conferences:

- the United Nations Conference on Human Settlement (HABITAT) held in Vancouver, British Columbia, Canada in June 1976 which adopted a Declaration of Principles and a series of recommendations to meet the urgent needs of housing shortages, the constraint crisis of urban and rural communities, the problems of proper use of land and access to essential services, and the creation of public involvement in remedial actions;
- the United Nations Water Conference in Mar de Plata, Argentina in March 1977 which established the goals for the Water Decade and formulated Action Plan for community water supply;
- the United Nations Conference on Desertification held in August 1977 in Nairobi, Kenya which was the outcome of a resolution passed in the General Assembly of the United Nations in 1974 calling for international co-operation in the attempt to stop 'desertification' which is the process of the spreading of arid lands as a result of the interaction of the ill-considered activities of man and an adverse environment.

UNEP is a co-ordinating, catalytic agency of the United Nations System through which all its programmes are executed in co-operation with other Untied Nations organizations such as UNDP, UNICEF, FAO and WHO. Priority projects with WHO involvement have been in human settlements, endemic diseases, the environmental health effects of pollution, risk assessment, monitoring and pollution control. Arrangement regarding an international registry of potentially toxic chemicals is being updated, and projects relating to the pollution of the Mediterranean coast,

Zambezi River basin, human settlement and other subjects of health interest have been formulated for implementation by participating member states.

The Food and Agriculture Organization

The Food and Agriculture Organization (FAO) of the United Nations was founded in Quebec on 16 October, 1945 and has its headquarters in Rome, Italy. The preamble of FAO's constitution states that the organization is aimed at raising the levels of nutrition and standards of living, improving the production, processing, marketing and distribution of all food and agricultural products from farms, forests and fisheries; promoting rural development and improving the living conditions of rural populations thus eliminating hunger. In carrying out these aims, FAO promotes investment in agriculture, better soil and water management, improved yields of crops and livestock, and the transfer of technology to and the development of agricultural research in developing countries. It promotes the conservation of natural resources (particularly plant genetic resources, and the rational use of fertilizers and pesticides) fisheries and of new and renewable sources of energy.

FAO's role and its activities have held in the creation of specialized international bodies, such as the Codex Alimentarius Commission, the Consultative Group on International Agricultural Research, the World Food Council, The International Fund for Agricultural Development, and many others. Its own major activities are decided upon from the headquarters office and are dedicated to providing technical assistance to developing countries. It acts as the lead agency for rural development in the United Nations System, and it gives individuals and organizations the opportunity to participate in rural development through the Freedom from Hunger/Action for Development programme. Co-ordination with WHO in water resources development has been strengthened with particular emphasis being laid on water-supply and sanitation for rural population, and on the prevention of the health risks associated with certain agricultural developments, particularly irrigation.

The International Labour Organization

The International Labour Organization (ILO) was established in 1919, under the Treaty of Versailles, as an autonomous institution associated with the League of Nations. An agreement establishing the relationship between the ILO and the United Nations was approved on 14 December, 1946, and it became the first specialized agency associated with the United Nations. The ILO works to promote social justice for working people everywhere. This promotion is unique because workers' and employers' representatives have an equal voice with those of governments in formulating its policies. One of ILO's most important functions is the adoption of conventions and recommendations which set international labour standards in such areas as freedom of association, wages, hours and conditions of work, workmen's compensation, social insurance, vacation with pay, industrial safety, employment services and labour inspection.

Through the organization's programme of technical co-operation, ILO's experts assist member countries in such fields as vocational training, management techniques, manpower planning, employment policies, occupational safety and health, social security systems, and co-operatives and small-scale handicraft industries. One of the main tasks of the ILO experts, which is also common to the staff of other UN specialized agencies, is to train counterpart personnel to take over and expand the activity of each individual project when the international team leaves. ILO collaborates with the WHO in relation to migrant workers and to the establishment of maximum permissible limits for physical and chemical agents in the working environment – ILO focusing on application and WHO on evaluation and assessment.

United Nations Educational, Scientific and Cultural Organization

The constitution of the United Nations Educational, Scientific and Cultural Organization (UNESCO) was prepared by a conference convened in London, England in 1945. UNESCO came into being on 4 November, 1946 and has its headquarters in Paris, France. Its primary aim is to contribute to peace and security in the world by promoting collaboration among nations through education, science, culture and communication. To realize these aims, UNESCO expands and guides education so as to enable people of every country to take their own development in their hands more effectively. It also helps in establishing the scientific and technological foundations through which every country can make better use of its resources; it encourages national cultural values and the preservation of cultural heritage. It also develops communication for a free flow and a wider and better balanced dissemination of information.

In education UNESCO combines literary programmes with a drive to make primary education universal and eliminate illiteracy root causes. In the natural sciences, its programmes include Man and the Biosphere; the programme of the Intergovernmental Oceanographic Commission; and the International Hydrological and International Geological correlation programme. In the social science, UNESCO has produced studies on such subjects as tensions leading to war and racism, the socio-economic factors of development, and the relationship between man and his environment. Its cultural activities are concentrated chiefly on the stimulation of artistic creativity, the study and development of cultures, and the conservation of the world's inheritance of books, works of art and monuments as well as the preservation of cultural identities and oral traditions.

References

Accelerating the Achievement of Health for All Africans – 'The Three-Phase Health Development Scenario' by Dr. G.L. Moneksso Regional Director WHO, Regional Office for Africa, Brazzaville – January 1989.

Basic Facts about the United Nations (UN) Department of Public Information, New York DPI/869. 1985.

'International Drinking Water Supply and Sanitation Decade'. 2nd Edition 1984. Publication of *World Water Magazine*.

Maxcy-Rosenau (1963) *Preventive Medicine and Public Health* (9th Edn. P.E. Startwell pp. 1036–45).

World Health Organization (1976) *Introducing WHO*, WHO, Geneva.

63

Community Problems in Nutrition and Diet

F.J. Bennett

In Africa, the community doctor with responsibility for one or several villages may encounter the following nutritional problems:

1. Protein-calorie (energy) malnutrition (PCM)
   - (a) growth retardation or stunting
   - (b) mild to moderate malnutrition
   - (c) severe PCM–kwashiorkor or marasmus
   - (d) low-birth weight babies
2. Avitaminoses – lack of vitamin A
   - rickets
   - pellagra
   - megaloblastic anaemia
3. Iron deficiency anaemia
4. Goitre
5. Excessive intake of fluorine leading to fluorosis
6. Obesity

There are also additional conditions which can be attributed to dietary patterns or are associated with nutritional problems, viz: dental caries, alcoholism and ataxic tropical neuropathy. The virtues of traditional African diets need to be emphasized; and so one may add a final category of problems that stem from a change towards a so-called westernized pattern of diet. These include not only some of those already mentioned above, such as obesity and dental caries, but also where the exact aetiology or mechanism is debated. Hypertension, appendicitis, coronary artery disease, and a host of other conditions at present uncommon in Africa, but common in wealthy countries, are included here. Various theories have linked their aetiology with dietary patterns such as lack of dietary fibre, diets with different ratio of calorie intake from carbohydrates, fats and protein diets with high intake of animal fats, with high intake of animal protein, with excess salt intake, etc.

Village Surveys

The technique of rapid village nutrition surveys has been adequately described in several manuals and papers by Blankhort (1971), Jelliffe (1966), Bailey (1976), and the World Health Organization (1976). One of the most useful summaries is the one on Rapid Village Nutrition Survey Technique from the Brazzaville Office of the World Health Organization (WHO AFRO, 1977). The technique of epidemiological prevalence surveys has been described by Barker (1976). In this chapter only some additional points and those requiring special emphasis will be mentioned. The surveys described in the above mentioned papers put special emphasis on anthropometry and clinical examination; but the community doctor must not forget to obtain related information. This should include agricultural details: crops for food, cash crops, seasonal variations, frequency of failure of crops, and the reasons for the failure. The people's knowledge, attitudes, and practices in relation to food production, storage and use, and also to weaning, must be investigated using a suitably composed questionnaire. Data should also be obtained about infectious conditions (for example diarrhoea, worms, measles, whooping cough) and environmental conditions that are relevant to nutrition. The use of maternal and child health services should also be investigated; especially the degree to which nutritional surveillance and nutrition education are available.

A market survey to find out the cost of foods, and a calculation of the cheapest sources of calories and protein is also useful; and this would require the use of food tables, such as those of Platt (1962) or the FAO. Birth weights can be obtained from local health centres or maternity units, and are a useful indicator, in spite of being biased in that they probably do not represent a very large proportion of all births in the community.

Protein Energy Malnutrition

The most usual community diagnostic method is to take a random sample of children under five years, and to measure weight, length (height), and arm circumference, and relate these to age; and also to weight and height. In addition, clinical examination is undertaken to identify oedema, hair changes, and signs of avitaminosis and anaemia. Children found with severe malnutrition need complete examination, and usually need urgent medical care. It may be discovered that some cases have additional or underlying problems, for example, tuberculosis, urinary tract infection, sickle cell anaemia, or heavy infestations of parasites. At the same time, during the survey, a variety of factors can be investigated – family size, economic status of the family, weaning foods, age of weaning, and use of breast or bottle feeds, occupation of parents, etc. When all the data from the survey are analysed, it should be apparent how prevalent the severe syndromes of kwashiorkor and marasmus are, and what age groups they affect. It should also be clear what proportion of the children are underweight for their age, or merely stunted in height, or stunted and underweight for their age. The first condition indicating especially current acute malnutrition and the second chronic long-term malnutrition and the last being due to a combination of previous chronic and present continuing malnutrition. The well nourished and poorly nourished children can be compared statistically to see what the associated factors are. Such an analysis may suggest that, for example in a particular community malnutrition is chiefly associated with late introduction of vegetable protein or calories from the staple diet, or that it is related to family size or to the marital status of the mother.

Avitaminoses

Lack of vitamin A or carotenoids in the diet is common in many developing countries. This is often due to lack of meat, milk, or fish, or to lack of green and yellow vegetables and fruit. The different stages of deficiency are characterized by night blindness, dryness of the conjunctiva or xerosis, Bitot's spots, and finally keratomalacia, followed by blindness. Again the target group to be examined would be young children. Serum levels of vitamin A may also be determined if such laboratory facilities are available. The WHO Technical Report on Vitamin A Deficiency and Xerophthalmia (1976b) gives a good account of this nutrition problem, which carries with it the serious consequence of blindness.

Pellagra

This occurs mostly in areas where maize is a staple diet, and in groups in the community who have a restricted diet without green vegetables or other items to eat with their staple. This situation can occur in poor boarding schools, in prisons, in labourers' camps, and in migrant labourers living without their wives to cook for them. Pellagra also occurs in alcoholics. It is sometimes confused by auxiliaries with other skin conditions, such as tinea or even leprosy.

Anaemia Due to Folate Deficiency

This occurs in some areas with a restricted diet and is especially seen in pregnant women. It can also complicate sickle cell anaemia. Any condition with recurrent haemolysis (e.g. malaria in pregnancy) can lead to secondary deficiency of folate, and thus to a megaloblastic anaemia.

Rickets

In Africa, with its generous amount of sunlight, it might be expected that rickets would be rare. However it does occur occasionally in children, sometimes in Moslem societies where the mothers do not go out much and where the infant is only allowed out if it is heavily covered, to avoid being seen by someone with the 'evil eye'. This condition is dealt with in greater detail in the textbook edited by Beaton and Bengoa (WHO 1976a).

Iron Deficiency Anaemia

This may well be the most common nutritional disorder in many communities. It occurs in infants weaned late on to a diet low in iron or without animal protein. It occurs also in older children associated with a loss of blood resulting from an infestation of hookworms or schistosomiasis. It occurs in schoolgirls starting their menses, and also in pregnant women. Old people too get iron deficiency anaemia from a restricted diet; and perhaps also sometimes from their exposure to hookworm in traditional environments without latrines. A survey to find out how great a problem anaemia is in a community must have very good community acceptance and participation, because it involves taking blood. It is not sufficient merely to look for clinical anaemia, as this misses very many cases. It is necessary to perform haemoglobin estimations by a reliable method. The Spencer haemoglobinometer is an accurate instrument, easy to use in the field; and it requires only a drop of capillary blood. From the same stab a further specimen can be obtained in a heparinized capillary tube for testing packed cell volume; and, if the investigator is experienced, he can also obtain thick and thin blood films for malaria parasites and cell morphology. In an anaemia survey, it is necessary to investigate all the common causes, viz,: malaria, iron deficiency, megaloblastic and sickle cell anaemia. All of these require blood specimens. Malaria can of course also be measured in a community by the spleen rate. To identify that a hypochromic microcytic anaemia is due to hookworm requires stool specimens; and this too requires as much discussion with the community as does taking blood.

Iodine Deficiency Disorders
It is now recognized that goitre is the visible part of the much larger problem of iodine deficiency disorders. Less severe deficiencies and deficiency in utero produce growth and development retardation. Cretinism is the extreme form but there is a whole spectrum of retarded development which includes children who are dull and slow in intellectual development. The need for salt iodization or for the interim interventions of iodine injections or capsules should thus be considered by all countries when special blood, urine or goitre surveys have shown an iodine deficiency.

Fluorosis
Some areas of Africa have water containing a high fluorine content. This may occur in volcanic areas or in areas relying on water from deep-bored wells. This condition is not often apparent in deciduous dentition, but is seen especially in secondary dentition, where it produces brown mottling. In areas with high levels, there may be imperfect enamel formation, leading to excessive caries and early loss of teeth. The spine and other bones may also be affected if the level is exceptionally high.

Obesity
In many parts of Africa, obesity is an increasing problem in urban areas. It is due to a combination of comparative affluence, excess intake in the form of sugar in tea, gruel, fats and alcohol. Many senior officials suffer from an unsightly deposition of fat within ten years of obtaining high managerial posts, with their accompanying high-calorie social dinners, large cars and long sedentary hours. Because a certain amount of obesity has some status value, it is often not realized that an adult should try to keep a steady weight. The conditions associated with obesity – diabetes, hypertension, etc – are the same in Africa as elsewhere, and are probably due both to a changed life style and to diet. Once again the value of traditional diet, with its high fibre content and low calories to bulk ratio must be emphasized, as it usually limits the development of obesity. Obesity in a community can be measured by cross-sectional survey for weight against height, and by weight for age measurements; and also by skinfold thickness measurements, using a skin fold caliper.

Dental Caries
This condition is mentioned in this chapter as it is associated with changes in diet – some of them introduced by advertising, and some even by health staff. Advertisements suggesting the consumption of sweetened fruit juices as a means of obtaining vitamin C are totally unnecessary in Africa, where scurvy is rarely seen – such things given to children encourage them to demand more sweet things, such as carbonated drinks and sweets, which numerous studies have linked with dental caries.

Alcoholism
Alcoholic drinks were a normal part of the diet in many traditional societies in Africa. They were, however, usually controlled – who could brew, under what circumstances, and who could drink the fermented brew were usually questions with culturally prescribed answers. Alcoholism was rare and often confined to older men. Changes in society, the fact that alcohol became for some a source

of cash, and the introduction of distilling technology have changed the picture. Now alcohol is sold to anyone who has the money for it, and cheap concentrated liquor puts alcoholic excess within the reach of many, including women and young people.

The purchase of bottled beer has also become an undesirable status symbol in some parts of Africa. Many calories are diverted from children's and family nutrition into the production of alcohol-sugarcane, maize, sorghum, honey, bananas, sweet potatoes, etc., are all used; and an increase in the production of alcohol in a community is an ominous sign.

Ataxic Tropical Neuropathy

The last condition included in this chapter is an example of the sort of problems that may possibly arise from excessive use of one staple. The current thinking on this syndrome of sensory ataxia and optic atrophy is that it is due to the cyanogenetic glycosides in cassava (Makene and Lodha 1976; Monekosso and Wilson 1966; Osuntokun 1969). In some 'cassava cultures' there are many activities involving pounding into flour. Not only the roots are used but also the leaves. The stalks are also handled, as they form the cutting for planting. All of this handling and processing, as well as the actual consumption of cassava, may lead to the absorption of cyanates. It is especially when diet is based almost exclusively on cassava that this syndrome is seen, in both West and East Africa. However, this does not mean that cassava is not a valuable crop; it is one of the top producers of calories per hectare, and it is a valuable famine reserve. The leaves, compared with many other leaves, have a very high protein content. Condemnation of cassava for an epidemiological association would be much the same as condemning groundnuts as a food because of an association between aflatoxin levels and hepatoma. The methods of usage have rather to be modified.

Measurement of the Last Three Problems

Each of these is a specialized field, and the community doctor is advised to seek aid from a dentist, a psychiatrist or neurologist, or a physician if he really wishes to measure the prevalence of these conditions in a community. It is easier but less complete to record these conditions in outpatient clinics; in this case their relative frequency (but not actual frequency) may indicate whether they are possibly increasing problems.

Nutrition Programmes

Most of this chapter has been devoted to the diagnosis of nutritional conditions in the community. The doctor who actually goes out and does a survey in his community is of course finding out more than just frequency – he is also determining the burden of morbidity on the community, and thus the level of priority. With this type of knowledge he is better able to prevent and control nutrition programmes, and the need for an integrated approach through agriculture, health, education, etc., has been stressed. This same co-ordination is needed at the family level. National level approaches has been tried for many things: the making of a national low-cost high protein weaning food – for example, calories from a cereal staple, protein from the residue of groundnuts (after selling the oil), and a smaller amount of animal protein (dried skimmed milk after selling the cream). However, Jelliffe (1966) has emphasized the need for these same resolutions to the problem at the family or household level, where a similar type of 'triple mix' can be made more cheaply in the family cooking pot from home produce. Similarly, village health committees and primary health workers can probably do more with their understanding of local ecology than any number of expert committees sitting in ministerial conference rooms.

One local programme which could be initiated by a community doctor with hope of success is a nutritional surveillance and rehabilitation programme (advice suitable for all levels of health workers is well set out in King's book of Primary Child Care, King and Montodipoero, 1979). Increased use of small-animal protein sources for example, rabbits, fowls' eggs and goat's milk; improved food preservation; increased usage of legumes and green leaves (Domen and Grubben, 1977) for children; 'appropriate technology' storage for cereals and legumes; and marketing and buying food co-operatives are also all nutrition activities that can be initiated through Primary Health Care programmes. Improved maternal and child health programmes (especially those extended into the community by primary health care workers), including family planning programmes, all have great nutritional relevance also. The relationship between infection and malnutrition is well established; and diarrhoeal diseases, skin infections, worms, malaria, and measles are especially prominent in this group, among whom their prevention would lead to improved nutritional and health status.

The best thing the doctor can do is to make the community aware of its nutritional problems and their multiple causes; and then to work together with them to develop the most appropriate local programme.

Nutrition Programme

Nutrition programmes are usually multisectoral with health sector activities as well as activities based in agriculture, local government, community development, information, education and women affairs. Co-ordination is very necessary but few countries have a really well functioning co-ordinating body such as a National Nutrition Council or Food and Nutrition Institution. At the local level the community itself is the important implementing agency so the more communities are involved in their own assessment and planning for improved nutrition the more dramatic will be the improvements in nutrition status. Communities can be helped to organize their own growth monitoring programme with community health workers and mothers trained in weighing, plotting the weight on growth charts and analysing the results collectively. Community nutritional surveillance with community action can thus complement individual growth monitoring with relevant maternal and family action.

References

Bailey K.V. (1976). *Manual on Public Health Nutrition Docant* AFR/NUT79. WHO, Brazzaville.

Baker, D.J.P. (1976). *Practical Epidemiology Medicine in the Tropics Series*. Churchill Livingstone, London.

Blankhort, D.M. (1971). Outlines for a Survey of the Feeding and Nutritional Status of Children under Three Years of Age and Their Mothers *J. Trop. Paed 17*, 175, 196.

Domen, H.A. and Grubben, G. (1977). *Tropical Leaf Vegetables in Human Nutrition*. Communication 62. Department of Agricultural Research. Royal Tropical Institute, Amsterdam.

Jelliffe, D.B. (1966). *The Assessment of Nutritional Status of the Community*. WHO Monograph Series No. 53. WHO, Geneva.

King, M., King, F., Morley, D., Burgess, L., and Burgess, A. (1972). *Nutrition for Developing Countries*. Oxford University Press, Nairobi.

– King, F., and Montodipoero Soebagio (1979). *Primary Child Care–A Manual for Health Workers*. Oxford University Press, Nairobi.

Makene, W.J. and Lodha, S.M. (1976). Ataxic Tropical Neuropathy in Tanzania. In *Degenerative Disorders in the African environment* (ed. F.J. Bennett, A.M. Nhonoli, and H. Nsanzemichive). East African Literature Bereau, Nairobi.

Monekosso, G.L. and Wilson, J. (1966). Plasmathiocyonate and vitamin B12 in Nigerian Patients with Degenerative Neurological Disease *Lanceti*, 1062.

Osuntokun, B.O. (1969). Chronic Cyanide Intoxication and a Degenerative Neuropathy in Nigeria. Ph.D thesis, University of Ibadan.

Platt, B.S. (1962). *Tables of Representative Values of Food Commonly Used in Tropical Countries,* Medical Research Council Special Report Series No. 302. Her Majesty's Stationery Office, London.

WHO (1976a). *Nutrition. In Preventive Medicine*. Monograph series No. 62 (ed. G.H. Beaton and J.M. Bengoa). WHO, Geneva.

–(1976b). Vitamin A Deficiency and Xerophthalmia. *Tech. Ser. Wld. Hlth. Org. 590*.

WHO AFRO (1977). *Rapid Village Nutrition Survey Technique*. AFR/NUT 84. WHO, Brazzaville.

64

The Role of International Agencies in the Control of Nutritional Problems in Africa

K. V. Bailey

Mandates and Main Activities

The principal international agencies involved directly in nutrition-related activities in Africa are those of the UN system, and the Organization of African Unity.

Food and Agriculture Organization of the United Nations

The FAO's role in relation to food and nutrition is strongly expressed in its constitution:

'The Nations accepting this Constitution, being determined to promote the common welfare furthering separate and collective action on their part for the purpose of:

- raising levels of nutrition and standards of living of the peoples under their respective jurisdictions;
- securing improvements in the efficiency of the production and distribution of all foods and agricultural products;
- bettering the conditions of rural populations;
- and thus, contributing towards an expanding world economy and ensuring humanity freedom from hunger...'

In the execution of this mandate, FAO has always had a strong division of food policy and nutrition. The principal components of this division are:

- nutrition planning, assessment and evaluation service
- nutrition programme services
- food quality and standards service

Most African countries in FAO belong to the African Region (three belong to the Middle East region). The regional office for Africa is based in Accra, Ghana, and has a food policy and nutrition unit. The secretariat of FAO is strongly centralized. The FAO country representatives relate to the headquarters at Rome. Much of FAO's country budget comes through UNDP programmes at country level; the FAO programmes constitute the largest single component (often 30-50%) of the UNDP programme in most countries.

FAO nutritional activities are partly regional or intercountry, and partly at country level. In the sixties and seventies, many countries had FAO nutritionist staff members assigned but increasingly the tendency is for consultancy services relating to the above fields. Intercountry activities include seminars, workshops and training courses. Currently the main emphasis in nutrition in the African region is on the following fields of activity:

- food and nutrition planning
- food and nutrition surveillance
- integration of nutritional considerations in rural development programmes/projects (including fisheries and animal husbandry)
- promotion of under-utilized nutritious traditional food crops
- control of vitamin A deficiency and
- development of national food control services.

Since its inception, FAO has become more oriented towards the economic aspects of agriculture. At country level, its contribution is seen mainly in terms of improved food production, storage, processing and marketing, the reduction of post-harvest losses and promotion of food control through country projects, technical co-operation programmes and training programmes in these fields. However, the nutritional aspect is sometimes given more prominence e.g. in the context of World Food Day celebration (16 October). Small-scale projects having some food and nutritional benefits are supported through Freedom From Hunger Campaign and other NGOs. In the African region FAO carried out two major series of country studies, each covering about half the countries of the region, on the subjects of (i) nutrition teaching and training (mainly at tertiary level), and (ii) infant feeding, weaning practices and local production of weaning foods. FAO also carried out important activities through its global information and early warning system and it is actively participating in the development of food and nutrition surveillance in a number of countries.

UNICEF

The United Nations Children's Fund had, since its inception after the Second World War, a strong emphasis on child nutrition: initially mainly in the form of supplementary feeding programmes but in later decades through intersectoral applied nutrition programmes.

Currently the main focus of UNICEF's nutritional activities in Africa is on the following:

- growth monitoring and promotion
- food and nutrition surveillance
- breast-feeding and nutrition education, based on thorough analysis of the local situation, and particularly oriented towards the improvement of weaning practices and maternal nutrition, through social marketing approaches
- control of specific nutritional disorders (vitamin A, iodine and iron/folate deficiencies)
- related measures such as oral rehydration therapy and immunization strengthening nutrition education in schools
- multisectoral support to cushion the nutritional effects of structural adjustment, generate household income, and other activities related to household food security.

In the 1960s and '70s substantial efforts were made to promote the production of weaning foods on an industrial scale in a number of African countries. Some of these were technically successful (e.g. in Algeria, Egypt and Ethiopia) but as they generally hardly reached the most needy groups in the community, the emphasis now is on small-scale processing at village and household level.

The present policy is towards a multisectoral type of indirect support to nutrition and with more emphasis on maternal nutrition, health, education and income-earning capacity, and other general programmes of support and development for women, whose role in relation to food production, storage, processing and marketing is so crucial in Africa.

Generally, UNICEF's nutritional activities are in the context of support to MCH/FP and primary health care programmes, but also through programmes focussing on the improvement of the situation of women.

UNICEF is highly decentralized and the general shape and details of country programmes are decided essentially at country level. Nevertheless, UNICEF also supports a number of intercountry activities such as seminars, workshops, and training programmes and visits. It also applies research, with particular emphasis on the sociological dimension of nutrition. Thus, while there is certainly some support to nutrition in all UNICEF country programmes in Africa, the nature of this support is highly varied.

World Health Organization

For WHO, nutrition is an integral part of public health, for which WHO has technical responsibility within the UN family. The first session of the World Health Assembly requested the setting up of a joint FAO/WHO Expert Committee on nutrition.

Adequate food and nutrition constitutes one of the eight essential elements of primary health care – but regrettably, is one of the least developed of those elements in most countries of the region, especially at grassroot level. Globally and regionally, WHO's main objectives are to improve the nutritional state of vulnerable groups (particularly infants and young children, pregnant and lactating women) and to support programmes for control of specific nutritional disorders (nutritional anaemia, iodine and vitamin A deficiencies).

In the African region the current strategy is to develop district-based action for food and nutrition improvement in the context of primary health care, using intersectoral approaches as expressed in several documents (1-3). In WHO, programming is carried out at regional, sub-regional and country levels. Currently some twenty countries have reserved a part of their country budget for nutritional programmes. The main activities are:

- nutritional surveys and surveillance
- nutritional education and social mobilization with particular emphasis on breast-feeding, control of marketing of breast-milk substitutes, and development of local weaning food mixtures at household, community and district levels
- control of specific nutritional disorders
- training in district-level management of food and nutrition programmes
- applied research on nutritional problems at the local and district levels.

Since 1987, three sub-regional health development teams have been set up based in Bamako (Mali) for West Africa, Bujumbura (Burundi)for Central Africa and Harare (Zimbabwe) for Eastern/Southern Africa. These teams give technical support to countries, mainly in developing district-based approaches to health development, including food and nutrition. These teams help to develop food and nutrition training programmes, and problem-oriented research at the local level, e.g. on how to carry out community-based nutritional surveillance; promotion of production of local weaning food: modalities of control of specific nutritional disorders, etc.

Two activities currently given particular prominence are the development of nutritional surveillance based on growth monitoring of young children at village level, and the control of iodine deficiency disorders. In all of these programmes, the emphasis is on training of national staff, to enhance their capacities to tackle effectively the food and nutritional problems, and applied research at the local level, using a problem-solving approach. Considerable extra budgetary resources have been mobilized for most of these programmes.

Currently, the activities being supported in the countries and through intercountry meetings, are: food and nutrition surveillance (establishment of national systems and computerized data banks), control of iodine and vitamin A deficiencies, and educational activities. Among the latter is the development of national codes of marketing of breast-milk substitutes to prevent the erosion of traditionally favourable breast-feeding practices by aggressive marketing of breast-milk substitutes. A new sub-programme on control of anaemia is just beginning.

Control of iodine deficiencies is one field in which relatively rapid progress is being made in co-operation with UNICEF and the International Council for Control of Iodine Deficiency Disorders. This has permitted the mobilization of resources to support intercountry activities as well as national programmes. Thirty-four countries in the region have a significant IDD problem. A regional seminar was held on the subject in 1987 by both the African and Eastern Mediterranean regional offices.

UNESCO

UNESCO's mandate relates mainly to nutrition education, and the teaching of nutrition in schools – a field shared with FAO. Nutrition educational guidelines have been widely disseminated in the region and collections of educational materials made.

Organization of African Unity

The OAU has been involved in nutritional work mainly through the Joint FAO/WHO/OAU Commission, referred to below.

Joint Activities

Many activities have been undertaken jointly by the international agencies, of which only a few are cited here.

FAO/WHO Expert Committee on Nutrition

The Joint Committee continues to meet periodically to make reports and important recommendations on a wide range of subjects from national food and nutritional policy to energy and nutrient requirements, and the control of specific nutritional disorders. The United Nations University participates in some of these meetings.

Joint FAO/WHO/OAU Regional Food and Nutrition Commission for Africa

The Secretariat of the Commission was set up in Accra in 1964. Sessions of the Commission were held in 1974, 1981, 1983 and 1985. The main achievements were the publication of bulletins, briefs for administrators and special papers; and food and nutrition seminars for all countries of the region. Also national food and nutrition policies and programmes were drawn up as a collaborative effort with seven countries.

FAO/UNICEF/WHO Technical Group on Nutrition
This group, set up in 1987, has had two meetings, to foster closer co-operation in the types of nutrition programmes referred to above.

African Regional Task Force on Food and Nutrition Development
This Task Force had its first meeting in Addis Ababa in 1988. It made recommendations designed to promote district-focus food and nutrition development, particularly through combined action of those agencies represented at country level. Its second meeting was held in Niamey in September 1989.

Inter-agency Food and Nutrition Surveillance Programme (UNICEF/FAO/WHO)
This programme, whose secretariat is in UNICEF/New York, has mobilized substantial extra budgetary funds to support food and nutrition surveillance activities at intercountry and country levels. One workshop in the African region was already funded partly from this source in the African region (April 1988). Efforts are now being made jointly by the three agencies to develop country projects in food and nutrition surveillance, following guidelines recently agreed upon and distributed to the countries.

International Professional Associations
ICCIDD/WHO/UNICEF are co-operating in a very active programme of support to countries in the region. An IDD Task Force for Africa has been set up by ICCIDD which has designated a Regional co-ordinator and three sub-regional co-ordinators for the African Region of WHO and another for the Eastern Mediterranean. The main effort is toward supporting countries in developing technically sound comprehensive national IDD control programmes, which can then obtain donor support. About twenty countries have activities under way with support of international agencies. Several intercountry meetings have also been supported.

To some extent, a similar co-operation is developing between WHO and two other consultative groups: the International Vitamin A Consultative Group (IVACG) and the International Nutritional Anaemia Consultative Group (INACG), both based in USA.

WHO/UNICEF Joint Nutrition Support Programme
The Italian government generously provided funds for major support to nutrition programmes of an intersectoral community-based type in six countries (Angola, Ethiopia, Mali, Mozambique, Niger and Tanzania). Essentially these projects have operated in several districts of each country since 1984. One has been particularly successful in developing village-based growth monitoring and nutritional surveillance, and a wide range of activities all designed to improve the nutritional situation at the local level.

Belgian Survival Fund/FIAD/WHO/UNIEF/UNDP
Substantial funds voted by the Belgian parliament are being used in support of rural development programmes with primary health care and nutrition components in Ethiopia, Kenya, Somalia and Uganda.

Overall Strategy and Impact
The role of the international agencies is essentially to develop national capacities for analysis of their problems and the implementation, monitoring and evaluation of programmes to improve their situation. In the earlier postwar decades, teams of international staff operated in many countries

but as more and more nationals have acquired the necessary training and experience, the pattern of international co-operation is changing. Currently there are several trends:

- more short-term consultant services in specialized fields rather than long-term staff at country level
- more use of experts within the region for such consultancies
- more direct forms of programme support such as provision of equipment and supplies, support for programmes of training at national or local level, and grants to national institutions
- more support for training and applied research programmes.

The overall food and nutrition situation has been recently reviewed by the Sub-committee on Nutrition of the UN Administrative Committee for Co-ordination. While the figures seem to show some improvement on the nutritional situation, food supply has become more precarious in Africa with declining per capita food production. In many countries where structural adjustment measures are being implemented, there is some evidence of growing nutritional hardship.

Overall it would be difficult to demonstrate many success stories – although there are quite a few of them. What is certain is that the development of national capacities for tackling the situation would have been much slower, and the situation would have been correspondingly poorer but for the input of the international agencies. However, it has to be admitted that the efficiency, effectiveness and even the relevance of much that has been and is being done, is questionable. The current view of the agencies seems to be that one of the best ways for achieving progress will be through monitoring the situation at village level, by villagers, with reporting of the results to the village and district development committees, both of which take appropriate action at their levels according to their means. In some countries, this type of community involvement has been conclusively successful. At the same time, the formulation and implementation of national food and nutrition policies, strategies and programmes are also essential.

It is to be hoped that an effective forum could be established in the region, where these issues could be thoroughly reviewed on an inter-agency, intersectoral and interdisciplinary basis, and effective policies and strategies decided upon and implemented. The Task Force mentioned above could be such a forum. Ways must be found to alleviate the nutritional hardship which is currently spreading over most of the continent, and to reach adequate levels of food and nutrition security for the entire people. While this is one of the implied or explicit goals of all the agencies by the year 2000, the efforts to achieve this will have to be greatly accelerated if the objectives are to be attained. Perhaps the most that can be hoped for would be the elimination of all except very occasional cases of severe malnutrition in its various forms (protein-energy malnutrition and the specific nutritional disorders mentioned above). It is estimated that about five million children die annually in Africa, of causes related to malnutrition, and much larger numbers of children and women suffer serious disabilities. It may not be realistic to expect the elimination of all the moderate forms of under - and malnutrition, but at least it is desirable and feasible to aim for the elimination of the severe forms and the reduction of the moderate ones. Concerted action by all these partners, with national governments and non-governmental organizations will be indispensable for success. Malnutrition is the silent killer and crippler which is unfortunately glossed over in face of the more dramatic problems of the continent. The effects of malnutrition are so far-reaching on the physical and mental development of children that these problems must be given the priority they deserve in the struggle for health for all.

65

Protein Energy Malnutrition

John Patrick

Introduction

Protein energy malnutrition remains one of the foremost symptoms of under-development. One should point out that some surveys show that 30-50per cent of patients in the hospitals of the developed world are also malnourished. This underlines the inevitability of weight loss when serious illness develops. In the under-developed world, the problem is worse because not only are there serious endemic diseases, like malaria, but also the diarrhoeal diseases consequent upon inadequate water supplies and poor sanitation. Thus, a child growing up in the developing world spends much of its first five years infected and therefore not growing. In addition, the use of nutritionally inadequate weaning foods, such as cassava and plantain together with unhygienic food preparation practices make the transition from breast to ordinary food hazardous. Unfortunately, the resulting high under – five mortality rate is so much a part of life, that it is accepted as inevitable. In the view of the author, it is this acceptance of high infant mortality rates, which is the primary barrier to their reduction. No amount of money and technology can produce the results we all desire, until this barrier is removed. Thus the education needed is not just specific nutrition education but general education, which increases the confidence of the people in their capacity to alter their environment for the better. It is the motivations of the 18th and 19th century reformers, like Wilberforce, Shaftesbury and Fry which need to be transmitted. Before these leaders arrived on the scene, malnutrition and high infant mortality rates were as prevalent in Europe as they are now in Africa.

The present attitude to children in the villages of Africa makes sense in a situation where sick children inevitably died and where the survival of the village was dependent on healthy adult males. There is no reason why most of these children should not survive, with only modest changes in village life. However, whilst women still spend most of the day working in the fields, thereby limiting the opportunities to feed newly weaned infants, and whilst men continue to consume the best food, malnutrition of children will be inevitable.

The slow inexorable development of malnutrition and its socio-economic background has been well described by Mata in Guatemala. The essential features being poverty, illiteracy, poor maternal health and antenatal care, frequent infections, early cessation of breast feeding and weaning to fewer than the minimum necessary meals per day, which are often poor quality, inappropriate foods. The infants response to this process is first to stop growing and then to alter his metabolism in ways which can be viewed as adaptive because they conserve energy but they are adaptations purchased at some cost, almost certainly including the mortgaging of future intellectual development.

By the time protein-energy malnutrition (PEM) is fully developed and clinically apparent, it is a multiple deficiency state of which energy is the most important deficiency. Protein is of major importance only in areas using cassava (manioc) or plantain as the major weaning foods without significant contributions from other foods. Of the minor nutrients, vitamins and minerals; vitamin A deficiency is the major preventable cause of infantile blindness in the world whilst deficiencies of vitamins A, E and C, zinc, copper and selenium may be important in the causation of kwashiorkor. The role of anti-oxidants and free-radicals in the etiology of kwashiorkor is probably the most exciting area of active research into malnutrition at present. If the free radical hypothesis proves to be correct, it also has practical implications for the treatment of kwashiorkor, because it changes the emphasis from the traditional one of provision of protein to other aspects of dietary quality, especially the anti-oxidants, vitamins A, E, C and the minerals, Se, Zn, and Cu. The correlation between provision of protein and cure of oedema would be due to the fact that higher protein intakes are usually associated with better general quality.

The Diagnosis of Malnutrition

There are two approaches to the diagnosis of PEM that are applicable to the African situation.

1. The simpler system to us uses longitudinal weight for age data on the traditional road to health charts. Initially the Gomez classification used cross-sectional data to divide children into four categories; 90-110% of the fiftieth percentile was defined as normal and 75-89%, 60-74% and below 60% as malnutrition grades 1-3. The problem with this classification is that it does not distinguish between children who have failed to grow in height but are perfectly proportioned and children with weight loss who are thin and wasted. Only the latter group are in immediate need and they will only respond dramatically to treatment. One way round the problem is to focus on the shape of growth curves. A persistent flat curve or a failing curve should initiate attempts to increase meal frequency and energy density of meals. Unfortunately, many charts are very inaccurately plotted and many health care workers are content with filling in the card as though that were therapeutic in itself. There is little use in filling in the chart unless there is a possibility of doing something about it. If these charts are to become really useful, much more education of health care workers and better supervision are necessary. Furthermore, the clinic workers must be able to give advice that is possible for the mother, preferably including the capacity to sell cheap, appropriate, local foods.
2. The alternative is to use weight for height charts. Waterlow also classified children into categories using >90% of the median wt/ht as normal and 80-90%, 70-80% and <70% as the degrees of malnutrition. Unfortunately the use of this system usually requires a specially trained team because height is not measured with sufficient reliability, without such teams. Weight for height data can be rapidly acquired and processed, using a measuring team and a portable computer with appropriate software such as the CASP programme from CDC Atlanta USA. This is probably the way that supervision of health posts could be improved because it would identify instantly, those children immediately in need of nutritional supplements. There is not an absolute concordance between the two

methods because a child normally at the 95th percentile of weight for height could lose 10% of body weight and be in need of resuscitation and yet still be above –2 z scores for weight for height. The longitudinal data would show clearly that there was a problem whereas cross-sectional data would not. Thus for the village, longitudinal weight for age charts are best, if the data quality is good and the health care workers understand how to interpret them.

The basic concepts to be expounded again and again to health care workers are:

1. A child with a flat or falling growth curve needs to be checked for infection and after giving appropriate treatment, needs to have nutritional supplements to catch up again.
2. All children with reduced weight for height are capable of responding to nutritional supplements.
3. Children who are not growing in height properly, i.e. children who are stunted may have reduced weight for age but be incapable of rapid weight gain. Improvements in statural growth are much slower than improvements in weight for height and are probably dependent upon many factors associated with increased affluence. Failure to reach genetic potential for height is very common in Africa (40% in many places) and this leads to wrong diagnoses of acute PEM based on weight for age criteria. This in turn, contributes to disillusionment with weight for age charts because in such an area, 40% of the children who are below the ideal weight for age will be stunted rather than wasted and incapable of rapid response to supplements.

The Pathophysiology of Malnutrition

In experimental animals, it is clear that feeding a diet deficient in energy leads to a diminished expenditure of energy per kg of body weight i.e. the animals become more efficient. The addition of moderate protein deficiency impairs this response and provision of free access to a diet with an extremely low protein totally inhibits this response. The size of the response is still a subject of debate but it is of the order of 15-30%. From a biochemical perspective, a response of this magnitude must involve either protein synthesis or membrane transport of sodium; both have been shown to be reduced. Since these mechanisms underlie almost all physiological activities, one should expect consequent changes in all organ systems and coincidental potassium depletion. Diminished capacities to respond to cold because of reduced maximal cardiac function, to salt and acid loading because of reduced renal function, to glucose administration and feeding because of reduced insulin secretion, have all been demonstrated and are exactly what would be predicted, if the adaptive hypothesis is correct. The failure to respond adequately to infection is well known, although this appears to be dependent upon deficiencies of minor nutrients especially zinc rather than protein and energy.

The oedema found in kwashiorkor, despite statements to the contrary in most textbooks, is not explained by specific protein deficiency. The essential practical points are that the treatment of kwashiorkor and marasmus is identical and kwashiorkor, although clinically dramatic, is only 0.5-1% of the total malnutrition problem and should not be the major interest of public health policies. The essential defect in kwashiorkor is a failure of sodium homeostasis, particularly the capacity to excrete a sodium load. Sodium intake should therefore be restricted in kwashiorkor and in all malnutrition children not suffering from gastro-enteritis.

Treatment

From these research findings, a rational approach to treatment is possible. The primary principle for the initial treatment is to proceed slowly to avoid exceeding the limited homeostatic capacities of the child, which are a consequence of adaptation to malnutrition. In the malnourished child, if a little is good it does not follow, in the early stage, that more is better. The second consideration is infection. It is almost always the explanation of any rapid deterioration and in the severely malnourished, the usual signs of infection are missing and only very careful search will uncover the infection. If the infection is diarrhoeal, electrolyte problems will be added and because of the reduced renal function, treatment is difficult and must proceed cautiously, except for the correction of peripheral circulatory failure.

The treatment of severe PEM is similar for marasmus and kwashiorkor. It can be divided into three phases.

1. Resuscitation
2. Rapid Growth
3. Establishment of normal diet.

1. Resuscitation

Children with severe malnutrition usually present with a precipitating infective illness such as gastro-enteritis, pneumonia, meningitis or other infection. Often there will be no signs of infection, therefore a very high index of suspicion is necessary. Small bowel overgrowth with anaerobic bacteria has also been well documented; in the severely ill, it should be presumed to be present and treated with metronidazole (15mg/kg/d for 5 days). Malnourished children are also limited in the extent to which they can handle electrolyte disorders or acute changes in any system. Unless severe diarrhoea is present, no more than 2mmol of sodium/kg/day should be given. Provision of more will lead to sodium retention and it can cause both oedema and heart failure. In kwashiorkor, the sign of oedema implies an expansion of at least 15% in the extracellular space, i.e. in a 10kg child, approximately 0.5l of excess physiological saline or 75mmol of sodium – several days supply! It is best to treat all diarrhoeal diseases orally, unless peripheral circulatory failure is present.

The "normal" haemoglobin for a severely malnourished child is 7-8g/100ml. However, it should be noted that the only mineral of which malnourished children are not deficient is iron. Iron is not needed until growth commences. The low haemoglobin can be viewed as part of the adaptation to chronic under-nutrition. Because the chronically malnourished have a reduced lean body mass, they require less oxygen carrying capacity and therefore a lower haemoglobin is adequate. This has the additional advantage of reducing the work of the heart, because of the reduced viscosity of the blood.

Fluid Requirements: 1ml/kcal + replacement of any losses due to gastro-enteritis. Severe gastro-enteritis can deplete the body of 15% of body water before death. Fluid can be replaced rapidly to resuscitate a failing circulation but thereafter replacement must be slow.

Energy Requirements: 100 kcal/kg is a reasonable value to use for maintenance energy requirements in the usual 1-2 year old age group. The 1985 WHO approach to energy requirements is much simpler and uses only weight and age in the formulae.

Protein Requirements: during resuscitation the maintenance requirements are very low at 0.6g/kg/day. Provision of large amounts can be counter-productive because of the associated need to excrete the acidic by-products of protein metabolism, before the full recovery of renal function makes that possible.

Energy intake should also be limited to the requirement for maintenance of the current normally hydrated body. Provision of greater quantities can lead to growth and that can aggravate mineral deficiencies, because lean tissues have high concentrations of several important minerals including potassium, magnesium, phosphate and zinc. This increased requirement for mineral during growth is the reason that deficiencies of trace elements can usually only be demonstrated in growing animals.

If one meets the requirements for energy and protein from dried skim milk; for easy calculation it is reasonable to assume that DSM is 30% protein and contains 4 kcals/g.

Step 1: Calculate fluid requirements assuming the child is burning 100 kcals/kg/d i.e. needing 100mls/kg/d. Given in 5 feeds/day if possible.

Step 2: Start with a 1/4 strength solution of DSM and increase every day in the absence of significant diarrhoea (2-3 semi-formed stools are not a contra-indication to increasing concentration). Full strength milk can be 100g DSM made up to 100mls. The addition of 50-75g of carbohydrate and some vegetable oil will reduce the protein concentration to more reasonable levels (More than 2% dietary protein is rarely needed even in rapidly growing children). In rural settings, supplements of the local staple are easily integrated. Because they are usually high carbohydrate foods, it is reasonable to meet the maintenance protein requirements from a good source (e.g. DSM or Soya) and then use local foods to boost the energy intake. This has the important advantage of making the expensive components of the diet go much further.

Mineral Requirements: all malnourished children are mineral deficient; in order of importance (in brackets suggested daily doses), potassium (2-4mmol/kg), magnesium (1-2mmol/kg), zinc (1mg/kg), selenium (1.0 microgram/kg), copper (0.1g/kg).

Vitamin Requirements: a standard capsule of water soluble vitamins is appropriate, with additional thiamine in rice eating areas. It should include vitamin C and folic acid (5mg/d) should also be given. Vitamins D & K are not required in special amounts but vitamin A (150,000 units intramuscularly) should be given where vitamin A deficiency is endemic. Vitamins A and E should be given especially in kwashiorkor. Skin changes may be viewed as evidence of deficiencies in minor nutrients especially zinc.

2. Rapid Growth

This can commence when the child's appetite returns. It is appropriate to progressively increase the total intake and also the energy density of the feeds by adding up to 60mls of vegetable oil to each litre of milk. Where staffing levels permit, feeding can be up to eight times per day. Once rapid growth has started, rates up to 30g/kg/day can be achieved provided the composition of the feeds is appropriate (see Table 65.1). Occasionally at the start of high energy feeding, some children (up to 5%) can develop a syndrome characterized by the sudden onset of breathlessness, tachycardia, hepatic enlargement and watery diarrhoea. There is a rapid and effective response to intravenous frusemide and oral digoxin (half the usual digitalizing dose). Without rapid treatment these children can die in less than half an hour.

Until expected weight for height is reached, the children should feed voraciously, unless infected. Once they reach their own expected weight for height, they spontaneously reduce their intake and may commence the third stage. At this stage they may still be a long way below normal weight for age because catch-up growth in height is slow.

Table 65.1
Requirements for a 2kg Weight Gain in a 10kg Infant

Intake KCAL/KG/D	Maintenance Requirement KCAL/KG/D	Growth Energy KCAL/KG/D	Growth G/KG/D	Total Growth G/D	Time Cost for 2Kg Days $
100	100	0	0	0	Infinite
105	100	5	1	10	200/100000
110	100	10	2	20	100/50000
120	100	20	4	40	50/25000
140	100	40	8	80	25/12500
180	100	80	16	160	12/6250

This assumes that the maintenance requirement does not increase with growth, which is not true but makes only a small difference. The cost of growth is assumed to be 5 kcal/g which is acceptable for lean tissue but adipose tissue costs about 10 kcal/g. The cost of resuscitation is calculated using a nominal developed world cost of $500/day.

3. Re-establishment of Normal Diet and Follow-Up
This will vary from place to place but often receives insufficient attention. Minor changes in infant feeding practices could easily prevent marginal growth faltering from progressing into serious malnutrition. There is little appreciation of the slow development of feeding efficiency in children. They do not reach adult levels of feeding efficiency until about eight years of age. Thus the common practice of feeding once a day virtually insures a high prevalence of malnutrition and if combined with the practice of giving first choice to the men, the situation will be even worse.

Prevention

It is usual under this heading to list all the WHO Alma Ata objectives. Commendable as they are, they seem to this author to be culturally naive. For the poorest people who live entirely in the present preventive activity they are unthinkable. The problems with maintenance in Africa are a clear reflection of this phenomenon. It has been traditional to belabour the activities of missionaries in Africa but the anthropologists who have been largely responsible for this abuse are not concerned with the health of the people they have studied for their dissertations. The view of the world which made possible the growth of science in NW Europe was essentially Judeao-christian and the ideas of contingency and consequence, which were so necessary, were drawn from that source.

Conclusion

The treatment of severe PEM is now improved so that under ideal circumstances 95% of severely malnourished children can survive. Nevertheless the prevalence of PEM is unchanged. The next stage is to understand the cultural and social barriers, which are preventing the effective application of the modern knowledge of how to prevent and treat severe malnutrition. This is not just a developing world problem, the western world analogy is the drug abuse problem. Everyone knows that drug abuse is dangerous, yet a large proportion of the population continue to play with them and die because of them. We are not as free or rational as we like to believe.

Reference

Golden MHN, Ramdath D. Free Radicles in the Pathogenesis of Kwashiorkor. *Proc. Nutr.* Soc 1987; 46:53-68.

Mata L J. (1978). *The Children of Santa Maria Cauque*. Massachusetts Institute of Technology Press, Cambridge.

Samonds KW, Hegsted DM. Protein Deficiency and Energy Restriction in Young Monkeys. *Proc Natl Acad Sci.* 1987; 75:1600-4.

UNICEF. The State of the World's Children. Oxford University Press, 1982.

Waterlow, JC, Golden, MHN, Patrick, J. 'The Treatment of Protein-energy Malnutrition'. In *Nutrition in the Clinical Management of Diseases*, eds. Dickerson and Leem Edward Arnold, London, 1977.

Waterlow J. C. Metabolic Adaptation to Low intakes of Energy and Protein. *Ann. Rev. Nutr.* 1986; 6:495-526.

WHO. Energy and Protein Requirements. *Technical Report Series*, 724, WHO, Geneva 1985.

66

Modern African Nutritional Problems and their Control

Osafu Ogbeide

History of Modern Africa

In February 1961, the then Prime Minister of Great Britain, the Rt. Hon. Harold MacMillan declared in a historic speech in Cape Town that 'the wind of change is blowing through the continent.' This was a clarion call to other colonial powers to follow Her Majesty's Government in granting independence to their erstwhile colonies in Africa, having done so in India, Pakistan and Ceylon. Hence in quick succession, Ghana (1959), Nigeria, Ivory Coast (1960), Belgian Congo, Sierra Leone, Tanganyika (1961), and later a host of others became self-governing nations. In addition to monarchies of the Maghreb States, there are several self-governing nations in Africa, apart from Namibia that was, until recently, being administered by South Africa under the UN mandate. For the purpose of this work, modern Africa started with the end of the second world war, about five decades ago.

The pattern of events in the newly independent African states was similar. There was a relatively short period of tranquility during which all the fanfare and festivities which signified the transition were wound up. In retrospect, this crucial interval determined the course of the new state. Basking in the euphoria of the newly acquired personality, the leader's valuable planning time was dissipated in building up an inflated ego. To sustain this, the new administration often became preoccupied with rather extravagant paraphernalia of status symbols. Rather than apply available resources to productive welfare needs, expensive apparatus of propaganda to ensure external and internal security were over- emphasized. This was exasperated in most cases, by the limited educated human resources available to the new administration to effectively discharge their additional responsibilities. In the ensuing quandary, the new central administration could not exert an impact greater than the colonial ones being replaced. This period was usually marked by the absence of lucid government policies. This observed policy vacuum was shown in many developmental programmes in Africa including food and nutrition programmes.

Nutritional Problems

Nutritional problems result from either undernutrition, malnutrition or overnutrition. In many affluent countries, problems of overnutrition relating to excessive consumption of such food items as sugar and fat are most important. The nutritional diseases prevalent in these areas are obesity and arteriosclerosis. In the developing countries however, the problems are those of undernutrition and malnutrition relating to low intake of calories, protein, some minerals and vitamins. The commonest clinical manifestations of such deficiencies include kwashiorkor, marasmus, keratomalcacia, anaemia, rickets, pellagra, goitre and scurvy.

In trying to discus the nutritional problems in modern Africa, it will be pertinent to suggest that such problems as may be seen, may not be peculiar to Africa. However, these problems which are known to occur in the continent do so under certain prevailing circumstances.

Food production is very important. In many African countries, agricultural programmes for the production of cash crops such as cocoa, rubber, cotton, coffee, tea etc. have been prosecuted to the detriment of food production. The deliberate erroneous belief that food production activities can take care of themselves without any governmental intervention has been the official farm policy in many of these African countries. Of special interest here was the time lag between independence in Nigeria in 1960 and this realization in 1974, during which there appeared to be the lack of food production policy to feed the population.

However, food production and hence availability of it to the population are inextricably associated with nutrition. It has been observed that nutrition cannot be described solely by the adequacy of available food. In a dual economy, it is argued that where there is overproduction of milk, the resulting poor income from this commodity may prevent the milk farmer from purchasing other essential items of food. This starvation in the midst of plenty may be further aggravated by religious prejudices, cultural taboos, and other misconceptions which arise from the lack of nutrition education. In Africa, most of these conditions above could be compounded by myriads of religious sects and tribes whose observances are sacrosanct. What to eat, which parts are forbidden, when to eat become constant and nagging questions. In many instances, the solution to the problem cannot be reasonably explained on the basis of available food and optimum nutritional requirements.

There are also certain forces which are entirely outside the control of the African but play an immense role in determining the food available and hence nutrition on the continent. The promotion of the colonies to independent states lifted the umbrella cover previously provided by the colonizing power. The new status involved the emerging nation in financial commitment which by and large was not directly related to production e.g. defence. Coupled with this is the regular slump in commodities' prices, and instability in oil markets which are the life wire of Africans. Lately, the dreaded Structural Adjustment Programmes are sad symptoms of the whole scale of unemployment and underemployment that have dodged our economic aspirations of previous years. Any hope that the rest of the world will evolve a kindlier understanding of her woes is forlorn. Thus, about 90% of Africans today live below the 'poverty line'. Resulting from this chaotic situation, the gaps between the rich and the poor individuals and nations become unbridgeable canyons. The implications of this unwholesome situation are well documented. In a reflection,

Copaland said that 'people coulu ..ot benefit from even over production of food to improve their nutrition status as an increase GNP would not necessarily be reflected in the eradication of poverty and malnutrition due to 'poverty syndrome.'

The history of modern Africa is associated with wars, for example the wars of secession of Biafra from Nigeria, Eretria and Tigre from Ethiopia, Ogaden from Somalia, Kivu and Katanga from the Belgian Congo, and Western Sahara from Morocco. Some are factional wars for the ascendancy of ethnic or tribal groups as in Burundi, Congo Brazzaville, Equatorial Guinea, Mozambique, etc; and fundamentalist wars in Maghred. Perhaps the most obnoxious of all are the ideological wars like those in Angola, Namibia, Sudan, Ethiopia and Uganda, exported by the exponents of various institutional ideologies to Africa and other developing countries which become the testing grounds of modern arsenals and new war strategies. This undesirable situation has thrown a greater part of the African population in recent times into a perpetual state of flux. For many African countries, this war syndrome has become their major preoccupation, consuming their most valuable, limited resources in man and materials. There is no end in sight in these wars of attrition fanned by super power interests. Consequently, one can almost justify the existence in Africa of a generation condemned to a refugee camp citizenry. The UN High Commission for Refugees in Africa estimate about four million huddled together in camps where they are deprived and exist in a shameful pattern not entirely of their own choosing. These refugees depend on relief food supply in aid. Such aid can hardly scratch their needs. However, in considering the nutrition problems of modern Africa, they justly represent a part of the entire population of the continent to be adequately fed. In these camps, all the different manifestations of malnutrition and undernutrition are bound to exist in acute forms.

There is perhaps no expression most aptly representative of modern African malady in nutrition consideration as 'population explosion'. The population of Nigeria for example has been variously quoted as between 120 and 150 million. One must say that these figures are provisional. There has not been an accurate acceptable census conducted in the country, a condition which appears common to most other countries. This is due on the one hand to the enormous demographic requirements for an accurate census and on the other hand to the rate of population explosion which tends to invalidate data even before collation. Nevertheless, there is some element of acceptability in these figures as they are derived from the usual formulae. What is inescapably important here is that nutrition problems in Africa and other Third World countries is how to feed the huge upsurge in population to militate against self-destruction. This is the crux of the matter: the population is to be adequately fed and nourished. There have been erudite and convincing arguments on either side as to the real and total effect of population expansion on the problem of nutrition. Some consider that population growth poses problems only when the means of food production, land, labour and materials are not maximally exploited. The Malthusians see population growth per se as constituting an impediment to optimum food availability and hence nutrition. One ventures to think that in the light of experience in modern Africa, the arguments are academic. In the first place, there is already an uncontrolled population growth. Secondly, even in a planned population growth, providing for the addition constitutes an automatic problem. The question in Africa is which of these two sides of the argument carries more weight? Without endemic economic predicament, it seems that adequate food production cannot be achieved in the immediate future. Hence the incontrovertible conclusion is drawn that population explosion has come to confound an already complex nutrition problem. Recent studies estimate that world population will add another one billion by the turn of the century: four-fifths of this will be in the undeveloped countries of Asia, Africa and Latin America. There is no doubt that this colossal increase will threaten the foundation of our existence and stretch our ingenuity. Food aid, no matter how massive, may not be able to stem the force of this demand.

As if these social environments which tend to thwart nutritional programmes in modern Africa were not daunting enough, natural disasters also combine to ensure just this. Floods, usually in the growing season of the farm calender have been known to sweep away cultivated farms before the hapless farmers. Cases of complete washout of farms have been recorded in West Africa, East Africa and the entire season's crops were lost. Severe leaching, which seriously depletes soil fertility and destablizes a conducive ecosystem, are invariably associated with these floods. Of equally devastating severity is the flip side of the coin – drought. Calamitous cases of this drought which were reported in the Sahel region, in the horn of Africa at various times, wreaked havoc on crops, farmland, and livestock and left the entire population hopelessly without provision. Again, the shipment of massive food aid during such disaster has at best only been able to tide the affected areas over one year, whereas, it naturally requires a much longer period to rebuild the ecosystem before a reliable harvest could be expected in subsequent years. Of importance in the food situation in Africa is the absence everywhere of strategic reserve programmes, a common practice in most other continents.

There are other factors that should be mentioned when discussing nutritional problems in Africa. The synergistic relationship between undernutrition and infection generates a vicious cycle leading to accelerating deterioration of health, which is part of the 'poverty syndrome,' currently afflicting many parts of the world.

Malnutrition also contributes to high maternal mortality in developing countries including Africa. It has been computed that, in a developing country, one out of every 50 women in the reproductive age dies during pregnancy, and 15-20% of such maternal deaths are attributable to anaemia.

Control

To help Africa tackle its food and nutrition problems, meaningful attention is being paid to the biological environment. There is hardly any food crop and livestock indigenous to this region which has not been improved by better husbandry. These have led to outstanding yields and concomitant greater economic rewards that ought to upgrade the nutrition of Africa. This has regretfully not been realized. In an exhaustive treatment of overcoming institutional obstacles to food production in developing countries, Schickele states, 'what we obviously do not know is how to organize ourselves to make full use of our technical knowledge and production capacity, how to motivate people to do what is needed: how to shape institutional arrangements and organizational methods and administrative procedures to render people and governments willing and able – each in its particular sphere – to produce what is needed and distribute where it is needed in the interest of national and international human welfare'. In addition to 'what we do not know' are such other imponderables resulting from political instability and military participation in politics in Africa. This is a serious consideration in developmental strategy as meaningful agriculture can only be pursued in relative peace. From the foregoing, it appears, based on the history of our immediate past, that the road to our destination in nutrition is laboriously tortuous. An unprecedented long-sighted consideration and application of a sound agrarian policy is therefore needed. Definitely, what has been most obvious in the African scene, is that in many facets of our endeavour, there has been some serious limitations in our overview of the goals. In biological concept, this has lead to accretion, that is, growth without real development. This is most noticeable in our efforts at providing food for all at a reasonable cost. A substantial body of scientific information now available points irrefutably to that judicious combination of locally available inexpensive vegetable food, for example, cereal and legumes can largely satisfy both the calorie and protein needs. Also, many symptoms which were associated with subsisting on cereal and other carbohydrate base diets have been alleviated through dedicated research. Olayide highlighted the food and nutrition crisis in Nigeria while Aylward wrote a report for Ghana. Their messages are clear. While it is not possible to emulate the food habits of the Western World, it is possible to capitalize on the intrinsic love for vegetable diets to approach our nutritional needs. From all available reports, what has to be done is for Africa to understand a comprehensive nutrition education. It is cheap, reassuring and reduces our seemingly insurmountable nutrition problem to the simple language of education for a purpose.

However, it is reasonable to expect that the solutions to these nutritional problems in modern Africa should be multinational and multipurpose. There does not appear to be a unilateral solution to it. Some unrelated issues as the level of illiteracy and other factors have been found to influence the nutritional status. Under these excruciating conditions, any improvement in the nutrition of the people of Africa can only be affected by an overall socio-economic development bearing in mind these numerous factors which interplay to undermine nutrition.

Thus, apart from food production and relevant nutrition education of the populace, the most rewarding strategy in combating nutritional problems in modern Africa will be integrated programme. These should induce the following mutually reinforcing components of environmental sanitation, immunization, family planning, specific nutrition services and health education. It is expected that under the prevailing circumstances like floods, droughts and wars which exist in modern Africa, infection should be a major problem. Since malnutrition and undernutrition are inextricably interwoven with the problem of infection, all programmes of immunization and improvement in environmental sanitation will inevitably have a beneficial impact on the nutritional problems in Africa. With the problem of population explosion in Africa, a realistic birth control policy would definitely make a major contribution to the improvement of the nutritional status of mothers and children. Above all, a degree of improvement in our social and distributive justice should be universally pursued.

Fortunately, several nutritional problems of developing countries today can be mitigated, if not entirely solved, through currently available technological tools under the prevailing socio-economic constraints. The prevention and control of endemic goitre through iodinized common salt; the control of iron deficiency anaemia through the distribution of iron tablets to mothers and children at risk, or possibly through fortification of common foods with iron, the control of nutritional blindness through food fortification or through periodic administration of massive oral doses of Vitamin A to children at risk are examples of such measures.

The health sector has a major role to play in the implementation of these programmes, which can make an important contribution to the national uplift of poor communities under the present circumstances. In fact, the health sector is ideally suited to spear-head a 'nutrition movement' within the government, and to act as a watch-dog of 'nutritional interests' in programmes of national development.

References

Agricultural Development in Nigeria, 1973-1985 (1974). The Federal Ministry of Agriculture and Natural Resources. Joint Planning Committee, Lagos. P.11.

An Agenda for Comparative European Policy Research. European Workshop on Policy Studies, University of Strathclyde (1972).

Aylward, F. (1961). *Food and Nutrition: Report to the Government of Ghana.* ETAP. No. 1449.

Beaton, H.G., McHenry, E.W. (1961). *Nutrition: A Comprehensive Treatise, Vol. II.* Academic Press, N. York P. 385-434.

Bebler, A. (1973). *Military Rule in Africa.* Praeger Publication, Inc; New York. Botzasis, A. (1961). Brown, L.R. (1980). *World Population and Food Supplies.* Am. Soc. Agron. Spec. Publication No. 6.

Burns, J; McInerney, J; Swinbank, A. (1983). *The Food Industry, Economics and Politics.* Dept. of Agric. Econ. and Management, University of Reading, P. 51-66.

Carter, G.M. (1960). *Independence for Africa* . Thomas and Hudson, London P.6-11.

Cairncross, A; Puri, M. (1976) ed. *Income Distribution and Development Strategy.* Uwins Brothers Ltd.

Cook, J. (1976). *Diet and your Religion* Woodbridge Press Publishing Co; Santa Barbara, California.

Copaland, C. (1980). *Nutritional Problems in Developing Countries World Nutrition and Nutrition Education* Sinclair, H.M; Howart.

Communist Penetration in Africa. L.S.N.I. Lisbon.

Davidson, B. (1974). *Can Africa Survive: Arguments Against Growth Without Development*. Heinemann Educational Books, London.

Dubious, V.D. (1974). *The Drought in West Africa, Evolution, Causes and Physical Consequences*. American Universities Field Staff: Personal Communication.

Grang, J.P; Maxonni, S.M; Laraba, N; *et. al.* (1983). *Combating Malnutrition in a Sector of Algiers*. Assignment Children 63/4 P.101.

Glantz, M. (1976). The Politics of Natural Disaster: *The Case of the Sahel Drought*. Praeger, New York.

Gordon, J.E. (1966). Ecology Interplay of Man, Environment and Health. *Am. J. Med. Sci.* 252, 341-356.

Hayes, M.D. (1975). *Policy Consequences of Military Participation in Politics*. Cihiske, P. 48-49.

Heiser, Jnr. C.B. (1920). *Seed to Civilization*. W.H. Freeman and Co, San Francisco. P. 11.

Holt, R.T.; Turner, J.E. (1966) *The Political Basis for Economic Development*. Van Mostrand: Princeton; Pp. 72, 120-121.

Ibid P. 41

Ibid P.133

Ibid P. 49

Ibingira G.S.K. (1980). *'African Upheavals Since Independence'*. West View Press; Boulder, Colorado P. 221–251.

Johnson, B.F. (1968). *The Staple Food Economics in Western Tropical Africa*. Stanford University Press.

Kuper, L; (1977). *The Pity of it all: Polarisation of Racial and Ethnic Relations in Africa*. General Duck worth, London.

Kuznets, S. (1972). *The Gap: Concept, Measurement, Trends: in the Gap between Rich and Poor Nations*. MacMillian Press, London.

Leichter, H.M. (1979) *A Comparative Approach to Policy Analysis*. Cambridge University Press, P. 6.

Lowry, J.H. (1970). *World Population Food Supply*, Edward Arnold, London. P.110.

Mandle, P.E; Nelson, J. (1968). Pari-Urban Malnutrition, A Neglected Problem: Patterns and Approaches. *Assignment Children* 43 25-46.

May, J.M. (1970). The *Ecology of Malnutrition in East Africa*. Oxford University Press.

Moor Jr. B. (1976). *Social Origins of Dictatorship and Democracy*. Beacon Press, Boston. P. 317.

Ogbeide O. (1974). Nutritional Hazards of Food Taboos and Preferences in Mid-Western Nigeria. *Am. J. Cli. Nutr.* 27: 213-217.

Olayide, O. (1982). *Food and Nutrition Crisis in Nigeria*. Ibadan University Press.

Omiride, S.H; Ejiogu, C.N. (1972). *Population Growth and Economic Development in Africa*. Heinemann Educational Books, London, Ibadan, Nairobi. P.237.

Sederberg, P. (1972). National Expenditure as an Indicator of Political Change in Ghana. *J. of Development Areas, 7*, P.37-56.

Scrimshaw, N.S; Taylor, C.E; Gordon, J.E. (1968). *Interaction of Nutrition and Infection*. WHO Monog. Series. 57, 392.

The Rt. Hon. Harold MacMillian: An Address to Members of Both Houses of the Parliament of the Union of South Africa; Cape Town; in *Pointing the Way*. Macmillan Press, London (1972).

Thompson, A.R. (1981). *Education and Development in Africa*. Macmillian Press, London P.57.

Trowell, H.C. (1978) A National Food Policy for Prevention of Coronary Disease. *Postgrad. Med. J.* 54, 215.

World Food Production and Need (1967). Iowa State University Centre of Agriculture and Economic Development. Iowa University, P.13.

67

Public Health Aspects of Hunger and Malnutrition in Developing Countries

Miriam K. Were

Fourteen Key Words used in this Chapter
Famine, Disaster, Undernutrition, Malnutrition, Food, Production, Aid, Distribute, Health, Services, Population, Ideology, Expenditure, Preventive

Chapter Subheads

Issues of Famine, Undernutrition and Malnutrition.
- Is under/malnutrition a public health problem?
- Definitions
- Interactions between Nutritional Status and Infections
- The Magnitude of the Problem of Food Shortages

Famine and Health Services in Africa
- Food Production in Africa
- Food Aid
- Access to Health Services in Africa

Will the Vicious Cycle be Broken in Africa?
- Which comes first?
- Population Increase Vis-a- Vis Food Shortage in Africa
- The Ideologico-economic Riddle
- Reflections from Disturbances in Africa
- What Africa Needs

Modes of Food Distribution and Opportunities for Health Services
- Food Distribution Modes

Diagnosis of Health needs of Food Distribution Sites
Social Disruption
Mental Unrest
Disease and Disability
Approaches to Organizing Health services at Food Distribution Sites
Health Services at Food Distribution Sites.
The Need for Overall Orderliness
Disease Preventive Services
Regularity of food
Water and Disposal of Human Waste
Distribution of Vitamin A
Nutritional Screening/Surveillance
Promotion of Oral Rehydration Therapy
Immunization Services
Curative services

Conclusion to the Chapter

Issues of Famine, Undernutrition and Malnutrition

Is Under/Malnutrition a Public Health Problem?

One criteria by which a problem is considered a public health problem is when that problem affects or threatens the well-being and survival of a large population of people. In the under/malnutrition riddle, famine is the end stage, implying that those who experience famine are often the tip of the iceberg of those under/malnourished. The Swedish report on Disaster Relief For Development (Linner 1986) presents famine in clear terms when it states,

'No disaster causes more suffering and deaths than famine:

- Every year 15 million people starve to death, every 24 hours 35,000, every minute 24, of which 18 are children under five years of age.
- More people starved to death during the last two years than died during the two world wars.
- As many people die during two days as were killed by the Hiroshima bomb.
- The worst earthquake in modern history–in Chile, 1976–killed 250,000 people. As many starve to death every week'.

It is therefore clear that in terms of populations affected, famine is, indeed, a public health problem. As famine is the tip of the iceberg of under/malnutrition, those affected with under/malnutrition are bigger than this. From a public point of view, it is essential that once magnitude is established, the problem should be localized and possible intervention looked for. Examples are developments in immunization for prevention of victims of stroke. An attempt is made to take this approach in this paper.

Definitions

Famine is extreme scarcity of food to the extent that life is threatened. It is a severe form of undernutrition. In the absence of relief, widespread famine can be accompanied by huge numbers of deaths. As the Swedish report on Disaster Relief For Development (Linner 1986) puts it, 'Famine implies that permanently undernourished people suddenly have no access to food'. Famine as stated above is an everyday occurrence for someone somewhere. Under 'normal' situations, those who die are scattered. This does not make news and is therefore generally overlooked. However, the horror of large numbers of people starving does sometimes jar on the conscience of humanity on a large scale. Most people have seen pictures of corpses without flesh; corpses with skin hanging like a bag around bones. Indeed the world conscience was shocked into alertness with the tragic scenes from Ethiopia displayed on the world's television sets in the 1984/85 famine, to mention just one case.

In most settings, **undernutrition** is defined as 'inadequate intake of dietary energy whether or not any specific nutrient is a limiting factor'. While mild undernutrition may be passed for 'normal' severe forms result in pictures of 'walking skeletons' which in the final stages die from starvation. Most basic text books of psychology have accounts of how food deprivation affects behaviour which ranges from apathy, mild antisocial behaviour to extremes of violence as the animal survival instincts acquire prominence over the human and humane aspects.

Malnutrition often refers to forms of poor nutritional status arising from deficiencies of specific nutrients or from diets based on the wrong kinds or wrong proportions of food. Such may be the case of inadequate intakes of iodine, vitamin C, iron and vitamin A leading respectively to conditions of goitre, scurvy, anaemia and certain eye defects.

The Fifth World Food Survey states, (FAO, 1987) 'Developing country population groups suffering from undernutrition or malnutrition are likely to be more or less the same'. On the whole, this has also been the observation of this author. Exceptions may exist in situations such as in highland populations which may have sufficient food supply but due to severe iodine or other mineral depletion in the soil or other conditions goitre may be present in the population. In this paper, these two terms, undernutrition and malnutrition, will be used interchangeably.

Interactions between Nutritional Status and Infection

Undernutrition does not exclusively result from dietary-energy intake below minimum requirement levels alone. Other factors may contribute to undernutrition. The interaction between infectious diseases and nutritional status is well established in medical literature. The Fifth World Food survey report (FAO 1987) notes that, 'Diseases such as diarrhoeas, malaria and measles may increase dietary-energy requirements by raising the body temperature or the rate of catabolic nutrient losses . . . Diarrhoea may also reduce food-absorption efficiecny so that some dietary energy simply passes into the faeces and is lost.' Frequent bouts with infection, especially in children may lead to undernutrition.

The extent to which one is exposed to infections and the rate at which infection is experienced is related to a large extent to the degree of crowding in living quarters, the quality of the house, environmental sanitation and water supply. In circumstances of crowding within poor quality houses, surrounded by poor environmental sanitation and with unsuitable water supply, infections are rampant.

Even in circumstances of frequent infections, prompt therapy can ameliorate the effects of these infections and correct mineral and vitamin deficiencies. Therefore availability of effective health services could influence the extent to which under/malnutrition is experienced. And the analysis of food availability needs to be accompanied by an analysis of availability of effective health services for populations at risk.

The Magnitude of the Problem of Food Shortage

The preceding paragraphs have already indicated the magnitude of the problem of famine. The extent of undernutrition is of course much greater than famine, since famine is the iceberg on under/malnutrition. A lot has been said about undernutrition in recent years. Severe widespread drought accompanied by famine in the period 1969/73 was perceived as tragic by the international community. The 1974 World Food Conference resolved that, by 1984 'no man, woman or child should go to bed hungry' (FAO 1985). The 1974 World Food Conference, also declared that such tragedies will be history (ECA, 1985a). Unfortunately the situation by 1983/1984 was far from this possibility.

In *State of Food and Agriculture 1984*, FAO (1985) reports that in twenty eight countries with a population of 357 million people in 1980, there had been a decline in food supply and availability. These twenty eight countries fall into the low-income group and Africa alone contributes eleven of the twenty eight countries. Indeed this report refers consistently to the African situation. It states 'In terms of human anguish and the prospects of famine-sparked instability, Africa continued to be the focus of world attention in 1984'. Reference is made to the food shortages in some Eastern African countries and in the Sahel with particular attention of this problem assuming critical proportions in Ethiopia and Chad.

The Fifth World Food Survey (FAO, 1987) exposes relative states of undernutrition in the world as shown in Table 67.1.

The proportions of those malnourished as shown in Table 67.1 indicate a substantial decline in most regions of the world except Africa. It has been pointed out, Bell (1986) 'Tropical Africa (continental sub-Saharan Africa and the nearby islands) is likely to have food nutrition problems for several generations to come. There is no easy solution since the problems are complex and deep-rooted; they involve both human institutions and nature; and, in a large part, they are so specific to the African environment that the mere transfer of existing knowledge and techniques from other continents does not respond to the imperfectly understood African needs. Most of the obstacles arise from Africa's history, institutions, and climatic and geographical factors and can only be overcome or bypassed in the long run'.

Partly because of this and also because of the enormity of the task of trying to address the entire world of developing countries, most of this chapter will focus on the African situation.

Table 67.1

Undernourished population of developing market economies by region and economic group, 1967-71 and 1979-81

Region or Economic group	Total Population		Number of undernourished				Proportion of population undernourished			
			Alternative A		Alternative B**		Alternative A*		Alternative B**	
	1970	1980	1969-71	1979-81	1969-71	1979-81	1969-71	1979-81	1969-71	1979-81
	(Millions)		(Millions)				%			
Regions										
Africa	282	376	57	70	81	99	20	19	29	26
Far East	986	1232	208	210	303	313	21	17	31	25
Latin America	278	357	36	38	53	56	13	11	19	16
Near East	159	210	23	16	34	25	15	8	22	12
Economic Groups										
Less-developed	217	280	55	77	74	102	26	28	34	36
Low-income food-deficit	1200	1522	258	278	372	406	21	18	31	27
Low-income	913	1153	199	237	288	343	22	20	31	30
Middle-to-high income	795	1026	126	98	184	151	16	10	23	15
Total developing market economies (98 countries)	1708	2179	325	335	472	494	19	15	28	23

Source: The Fifth (1985) World Food Survey p.22

* Alternative A: Dietary energy requirements for adults and adolescents: 1-2 Basic metabolichrate (BMR)

** Alternative B: Requirement raised to 1.4 BMR in line with the recommendations of a 1981 Expert Consultation (FAO/WHO/UNU, 1985)

Famine and Health Services in Africa

Food Production in Africa

A 1985 report of the Economic Commission for Africa, (ECA 1985b) brings out the fact that the per capita food production in Africa is negative in practically all the subregions. Table 67.2 illustrates this point.

Table 67. 2

Index Numbers and Rates of Changes for per Capita Food and Agriculture Production in Africa by Subregions

(Index Number) Subregion	(1974-76=100)					Exponential growth rates						
	1980	1981	1982	1983	1984[a]	71/80	71/75	80/81	81/83	82/83	83/84	86/84
Agricultural Production												
North Western	97	84	91	86	88	-1.3	-1.3	-13.3	8.0	-4.9	1.9	-1.7
Western	97	97	97	87	90	-0.8	-1.3	0.5	-0.1	-10.0	3.2	-2.4
North Eastern	93	94	90	88	88	-1.2	-0.5	1.1	-4.4	-1.4	-0.2	-1.6
Eastern	93	93	92	89	85	-1.1	-1.3	-0.5	-1.0	-2.6	-4.4	-.2.1
Central	91	91	91	89	88	-1.3	-0.1	-0.4	-0.6	-2.8	-1.1	-1.0
Southern	86	88	85	80	80	-2.9	-2.0	2.2	-2.8	-6.6	-0.2	-2.4
Total/b/	94	93	93	88	88	-1.1	-1.0	-1.2	-0.1	-5.7	0.2	-2.0
Food Production												
North Western	97	84	90	86	88	-1.3	-1.3	-13.5	8.1	-5.0	1.9	-1.7
Western	97	97	98	88	91	-0.8	-1.3	0.2	0.4	-10.2	3.9	-2.3
North Eastern	94	96	91	90	90	-0.4	0.6	2.9	-5.4	-1.4	-0.2	-1.5
Eastern	93	93	93	90	85	-0.9	-1.1	0.3	-0.8	-3.2	-5.3	-2.2
Central	92	93	93	91	89	-1.0	-0.4	0.1	0.2	-2.1	-1.5	-0.9
Southern	84	86	84	79	79	-3.2	-2.3	2.7	-2.4	-5.8	0.5	-2.2
Total	95	94	94	89	89	-0.9	-0.8	-1.0	0.1	-6.0	0.3	-1.9
Non-food Production												
North Western	91	92	94	95	97	-1.6	-0.5	0.6	2.5	0.6	2.4	1.5
Western	84	93	79	77	59	-2.5	-1.2	10.7	-16.5	-9.7	-23.3	-8.5
North Eastern	88	79	81	80	80	-5.0	-5.8	-10.1	2.3	-1.2	0.2	-1.7
Eastern	92	87	85	86	87	-2.4	-2.2	-5.7	-2.4	1.6	1.6	-1.1
Central	69	61	69	54	61	-7.5	-3.8	-12.1	14.3	-21.2	12.2	-3.5
Southern	118	111	101	99	96	2.8	4.0	-6.3	-8.4	-2.2	-2.9	-5.1
Total	87	83	81	79	78	-3.7	-3.3	-4.6	-2.4	-1.7	-2.2	-2.6

Source: *FAO, ESS, Computer printouts on index number 11 December 1984 and FAO, ESS, Computer printouts on Exp. Growth rate production indices 1 December 1984*

a/ Preliminary
b/ All Africa excluding South Africa

It is therefore clear that on the average the population in Africa are having less rather than more access to food with the passage of time.

In 1985, the Secretary General of the Organisation of African Unity (OAU) (1985a) stated 'The twin spectre of drought and famine is currently affecting a total of 150 million people in Africa. Of the fifty two OAU Member States, about thirty six countries are affected, and out of these, twenty are said to be seriously affected. These twenty are: (1) Angola, with 500,000 people in danger; (2) Burkina Faso, 500,000 people; (3) Chad, 1.5 million; (4) Ethiopia, 7.9 million; (5) Mali, 1.2 million; (6) Mauritania, 1.1 million; (7) Mozambique, 2.5 million; (8) Niger, 2.5 million; and (9) Sudan, 4.5 million. The other eleven countries with fewer people are: (10) Botswana; (11) Burundi, (12) Cape Verde, (13) Kenya, (14) Lesotho, (15) Rwanda, (16) Senegal, (17) Somalia, (18) Tanzania (19) Zambia, and (20) Zimbabwe'. He further stated 'Of the twenty countries that are seriously affected, six of these, namely, Chad, Ethiopia, Mali, Mozambique, Niger and Sudan are critically hit. With the exception of Mozambique, all these top six countries belong to the category of the Least Developed Countries as identified by the United Nations'.

Serious food shortages have, as an accompanying factor, movement of people. As the Secretary General noted in 1985, (OAU, 1985a) 'Drought and famine have triggered off massive displacement of people who have been running everywhere on their own in quest for food for themselves as well as for their animals. Roads, railways, rivers as well as urban centres have, in the process, constituted special areas of attraction of these drought and famine victims. In all, these areas of convergence, the social infrastructure and amenities, particularly within the urban centres, have been stretched beyond breaking point'.

Food Aid

There are pros and cons about food aid which will not be entered into here. Suffice it to say that this chapter has dealt with food aid as a humanitarian response to alleviate the suffering and prevent death caused by famine. In the last few years, Africa has received large amounts of food aid, in fact, this had been in quantities disproportionate to the population of Africa in comparison to other areas, like Asia. Table 67.3 illustrates this point:

Table 67.3
Food Aid in Cereal by Recipient in Low Income Countries

Country		1979/80*	1984/85*	1986/87*
Asia	Population in '000	2,583,892	2,818,214	2,913,191
	Food Aid in '000 tons	3,523.8	2,858.5	3,672.3
Africa	Population in '000	479,457	554,928	589,208
	Food Aid in '000 tons	3,422.8	7,247.4	5,484.8

* The year for which Mid Year Population is shown

Source: *Contribution of data from Food Outlook, 1987 (Statistical Supplement) and World Populations Prospects, 1986*

The population of Asia is far greater than the population of Africa, and yet Africa received far greater quantities of food aid than Asia did. The per capital importation of food to Africa is therefore much higher. Food import figures were 24.6 million tons in 1982, 28.7 in 1983 and was estimated to be twice this much in 1985, that is about 57.4 million tons (OAU 1985b).

Because of weak handling capacity at most African ports, poor road/railway infrastructures within countries, and scarcity of trucks to move food around, the food imports do not have the maximum effect they could have. As per the O.A.U. statement, those declared to be under famine in Africa in 1985 were about 150 million out of a 1985 mid year population of 554,928million; just under 30%. If one estimates those undernourished, this would be at least double this number. Therefore the undernourished in Africa constitute somewhere close to 60% of the continent's population.

Access to Health Services in Africa

Given that those undernourished in Africa may constitute anywhere up to 60% of the total population, and given the interaction between poor nutrition and infections, it is implied that most of these populations are prone to infections. And how is the continent equipped to handle this serious problem? From the available (UNICEF 1988) figures, the health service picture is dismal.

Less than 50% of the countries looked at have more than 60% of their population with access to health services. Less than half the countries have protected 50% of the children against tuberculosis, polio, whooping cough, measles and tetanus. The strategy of protecting expectant mothers and their new borns through tetanus toxoid immunization as applied by trained health personnel ranges from 2% to 89%, with the median in the 20-30% range. Given these levels of services in a precarious food situation, it is hardly surprising that the percentages of children aged under five years suffering from under/malnutrition is as high as 60% in some countries with concomitant high infant and child mortality rates.

The conclusion one is forced to make is that from the point of access to a stable food supply and access to health services, African populations are in a very precarious position. That Africa was in 1985 (UN 1986) declared a continent in crisis is not surprising given the compounding relationship between low access to food and health services.

Will the Vicious Cycle be Broken by Africa?

Which Comes First?

All data point to the constraints of development that Africa is going through. The continent seems tied up in a dismal economic situation that has repercussions all round. To farm in a better way requires implements and cash resources that are often beyond the majority of those who are responsible for most of food production in African countries. This cash shortage is tied up with low productivity which of course leads to the need to import food. This in turn leads to the need to bear the additional handling and transportation costs. These in turn take away whatever foreign exchange countries have and so they can not invest more in agriculture. Negative rates of food production continue. The situation is an extremely complex one. One of the factors that complicates this picture is the issue of population growth.

Population Increase Vis a Vis Food Shortage in Africa

An atlas of African Agriculture (FAO 1986) points out, 'Africa's population is growing faster than that of any other region. With an annual population increase of about 3 per cent, the continent is adding more than 14 million people to its population every year. In many African countries, the rate of population increase will not even peak until 1995 or later. In other areas of the world – developed and developing – the rate of population increase has already peaked, and population growth rates are now declining. In Africa, they are increasing. The rate at which they are doing so poses severe problems for African agriculture. Between 1970 and 1984, agricultural production in Africa was increased by 30 per cent. But the number of people rose by 50 per cent. The result was a decline in per caput agricultural production of 13 per cent'.

This analysis often makes people react as if controlled population growth must be the priority at all costs. No one is however clear on how to institute enforced fertility control. Most public opinion is against state-enforced fertility control; once pushed in India. So there are difficulties along the path of enforced planning of families.

In a historical perspective, the fact that rates of population increase in Africa are high is not unique to the African situation. Certain continents were saved from overcrowding and consequences of population growth not so much by 'disciplined population control' but by 'pouring out' into the 'new lands'. Let not this be forgotten.

When the difficulties inherent in attempts to have quick fixes for controlled population growth are pointed out, conclusions are often made to the effect that 'even educated Africans are negative with respect to population issues'. Let it be clear that even without the issue of regulating population, planned parenthood has recognized well-accepted benefits. As James P. Grant (1987), Executive Director of UNICEF has stated: 'The growing awareness is that birth spacing is one of the most powerful ways of improving the health of children and their mothers; noting also that when family planning is effectively included with other low-cost measures to improve the health of children and mothers, a survival revolution can be expected in most developing countries'.

The issue is how to go about creating the atmosphere that will facilitate this being adopted in an informed and sustainable manner. Grant (1987) further notes, 'A principal problem is, as we are all aware, that the gap between modern medical knowledge, such as family planning techniques, and its actual use in the community by those persons for whom it will make the vital difference, has historically been a formidable chasm'.

This chasm is often ignored. The 'experts' fail to appreciate that perceptions, even on the issue of growing population differ when seen from different positions. A respected village elder once took a medical doctor to task in a village discussion, (Were 1982) 'My child' he said, 'you tell me that these days there is more health and fewer deaths. But when I was young, I used to attend a funeral once every month or at longer intervals. Now there is a death almost every week. How can you not see that death is on the increase?'

For this kind of audience which makes up most of the current African populations, one gets nowhere by rattling off numbers indicating decreasing mortality rates. To communicate the concept of perceiving in units needs 'talking time' in order to communicate that when there were 10 families in a village,a death every month was more than when there are 100 families with a death every week. This understanding can only come about in a positive interactive process which helps people to see it as 'truth' rather than 'trickery' to be feared and avoided.

Another factor that is often ignored by experts is the reality of the high infant and child mortality rates in most of Africa. Most women have lost a child, a nephew/niece or seen a friend's child die. Death of infants and children is a personal experience today in most of Africa. Would it be rational for those deeply interested in being survived by their children to limit the number of their offsprings in these circumstances? And this is not just 'a steak position' in Africa. It is the reality of human experience. Grant (1987) has stated: 'The bottom line is that there has never been a significant and sustained fall in birth rates which has not been preceded by a significant and sustained fall in child death rates'.

Grant (1987) has quoted the President of the Population Council of New York as saying in 1986 'There is no example in contemporary societies where fertility decline has preceded declines in infant and child mortality. Thus, among high mortality societies, an emphasis on infant and child survival should be an important element of population-related policies, as well as a goal to be pursued for its own sake.'

Grant (1987), further quoted the U.S. Academy of Science statement, 'Policies and programmes aimed at reducing infant and child mortality considerably below present levels may be an essential underpinning of government programmes for fertility control, as death rates are brought below 10-15 per thousand in present high-fertility, high-mortality countries birth rates should be correspondingly reduced.'

It seems there is no escaping from the reality that current high infant and child mortality rates are contributing to the population increase, no matter how 'illogical' that relationship may appear. Countries themselves and the international community need to be concerned with child survival issues in Africa rather than appear as if they want to zero in to 'snuff out' children in what is perceived as anti-child, indeed anti-African, manoeuvers.

The Ideologio-economic Riddle

It is sometimes alleged that Africa is having problems in food production because of 'too much involvement by the public sector'. It sometimes seems as if Africa's food problems would be diminished with more privatization and less public sector involvement. However an analysis by the Economic Commission for Africa in 1984 brought out the facts in table 67.4 (ECA 1984):

Table 67.4

Average Annual Growth Rates of Total Public Expenditure for all Sectors and for the Agricultural sector at Constant Prices

	All Sectors					Agriculture				
	1979	1980	1981	1982	Average 1979-82	1979	1980	1981	1982	Average 1979-82
North Africa	6.1	4.0	-6.0	3.6	1.8	-6.3	2.2	-0.3	-5.8	-2.6
West Africa	9.1	-15.7	-18.4	-1.7	-7.3	-10.4	18.9	-5.4	8.0	2.1
Central West Africa	20.3	-3.0	3.1	-8.8	2.4	68.7	-7.5	-34.2	-34.5	-9.5
Central Africa	–	–	–	–	–	-13.5	-48.6	10.0	39.1	-9.2
East and South Africa	14.5	-3.9	-11.0	-18.7	-5.5	27.0	4.9	–1.1	-30.7	-2.2

Source: FAO, 1983: Public Expenditure on Agriculture Computer Print-outs 13/12/83, Rome.
As quoted in E/ECA/CM.10/21 of February, 1984.

It can be seen from Table 67.4 that public expenditure on agriculture has been negative rather than too much. If anything, the cry is for more public expenditure in agriculture. However the low level of public expenditure in agriculture may simply be a reflection of the overall depressed economic situation. As has been stated, (Bell 1986) 'The disappointing economic progress of sub-Saharan Africa also characterizes and affects the food and nutrition sector. Low export earnings, for example, hurts agriculture. Farmers are deprived of needed inputs purchased from abroad – even hoes in some countries are hard to come by. Processing and transport capacity break down. The goods that farmers would like to buy are scarce, and they lose the incentive to produce crops to sell on the market'.

Those who push the argument of too much public involvement do so mainly to point out the often pushed view that free enterprise/free market and 'strengthening of the private sector' are to be preferred to strong government involvement. These views are presented as if a strong private sector has people's development as its priority. Can multinational corporations, as an example of free enterprise, be said to always work in the interest of the development prospect of the average person? Is the bank account of the corporation not, in the long run, the determining factor of what is done? Need one go into reciting examples of degrading that took place in the developing countries, for example in the Amazon forest, to hint that free enterprise as currently practised in dominant Western cultures isn't always positive?

On the other extreme there are other protagonists of various forms of dictatorship as the answer to Africa's current problems. What is inherently different from dictatorships of kings vis a vis dictatorship of any other clique? Isn't the only difference the fact that kings don't usually claim to be speaking on behalf of the people (How can they? They are divine!) while other dictatorship cliques claim to speak for the people because 'we come from the rank and file'? Haven't some people in history acquired the title of 'king' after rising from the rank and file and 'planting the title on their own foreheads'? How do these dictatorships differ in terms of what is done to the people's development and self-sufficiency?

Africa is being suffocated to death between those who see it in terms of the making of a free-wheeling, free enterprise market and those who would rather turn the continent into a series of dictatorships. It is difficult to understand why both groups don't see that what they are pushing is oppressive to the development and self-sufficiency of the people. They use different methods, of course but their messages are the same. 'We know what's good for you. We want to do it for you. In fact we have to do it for you!'. And there is hardly a chance to speak back. How does one speak back to a television set and other mass media techniques that keep telling you day in and day out what you must 'consume' to be normal? And what access does the average person have to react to the pronouncement of august committees?

So much of Africa is caught up in externally engineered ideological games that have no relevance to the African situation. Yet what is required is an African answer arising from an interactive process amongst the people of Africa. Bell (1986) has noted that 'There is no easy solution since the problems are complex and deep-rooted; they involve both human institutions and nature; and, in a large part, they are so specific to the African environment that the mere transfer of existing knowledge and techniques from other continents does not respond to the imperfectly understood African needs. Most of the obstacles arise from Africa's history, institutions, and climatic and geographical factors and can only be overcome or bypassed in the long run.

Reflections from Disturbances in Africa

It is unfortunate that the frequent changes of governments in Africa and the atrocities reported by in-coming leaders about the out-going ones, particularly after each coup d-etat point, in most cases to unacceptable excesses in the management of affairs of state. One can understand how a single individual can lose balance and get derailed. But it is a puzzle that this goes unchecked by members of cabinet/Council of Ministers. It is most distressing when it is realized that many of the politicians in positions of influence have got there through some elective procedure.

It would seem that recent historical factors and international ideological warfare are still taking their toll within Africa. However, there are positive indications that adjustment to the realities is taking place which may result in overall improved management of the affairs of state in Africa. It is encouraging that African leaders are getting together and seriously reviewing the circumstances on the continent. These meetings have produced important pointers to the future in the form of LAGOS PLAN OF ACTION (UN 1980) and the O.A.U. document entitled AFRICA PRIORITY PROGRAMME FOR ECONOMIC RECOVERY 1986-90 (OAU 1985c), the basis of the U.N. Resolution A/RES/S-13/21 of June 1986.

The next section presents one situation in which people can respond to meet the needs of relief and also help to contribute to development by helping people survive the disaster of famine in as sound a state as possible.

Modes of Food Distribution and Opportunities for Health Services

Food Distribution Modes

Presence of famine goes hand in hand with displacement of people as they search for food unless food is provided early. Sometimes, people get to a food distribution site in an advanced state of starvation requiring intensive therapeutic feeding. This is best done in a shelter situation which includes providing residential facilities requiring provisions, equipment and other supplies for total needs of the residents. This is expensive. Besides, residential arrangements have to be such that the shelter does not become a disease – breeding site that it could so easily become. Cooking facilities, and all other public health aspects of food handling have to be properly established, as an approach to providing food in famine shelters should only be a last resort. It is an approach to be avoided by all means possible, especially by distributing food before displacement of people takes place. It is crucial that food aid comes early in a famine emergency.

Food distribution to people who are non-resident is generally referred to as dry ration. Dry rations can be provided close to the home; that is within the village/community for relatively small populations. Or this can be done for fairly large populations in a centralized manner. This centralized manner means that people have to travel, usually walking, over long distances to collect food. In most cases, people coming for rations at food distribution sites are undernourished. Unless food distribution started before the state of undernutrition in the population, the experience is that people coming to food distribution sites have health needs that should be looked after. Because of the special circumstances of these people it is considered helpful to have a closer look at them and the kinds of needs they have beyond food rations. The rest of this chapter deals with that.

A Diagnosis of the Health Need at Food Distribution Sites

The WHO definition of health states that health is a state of complete physical, mental and social well-being and not merely the absence of disease or infirmity. This definition is the foundation on which the following remarks are built. How is the health of the people affected in circumstances where they have to go for food at distribution sites? A diagnostic look at the three dimensions of health: social, mental and physical may put some light on this.

Social Disruption: The people found at food distribution sites are often experiencing a state of social disorganization at various levels. This is at least true at the individual and family levels since individuals have to break away from their routine patterns of life to go to the food distribution sites on schedules organized by others. Community social events such as get togethers at coffee ceremonies (a beautiful Ethiopian custom) have to be abandoned. Weddings may have to be put off. If death occurs, the community support that is usual is often lacking as everyone is involved in a basic struggle for survival. In circumstances where people leave their homes and communities in a desperate search for food especially without a clear idea of where the food may be found, entire communities have been known to disintegrate as each one takes off in a different direction, many of them not to return as happened in Ethiopia in 1983/84/85. Animals on which many people depend for their livelihood often die or are sold in a desperate search to have something with which to buy food. People have been seen to sell core items from their houses and sometimes the wood used to build the roofs of their houses may be torn out to be sold. It is important, therefore to recognize that in dealing with those at food distribution sites, one is dealing with those whose social well-being has been disturbed. The greater the distance one has to walk away from one's village to the food distribution site, the more days are spent in walking etc. the greater the experience of social disruption.

Mental Unrest: It is difficult to be in a state of mental calmness if one is experiencing disruption in the basic patterns of one's life. It is even more difficult when in a previous famine the same people have seen members of their communities starve to death. They have seen their neighbours die. They have seen husbands and wives die. Their children have died in their arms. Perhaps the greatest state of restlessness and mental torture comes from feeling that this can happen all over again and the individual has no means to stop it. There is an inner state of restlessness in the gathered group as they wait for food, especially if there is uncertainty of whether there is food today and whether there will be food next time. Most adults in most societies of the world are brought up to feel responsible and to have a certain amount of control in the way one's life and one's family proceeds. To lose this sense of control completely leads to high levels of anxiety.

Both social restlessness and mental unrest are made worse when, in addition to a state of natural calamity, one is also dealing with problems of security. Situations such as what is happening in Mozambique, for example, where fighting is taking place in communities which are already hit by drought, insecurity compounds the famine problem. The people who receive food may not even be sure that the food will be theirs, as fighters may snatch it from them. In a nut-shell one can say that those at food distribution sites may be in varying degrees of mental unrest or anxiety as well as being in a disrupted social fabric.

Disease and Disability: A walk in the crowds waiting for food may reveal certain states of disease or disability. There may be wasting due to the effects of famine. In some situations, people say that they have had to walk for more than five days to get to the food distribution sites. In these long walks, often accompanied with young children, they may have had no water either to drink or to wash their faces or hands. They are thirsty and their faces are unwashed and a large proportion develop severe eye infections. In these long walks, people are exposed to the natural elements of wind and chills and many of them develop fevers and coughs. Many of the people complain of abdominal pains and diarrhoea. Many complain of heart burn and severe headaches, and many have chronic illnesses they have had for a long time due to the poor health infrastructure in most of these affected countries. One finds people coughing up blood while others have chronic tropical ulcers.

One also finds children and adults with burns resulting from makeshift cooking arrangements that are done in the open. One has seen people with severe bleeding from a fall or a cut on the scalp in this struggle for survival. And then, there are special risks of disease outbreaks due to the crowding. In particular, poor nutritional status predisposes children to fatal attacks of measles and diarrhoea.

It is clear that there is a need for health services at most food distribution sites. Those organizing health services need to have a clear perspective of the whole situation being faced. It should be noted that organizing health services is greatly affected by the food distribution process and how the location of the sites is undertaken.

Health at Food Distribution Sites

The Need for Orderliness and Reassurance of the People: On the basis of the social disruption referred to earlier on, one of the needs of the people to be responded to is to provide an atmosphere of orderliness and reassurance at the food distribution sites. This has to do with the way events are organized from the time people arrive at the food distribution site. This organized atmosphere helps to reduce the stressful feeling that the people have as they get the message that things are under control. It is often difficult to have an atmosphere of orderliness and reassurance with large groups of people. This points to the need to establish, where possible, food distribution sites close to where people live, within communities and villages.

In most situations of food distribution, there is waiting time. This time can become a period of stressful speculations. If health education sessions/demonstrations can be organized during this time, the waiting time can be changed to a time of learning or at least 'positive diversion'. The central aim of this activity should be to establish a sense of hope and a feeling of confidence and a dignity among the people during this difficult time. People need to be assisted to continue to feel good about themselves and their role in society.

In order for those distributing food and providing health care to carry this out well, it is necessary for the workers to have a time of training/orientation/preparation so that they themselves are reassured and confident enough to reassure those they are serving.

Disease Preventive Services: The first 'treatment' at food distribution sites is therefore the assurance of the *availability of food regularly*. To achieve this the national and international agencies have a major responsibility to ensure that people get the essential supplies regularly. Again the further away people come to get food, the greater their anxiety if they have to return without food.

Water to Drink, Wash Hands/Eyes and Facilities for Disposal of Human Waste: These are needed at food distribution sites. Organization of disposal of *human waste* is difficult in populations unfamiliar with even latrine use. But this must be established to reduce the hazards of spreading disease in large populations. Both of these headaches are avoided if food is distributed close to the homes.

Vitamin A Intake has an effect of strengthening the body linings including the lining of the eye and the lining of the gut that protects against damage. Its administration has been found to contribute to the survival of children under stress from lack of food. The Vitamin A capsule can be distributed by lay people. To avoid multiple doses with a risk of toxicity, a recording system needs to be established and linked with existing record systems for dry ration distribution.

Nutritional Screening/Surveillance: This can be an important activity at food distribution sites and can help the workers to calculate the percentage of those who fall in the high risk groups. This can help guide when to start and stop food distribution. In the Ethiopian setting, Save the Children Fund (UK) have established this at food distribution sites. It is simple and fast such that no delays occur to the flow of distributing food.

Promotion of Oral Rehydration Therapy (ORT): ORT demonstration at food distribution sites seems to be a good investment. One of the remarkable findings during the 1987/88 emergency in Ethiopia is from the area where Save the Children Federation (USA) supervised food distribution in the previous drought. Mothers were taught the importance of cereal-based ORT for saving lives from diarrhoea during the 1983/85 drought/famine by demonstration. It has been found that during the 1987/88 famine, more than 90% of the mothers have kept to this practice since they adopted it. This simple life saving therapy can be demonstrated at all food distribution sites using ORT packets that can be obtainable through UNICEF, WHO and other agencies.

Immunization Services: Especially administration of *measles* vaccines in children nine months to five years has been shown to reduce mortality during famine when the nutritional status is compromised. This single injection procedure should be routine at all food distribution sites using the same record as the food distribution register to avoid repeated doses. The other five antigens in the EPI programme have also been administered in the context of food distribution in Ethiopia. In the 1983/85 famine a church NGO was able to achieve full immunization status in all children under five in an area of about 100,000 people. If this had been the practice at all food distribution sites, the level of immunized children under five years would have been considerably higher than the 5% in Ethiopia in 1985.

Curative Services: Whether or not to provide curative services at food distribution sites leads to debate because of the potential to encourage people to stay and turn a food distribution site into a shelter. In the current food distribution activities in Ethiopia, the Ministry of Health has taken the pragmatic position of establishing first aid services at large food distribution sites or those sites located far from the health centres/stations; otherwise, the sick are encouraged to go to the health centre/health station near the food distribution sites. These health facilities in the drought-affected areas are being strengthened with additional drugs and equipment supplied by UNICEF and some NGOs with donations from the international community.

Conclusion to the Chapter

The central conclusion of a review of public health aspects of famine and malnutrition is that famine maims and kills and the problems of hunger and under/malnutrition are 'immense'. The challenge to the national and international communities is enormous.

It has been heartening to note that given a large starving population, people have responded to end this inhuman state of affairs. The response of the international community, once the *people* are made aware of the problem has given reason for hope.

However, it is to be noted that people get tired of being required to respond to these disasters often; and so they need to be informed that recurrences are not due to carelessness on the part of the people they assisted previously. People need to be made to realize that without sustained assistance these recurrences are unavoidable. African countries will remain fragile since African governments and people cannot immediately reverse the underlying causes of drought alone. It is therefore essential that people who donate for relief be made aware that they could help stop these recurrences through a donation to development/rehabilitation efforts. Governments which are not experiencing similar misfortunes need to look at these circumstances with empathy. It is a common practice that in addition to direct contributions to governments, other channels are also utilized. These include the UN system and Non-Governmental Organizations (NGOs). In Ethiopia the Emergency Prevention and Preparedness Group (EPPG) of the UN, the World Food Programme, UNDRO, WHO and UNICEF are working closely in efforts related to the current emergency. Examples of NGOs are Save the Children Fund, UK (SCF/UK) and Save the Children Federation, USA (SCF/USA). SCF/UK and SCF/USA are contributing in the Ethiopian setting both to relief and rehabilitating activities in some areas. These are examples of what International NGOs can do. The Ethiopian Red Cross Society is assisting rehabilitation in another area of the country. People can reach out to people in the spirit of the People-to-People movement if that is the preferred route.

It is essential that people find ways to express solidarity for survival. Linking development into relief has the greatest chance of success when food distribution is close to home. Left alone, African governments cannot provide the required logistic support to distribute food to the community level due to financial constraints. Yet this is the preferred path if these recurrences are to end. The support of the international community, the world's people, is crucial.

In some Kenyan villages, they say 'food is health', and without healthy populations, it is impossible to achieve much. Dr. H. Mahler the past WHO Director-General has stated, 'health is not everything but without health we have nothing'. Investments required for health development are shunned because it has been erroneously said, 'Health is a bottomless pit'. This is false. Establishing a viable health care infrastructure is not a bottomless pit. Perhaps demand for health services is a bottomless pit. And no one is talking of demand. The issue is that the countries of the world need to have viable health infrastructures in place in order to meet the kinds of needs that arise in situations of disaster. This necessity needs to be addressed seriously by both national and international communities. When a country has 15% of the population with access to health care, should this only be noted and bypassed? It seems the answer should be NO. Is it NO?

References

Bell, D. E. and Reich, M. R. (Eds). 1986. *Health Nutrition and Economic Crises.* Published by Auburn House Publishing Co. Dover MA for the Havard School of Public Health.

Economic Commission For Africa. 1984. *Apparent Discrepancy Between Increasing Resources Allocation to Food and Agriculture in Africa and the Declining Performance of the Sector.* E/ECA/CM. 10/21. Addis Ababa.

Economic Commission For Africa. 1985. *The Situation of Food and Agriculture in Africa.* E/ECA/CM. 12/12/Rev. 1. ECA. Addis Ababa.

Economic Commission For Africa 1985. *Africa's Food and Agriculture Crisis Prospect and Proposals for 1985 and 1986.* (E/ECA/CM. 11/29). ECA. Addis Ababa.

Food and Agriculture Organisation (FAO) of the United Nations. 1985. *The State of Food and Agriculture 1984*. FOA Agriculture Series No. 18, Rome.

Food and Agriculture Organisation of the United Nations. 1987. *The Fifth World Food Survey*. Rome.

Food and Agriculture Organisation of the United nations. 1986. *Atlas of African Agriculture*. Rome.

Grant, James P. 1987. *Fewer Deaths/Fewer Birth: A Virtuous Circle*. An address by James P. Grant, Executive Director of UNICEF to the International Conference on Better Health for Women and Children Through Family Planning, UNICEF, New York, NY.

Liner, S. 1986. *Disaster Relief for Development*. Stockholm, Sweden. A Study Commissioned by the Foreign Ministry of Sweden and SIDA.

Organisation of African Unity, 1985. *Drought and Famine Have Triggered Off Massive Displacement of People*. African Refugees Issue No. 7 June 1985.

Organisation of African Unity 1985. R*eport of the Secretary General on the Visit to Drought Affected Countries*. CM/1308/ XL III O.A.U. Addis Ababa.

Organisation of African Unity 1985. *Africa's Priority Programme for Economic Recovery 1986-1990*. OAU, Addis Ababa.

United Nations Children's Fund. 1988. *State of the World's Children 1988*.

United Nations Programme of Action for African Economic Recovery and Development, 1986–1990 (A/RES/5-13/2 of June 1985).

United Nations General Assembly. 1980 A/S-11/14 *Annex 1: Lagos Plan of Action for the Implementation of Monrovia Strategy for the Economic Development of Africa*. New York. NY.

Were, Miriam K. 1982. *Organization Management of Community-based Health Care*. UNCIEF, Nairobi.

68

Information Resources For Health Workers

B. Weintraub and L. Frenkiel

Seeking knowledge from the medical and health literature is like a game. You can win if you understand and follow specific rules and guidelines. If you master the skills needed, in the course of your work you will be able to draw upon the world's accumulated recorded experiences and knowledge. Your library, whatever its size, should be your most important 'ally' in this task. Besides its archival and traditional role of storing books and other written material, the library has become an information centre providing the user with the information needed.

This brief guide is intended to familiarize the student with some of the basic services available and some of the vocabulary encountered in the medical library. The library should be considered as the place to go for specific information and as a life-long learning centre.

The Information Chain

One of the ways that information sources have been classified is the following:

1. *Primary Sources* are where you find the most recent and original information: primary sources include journal articles and original books. Taken all together, these materials form the archive or permanent record of the progress of science.
2. *Secondary Sources* provide keys to information: these are indexes, bibliographies, etc. For example, a card catalogue is a key to the book collection; an index in the back of a book or journal is a key to its contents; a specialized index like the *Index Medicus* is a key to gain access to the mass of medical periodical publications.
3. *The Tertiary Sources* provide a composite of existing information. Information is not original in itself and authors are reporting what is already known and understood: these are textbooks, encyclopaedias and handbooks.

As a student you will probably need tertiary sources more than anything else but as your knowledge and expertise grow you'll move naturally to primary sources to find out 'what's new?' and to secondary sources such as indexes to find the location of information you want.

Of the primary sources, periodicals are the most important for the medical or health researcher. They report within a relatively short time discoveries and experiences which could not be published in book form for several months or even years. They are the vehicle for the publication of articles, reviews of progress in research, case reports, correspondence,etc. Journal articles focus on a relatively narrow subject and should supply details covering all of the aspects of the work (methodology, process of research, conclusion and discussion).

Databases and Electronic Information Transfer

Information for the health care worker comes in a variety of forms. Primary and tertiary sources are still most readily available in print versions. Books and journals in this form are referred to as *hardcopy*.

Secondary Sources are available in hardcopy and also in two *electronic forms – online* and on *computer disks or diskettes*. The indexing and abstracting services are becoming less and less available in printed form. Where hardcopy does still exist, it is generally less complete and not as up-to-date as the corresponding electronic version.

Online

Online retrieval means *accessing* information that is stored in a computer in a different location – often in a different city or on a different continent. Many *databases* are *loaded* onto a big computer, which is referred to as the *vendor*. When information is needed, the vendor is accessed from a *computer terminal* via a *modem*. A modem is a device that converts *digital data* from the computer into *analog* signals that can be carried over ordinary *telecommunications lines*. When the analog signal reaches its destination, it is then reconverted by a modem back into digital format.

In this manner, an *interactive* conversation can be conducted between someone seeking information sitting at a computer terminal and a vendor in a far way location. Questions are asked in a *structured language* and the distant computer is searched for the relevant information. The answers are then relayed through telecommunication lines back to the requester. One can research many millions of bibliographic references and receive an answer almost immediately.

Diskettes and Cd-Rom

Another way to access databases is to have them available at your location. Databases are purchased or rented and accessed from one's own microcomputer. The information arrives by regular mail at certain set intervals, monthly for example, each time that the database is updated. The database is supplied either on computer diskettes or on *cd-rom disks*. Cd-rom is an acronym for *compact disk-read only memory*. This name reflects the fact that these diskettes serve as a store of information (memory) but cannot be altered, added to or deleted by the user (read only).

One cd-rom is capable of storing 550 megabytes of information. A cd-rom can hold the equivalent of about 200,000 printed pages of information, or the equivalent of about 200 textbooks. Each one comes in a plastic container of dimensions 14cm x12.5cm x 1cm. The amount of information that can be held on this medium and stored in an area the size of one room is by far greater than the amount of information held by the worlds greatest libraries collectively.

In order to extend the use of a given cd-rom to many terminals simultaneously, some hospitals and universities have set up *lan's (local area networks)*. A lan enables many users to access a database at the same time from different close locations.

A cd-rom has the advantage of being independent of the telecommunications infrastructure. To access databases locally on cd-roms, one needs a subscription to the databases, a suitable microcomputer, a source of electricity, and a more or less reliable postal service. An advantage of the online systems over the cd-rom subscription is that of being independent of the postal service.

The range of electronic services available has been expanding rapidly. The most important services available in the health field at this time are secondary sources of information. All of the examples mentioned below are available in hardcopy, online, and on either cd-rom or diskettes. Examples of output of some databases are shown in the accompanying figures 68.1. 68.2 and 68.3.

Medline

Medline is the world's foremost medical database. The subject coverage is all areas of medicine and allied health, veterinary medicine, and the basic life sciences. Due to its comprehensive coverage and low cost, Medline is usually the database searched when looking for references with abstracts to the medical literature. Its print counterparts include *Index Meicus, International Nursing Index,* and *Index to Dental Literature.* Medline covers medical literature contained in 3,200 journals from more than 70 countries. It is produced by the United States *National Library of Medicine. (NLM)*

Embase

Embase is the second major biomedical database. It provides citations with abstracts on all aspects of human medicine and related disciplines. Its coverage does not include veterinary medicine, nursing or dentistry. The journals screened are published in 100 countries. Embase is particularly strong in the areas of pharmaceuticals and environmental health. There is a marked bias towards non-USA journals.

Comparison of Medline and Embase

When is each one searched?

The overlap of Medline with Embase for an average search is about 40%. This surprisingly low figure results from different selection policies of the two producers. When an exhaustive search of the medical literature is desired, it is necessary to search both of these sources. In fact, however, due in part to the higher cost of Embase, most medical searches are run only on Medline.

Embase should be searched in addition to Medline on those occasions when drug or environmental information is sought; the information might be better covered in non-U.S. journals, a particular question needs to be checked completely without any doubt as to the thoroughness of the search, or when Medline fails to satisfy the information needed.

Biosis including Biological Abstracts

Biosis online is the major database serving the entire field of biology. Over 9,300 serials published in over 100 countries are covered. Included are patents, conference proceedings, books, dissertations, reviews and research reports. Biosis can be useful to the health worker in that its indexing system allows searching by biological concepts and taxonomic groups.

Current Contents

Current Contents is an updating service. It provides copies of the table of contents pages of current journals. This tool can be of particular value to the health worker at a location where many journals are not available locally. It enables one to keep abreast of the latest happenings in the professional literature.

Science Citation Index

Science Citation Index is a database that contains citations to articles in all fields of science and engineering – including medicine. This tool is not, in general, as useful for the health care worker as are the databases devoted specifically to the fields of health. It is noteworthy in this discussion for one special feature that is not available with the other databases discussed. It can be searched by article cited. This feature enables one to follow up a particular article after it has appeared in print – to find where it has been cited in later works.

Other Services Available

Hundreds of health related databases are available covering just about every area of medical specialization imagineable. For most work, the databases mentioned above are more than adequate to meet the information needs. Some health workers, depending on their type of work and specialty, might find it advantageous to refer to the more specialized databases. Examples of topics covered by specialist databases are AIDS, cancer, drug and alcohol addiction, child abuse and neglect, gerontology, mental health, nucleotide sequences, occupational health, population and demographics, nursing, psychology, sociology, toxic chemicals registries and so on . A medical librarian should be contacted to clarify which databases will best meet the needs at hand.

Regional Databases

National and regional databases are available. These may cover the literature of a particular country or geographical area, deal with the special needs in one part of the world, or draw heavily on the literature of local languages. Indigenous sources of information can supply important information of use locally that may lack relevance to the larger international market.

As an illustration of the above, much of the information dealing with malaria or malnutrition may not have significance to indexes aimed primarily at meeting the needs of the developed countries. More generally, experience gained from dealing with problems resulting from a combination of illiteracy and poverty can be expected to be poorly represented in the big international databases. On the other hand, these databases do contain large amounts of material which might otherwise be overlooked if only local databases were to be accessed. Thus, both regional and international databases should be consulted when relevant.

One example of regional database is *Lilacs*. Lilacs contains bibliographic citations and abstracts from the health-related literature published in Latin America and the Caribbean regions. The interface software is available in Spanish, Portugese and in English. Lilacs covers 250 Latin American journals, as compared to Index Medicus' coverage of 44.

The Role of the Medical Librarian

Some databases are designed for the health care worker to search without the help of an intermediary. One such example of this is Current Contents. Other databases, despite claims to the contrary by the producers of some of these products, are designed to be searched by professional librarians. Medline, Embase, and Biosis are examples of such databases.

Artificial Intelligence computer programmes are called *expert systems* when they are designed to mimic the manner in which human experts reach decisions. The science of expert system has not yet reached the level of sophistication necessary to translate an information need into the structured language required for searching most databases.

Medical libraries provide a wide range of inter – library loan services that enable one to obtain just about any piece of literature that is available anywhere. Some of these services are run by private companies, government organizations, groups of libraries, and the World Health Organization.

If you do not have access to a professional medical librarian, then you might need to learn for yourself some of the more advanced skills needed for access to the world's literature. There are some health care workers that search databases themselves and are pleased with their results – without being aware that they are missing most of the literature relevant to their topic. Searching properly is a trained skill that needs to be studied and practised in order to be mastered.

Accessing information is a sophisticated and rapidly changing field. It is best to consult with a professional medical librarian to gain an understanding of which resources are available at your location to best meet your specific needs.

References

Grogan, Denis, *Science and Technology: An Introduction to the Literature*. 3rd Ed. Rev. London: Linnet, 1976.

Panel On Information Technology and the Conduct of Research (U.S.) *Information Technology and the Conduct of Research*. Washington, D.C.: National Academy Press, 1989.

Medical Libraries: A User Guide. London: British Medical Association, 1987.

Medical Libraries–One World: Resources, Cooperative, Services. 5th International Congress on Medical Librarianship. Proceedings. Tokyo 1985.

Morton, L.C. and Godbolt, S. (eds.) *Information Sources in the Medical Sciences*, 3rd Ed. London: Butterworths, 1984.

Online Databases in the Medical and Life Sciences. New York: Caudra/Elsevier, 1987.

Poland, U.H. (ed.) *World Directory of Biological and Medical Sciences Libraries*. Munchen: Saurs, 1988.

Roper, Fred W., and Boorkman, Jo Anne, *Introduction to Reference Sources in the Health Sciences*. Chicago: Medical Library Association, 1980.

The following journals published by Pemberton Press were consulted during the preparation of this work:

Database
Cd-rom Professional
Online

Fig. 68.1

A sample Medline entry. Data fields are the title (ti), author (au), address (ad), literature source of the article (so), language of the article (la) and country of publication of the journal (cp).

TI:	Parasitology survey of *Onchocerca volvulus* infection in the Nimiyama Chiefdom, Kono District, Sierra Leone
AU:	Gbakima–AA; White-PT; Bockarie-A; Komba-Kono-G
AD:	Department of Biological Sciences, Njala University College, Freetown.
SO:	Trop-Georgr-Med. 1989 Jul; 41(3): 201-7
LA:	ENGLISH
CP:	NETHERLANDS

AB: Infection due to Onchocerca volvulus was investigated in the Nimiyama Chiefdom, Kono District, Sierra Leone, where *Simullium damnosum* s.l. is known to breed but no data on the prevalence and intensity of *O. volvulus* infection exists. Of the 735 individuals sampled by the skin snip method in five villages, 471 (64%) were infected. The infection rates for males was significantly (p less than 0.05) higher than that of the females. Two hundred and ninety-one (70.0%) of the 416 males skin snipped and 180 (56.0%) of the 323 of their female cohorts were infected. The intensity of infection increased with age, with the younger cohorts presenting lower microfilarial density (MFD). Palpable nodules were observed in 230 (48.4%) of individuals found positive for skin microfilariae and in 37 (5.0%) individuals found negative for skin microfilariae. It is concluded that *O. volvulus* infection is mesoendemic in the Nimiyama Chiefdom, with the intensity of infection increasing with age.

Fig. 68.2

Sample record from Current Contents on Diskette. Data fields shown are author (au) title (ti), language, (la), address of the author (ad) and literature source (so).

AU:	Dadzie KY
AU:	Remme J
AU:	Alley ES
AU:	Desole G
TI:	Changes in Ocular Onchocerciasis 4 and 12 Months After Community – Based Treatment with Ivermectin in a Holoendemic Onchocerciasis Focus.

LA: English
AD: KY Dadzie, Onchocerciasis Control, Programme W. Africa, Bp 549, Ouagadougou, Burkina Faso
SO: T RS TROP M 1990 JAN-FEB; 84(1): 103-108.

Fig. 68.3

Sample record from Biological Abstracts. Data fields shown are title (ti), author (au), corporate source (cs), publication year (py) and language of article (la).

TI: Seasonal population changes and malaria transmission potential of *Anopheles pharoensis* and the minor anophelines in Mwea Irrigation Scheme, Kenya.
AU: MUKIAMA-T-K; NWANGI-R-W
CS: Dep. Botany, Univ. Nairobi, P.O. Box 30197, Nairobi, Kenya
SO: ACTA TROPICA 46 (3): 181-190
PY: 1989
LA: English

AB: A study in 1984 and 1985 showed that *Anopheles gambiae* s.l. and *An. pharoensis* were the major anophelines in Mwea Irrigation Scheme, Kenya, constituting 83.86% and 15.69%of the catch respectively. Four minor species made up the remaining 0.45%. The irrigation phase of the rice cultivation cycle in August, which linked the flooding effects of the two rainy seasons, resulted in major population increases of *An. pharoensis* and enabled continuous breeding for up to 9 months per year. The average of mean monthly proportions of unfed, bloodfed, and gravid females was 26.6, 58.8, and 14.6% respectively. The Plasmodium falciparum sporozoite rates for *An. pharoensis* were 1.3% by ELISA and 0.68% by dissection, while those for An. funestus were 1.7% by ELISA and 1.25% by dissection. An. pharoensis can contribute to the epidemiology of Malaria in the Mwea area.

69

Health Education: The Role of the Public Health Doctor

F.J. Bennett

We can assume that all medical students in Africa now have adequate training in the behavioural sciences, and have an actual course, together with some practical periods, devoted to health education. What is lacking, however, in many countries is adequate experience of the problems of working in a community, perhaps with primary health workers and several health units, such as a small hospital, health centres, and dispensaries. This chapter aims at giving some practical guidelines to the young doctor who realizes the need for health education in his community but is not sure either how to start programmes or how to rejuvenate ineffective ones.

Information: The Starting Point

The easiest and most relevant starting point lies in obtaining information about the clinical problems flowing into the outpatients department and wards. An analysis (or a new and critical look at the routine analysis) will show which problems are greatest in terms of frequency or increasing frequency, mortality, disability, social consequences, and recurrent epidemics. This can be done by reviewing each area of work that keeps records: the adult outpatients, the MCH clinic, the maternity wards, paediatric wards, the gynaecology clinic, etc. These figures of course reflect demand, and do not necessarily indicate true community needs.

Another starting point is to examine the returns of various services that can actually be related to population denominators. How many immunizations have been done and how many children still require them in the population? How many antenatal cases are seen out of a calculated number of pregnancies? How many births receive skilled attention out of the number of total births calculated from the birth rate? How many latrines are built, compared with the proportion of the population without latrines? What proportion of the population use piped water supplies?

Yet another starting point is the needs of the people. This is more difficult, and implies a prior morbidity survey, perhaps on a random sample of the population, or perhaps on a stratified random sample. This is getting closer to the concept of a prior 'community diagnosis'. In fact, one of the reasons for a community diagnosis is to enable all health services, including the health education component, to be planned realistically.

Another less used but more effective starting point is from the desires, wants, and felt needs of the community; and this also takes cognizance of their priorities. Felt needs could come directly from a health committee, or even a questionnaire administered to a representative sample of the community.

It can be seen that some of this basic information about problems may be available, but perhaps has never been analyzed in a way that gives some estimate of the size of each problem or of their distribution in the community. The methods most useful are those of epidemiology, as has been suggested by Barker (1976).

Having ascertained the major problems (for example, tuberculosis), causes of diseases (for example, lack of latrines) it is then necessary to seek further information on the reasons why there are problems. The most useful method is the K.A.P. (Knowledge, Attitudes, Practices) questionnaire. *Knowledge* of a condition may relate to recognition of signs and symptoms, diagnostic methods, complications, treatment and prevention. *Attitudes* involves people's feelings about a problem, and can relate to the degree of perceived personal threat, the seriousness and treatability or the ease of prevention of a condition, the degree of social stigma attached to it, or to a wide variety of other qualities that people may perceive. Attitudes can be rated on a scale that ranges from one extreme feeling to the opposite. Thus, one mother may feel poliomyelitis is a great threat to her child; whereas another may feel that it is a negligible possibility. One person may hold the attitude that gonorrhea is a trivial, easily treated disease; and another may feel it is a very serious disease, which is difficult to treat. *Practices* are what people do: and questions to probe this area should ask about what is done on first suspecting an illness, what health facilities are used, whether children are immunized, whether a latrine has been built and is used, what food is given to children,and so on. In analyzing a K.A.P survey, it is useful to break down the replies by age, sex, socio-economic or educational status, and locality and ethnic group. This then defines the target groups most in need of health education: because it will be found that health knowledge, attitudes, and behaviour are not uniformly distributed.

Thinking About the Information

The next step in preparing for health education is to use all the information gathered for making a health education diagnosis. Or perhaps it would be more accurate to say a behavioural diagnosis; because the process is to first define the behavioural correlates of the priority diseases or health problems, and then to decide on what health education has to be given to correct that behaviour. Health education is here considered in the broad terms stated by WHO (1969), viz. it concerns all those experiences of an individual group or community that influence beliefs, attitudes, and behaviour in respect of health, as well as the processes and efforts necessary for producing change, when change is necessary for optimal health.

This process of thinking or planning is best done as a group exercise with all the staff involved and also with representatives of the community, such as health committees and primary health workers. In many countries of Africa, there are cadres of health education workers. These may be at degree, diploma, certificate, or even so-called grass-roots levels. Their actual contribution to surveys and planning depends on their level of training; but they must always be involved, if they themselves have not been prime movers.

An example might make the process clear. In one nutrition survey in East Africa, it was found that 30 per cent of children under five years had low weight for age, representing a mild form of protein-calorie malnutrition, and 2 per cent had actual marasmic kwashiorkor, marasmus or kwashiorkor. Most of these malnourished children were in the second year of life. It was also clear that mothers only took their children regularly to the MCH clinics during the first year of life, so as to get injections (immunization); and that after that the infants were too heavy to carry and too small to walk. Mothers did not realize that the second year of life is a danger period, nor the value of nutritional surveillance by weighing; nor did they expect to get any nutritional advice from young nurses. There was a long history in the area of inappropriate advice from health workers, who previously emphasized the use of milk and eggs and other expensive or difficult-to-obtain forms of protein. In their homes mothers either relied too much on the breast and delayed introducing other foods, or were weaning babies increasingly early. Thin maize gruel, diluted to be given by bottle, was being introduced, and was very low in calories. Beans and green leaves, which were available, were seldom introduced early enough into children's diets. Episodes of diarrhoeal disease were common, as a result of poor food hygiene, contaminated water supplies, and increasing bottle feeding. Intervals between births were relatively short. Husbands were often away as migrant labourers in the towns; leaving wives to do the cultivation of the fields, and with little time to tend the small infants, who were often left in the care of older children. Previous attempts at nutrition education had been limited to talks and demonstrations by nutrition educators, given at MCH clinics and sometimes to groups of women either in the markets or at a meeting.

Discussion between health workers and women in that community using the above facts would probably emphasize that malnutrition affects a large number of children, and so is really a big community problem; that it contributes to deaths of children in the community; and that the clinics are not seeing these children frequently enough to make an impact on the problem. (The good immunization coverage in the first year of life, however, helps considerably). In addition, future dietary advice should be given nearer to people's homes, and must be realistic; and the trend towards early weaning should be halted. Gruel should be made less watery, and it should be fed with a cup and spoon; and beans and green leaves could be introduced earlier. Simple measures should be taken to ensure adequate fluid intake when children get diarrhoea. There is, lastly, a need for family planning; although there is as yet no demand for it.

Health educators could spend a day in discussing the details of the content and the strategy of education required to deal with the above points. And then it would also be necessary to plan the method, work out audio-visual aids, and train workers.

In many parts of Africa, this process does not go on exclusively in the far-off rooms of the Health Education Unit of the Ministry of Health. Nor does it just go on in the Medical Officer of health's office at local level; nor is it the exclusive province of a professional health educator. It is now a process which should be worked through by the mothers and fathers themselves, with assistance from more trained educators who have the scientific knowledge (but no prerogative right to that knowledge) which can always be simplified down to the essentials that anyone could grasp. Recently attempts have been made to have child-to-child health care and education, and thus even school children have become involved (Aaron and Hawes 1979).

Details of Content of Education

Knowledge and ideas change, and some of what was considered essential to teach the general public twenty years ago is now regarded as wrong, inaccurate, harmful, useless, or immaterial. It is now difficult to eliminate previously introduced ideas about the need for expensive vitamin preparations, or dried milk powder, or the idea that immunization is only advisable for completely 'well' children, and so on. The doctor who wants to introduce new ideas into his community must therefore be very sure of the permanent value of what he is doing. It is safer to adapt or re-emphasize ideas and practices that are already in the community, but which may only belong to certain healthy groups. In nutrition work, for example, it is more reasonable to ask 'in this community, what are the ideas, attitudes, and practices of the mothers of the well-nourished children? They are the people who can describe the most applicable content for local education better than any textbook.

Method of Changing Behaviour and of Ensuring Effective Communication

Much has been written on motivation for change, and on communication and on the problem of different people's perception of a given message (Scotney 1976; Morley 1973). The practising doctor on the whole will have to deal with three types of situations. The first is the ongoing routine contact between his staff and the community for example, maternal and child health clinics and health visiting programmes. The second is where he branches out into a new and specific programme. The objectives and targets, for example a campaign against an outbreak of cholera, or a project to deal with an upsurge of sexually transmitted disease in secondary school students. The third is where he and his staff act as stimulators, motivators, facilitators and resource people to a community-generated and community-executed primary health care programme.

The first is difficult, and the most likely to be congealed in dead routines – a fifteen minutes harangue by a nurse at a group of pregnant women sitting in rows, and giving the required responses to the usual rhetorical questions. If a health education review is held once a month at a team meeting then staff members can discuss their feelings about such programmes. Usually new ideas are suggested. The doctor may have come across some innovative method being tried elsewhere. The nurse giving the talk or leading the discussion will welcome these suggestions.

The second situation is fairly precise and easy to work out. The target groups are defined. The educational objectives can be worked out precisely. Evaluation, before and after, can be built into the programme. The timing, place, and staff required can be planned. Suitable audio-visual aids can be made or obtained from many sources; and they can also be pretested to ensure correct perception of their intended messages.

The third approach, through health workers (PHW) drawn from and chosen by the villages and working in the villages with self-organized groups, seems to be the latest direction taken by rural health work. PHWs can get primary friendship groups together to discuss and work out their own problems, and can call in additional health workers as resource people or facilitators. The doctor invited to such a group meeting can explain what he sees as the problem, breaking it down to simple levels of behaviour, and can elicit solutions, and perhaps discreetly guide the discussion. The doctor can also stress various incentives, and the advantages gained from certain behaviour. The final decisions about implementation remain with the people. Aids to discussion depend on the local culture and the doctor's imagination – a visit to the market, a strip of X-ray film for measuring arm circumference, a beer bottle filled with water for making up the salt and sugar solution for oral rehydration, a picture (or perhaps a poster) showing some clinical signs, immunization material for a demonstration, and so on. More often the doctor will be in the background, just sparking off the imagination of his workers, who in their turn supervize the primary health workers.

One of the reasons why the doctor has been mentioned is that he should occasionally try out methods, media, and aids himself, so that he can participate in staff discussion with a greater insight into what is useful and what is not.

Training of Staff

Fortunately in most parts of Africa, there is now a cadre of health educators trained to a level where they can train others. So many districts can have regular refresher courses on health education. This is necessary as refresher courses in clinical medicine or orthopaedic surgery; and any district that has never attempted to improve the health education it provides by improving the training of its workers should start immediately. These refresher courses usually lay stress on group dynamics, personal interaction, and establishing true helping relationships. They then go on to processes of working with people, defining educational objectives, giving skills in preparation of material and aids to learning, and perhaps to setting up simple criteria for evaluation.

Review of Programmes–Evaluation

Scientific evaluation of health education programmes is difficult and time-consuming, and needs adequate control and sample size if it is to be valid.

However, evaluation can also go on at simpler levels, and can provide a useful feedback for modifying programmes. The original starting points mentioned for example, a high prevalence of disease or a low proportion of children being immunized, can be kept under review to see if there is improvement. If target groups have been defined – for example, immigrants to town – these can be specifically surveyed, or records can be kept. KAP surveys can be done periodically on samples of the population. Immediate feedback on group discussions can be obtained by recording the questions asked and the answers given to the questions. Follow-up records of home visits can sometimes show changes, if these are specifically looked for. For every phase or facet of health education in the district the health staff should aim at having at least one criterion for evaluation that is valid and easy to obtain. A yearly timetable should specify definite dates for review of this information. Evaluation and analysis of records is only useful if it improves the actual effectiveness of the health education.

Resources, Allies and Co-workers

Fortunately, improvement of health through educational means does not only come about through the activities of health educators. The workers in agriculture, education, community development, and other departments are also striving to change people's behaviour in some ways; often in the direction of improved standards of living and improvements in health status. Religious organizations (such as missions) also often have much the same objectives, and are now increasingly involved in group work in the community, sometimes even to the point of training primary health care workers. All of these resources in the community need co-ordination, and sometimes technical guidance. This could well come from an enthusiastic, dedicated, and energetic doctor. However it takes energy and time to co-ordinate a variety of agencies, and not every doctor is capable of this extra outlay of effort – but it is a challenge.

Summary

The doctor's role in health education includes:

(1) the acquisition of relevant information about diseases and their causes which are related to behaviour;

(2) the analysis of these data in a manner that can be used for planning health education;

(3) ensuring that the community is actively involved in the planning process with the health workers;

(4) guiding people as to the possible methods, media, and aids that are available through health channels, and trying to stimulate workers to explore new methods;

(5) training and organizing refresher courses for community workers, health workers, and others;

(6) helping with the co-ordination of different cadres engaged in health education; and

(7) evaluation of health education by criteria that can be obtained through health services or health-service-organized surveys, or by the communities themselves if there is a primary health care programme.

References

Aaron, A. and Haves, H. (1979). *Child-to-child*, Macmillan, London.

Baker, D.J.P. (1976). *Practical Epidemiology Medicine in the Tropics Series*. Churchill Livingstone, London.

Morley, D. (1973). *Paediatric Priorities in the Developing World*. Butterworth, London.

Scotney, N. (1976). *Health Education–A Manual for Medical Assistants and Other Rural Health Workers*. African Medical and Research Foundation, Nairobi.

WHO (1969). Research in Health Education, *Tech. Rep. Ser. Wld. Hlth Org. 432*.

70

Section A

The Principles of Health Education

Z.A. Ademuwagun

What is Health Education?

The concept 'health education' has meant different things to different people. But there are general areas of agreement among professional health educators about the functional role of health education in health, education, and other social welfare programmes.

Health education in this text is a term embracing knowledge, attitudes, and practices (KAP). It is concerned with the study of consumers' behaviour towards diseases and health problems, as well as their reactions towards health programmes and the dispensers of health services in the consumers' total environmental setting. It is also concerned with the use of educational processes, including consumer participation, and of motivational, facilitating, and helping methods and techniques paying particular attention to the total setting of the consumers, to bring about positively healthy behaviour.

Health education as a process of positively influencing, changing or reinforcing people's health knowledge, attitudes, and practices has long been recognized as an integral part of all health programmes. To this end, it is concerned with *learning* and *change* in health matters. However, many previous text books have associated health education solely with *changes* in people's health behaviour. This is an over narrow approach to the mechanics of health education, and based on the wrong assumption that all consumers' existing health behaviour is negative in its effect.

Health education is concerned with health problem analysis and health programme planning. It is a dynamic and vitalizing force, whose constant focus is on how to make the programme acceptable, available, and accessible to the health consumers. Thus, health education is consumer-oriented in its operational processes. Through operational research, it seeks to identify those things which block the achievement of the objectives of health programmes, and then plans for their removal or circumvention. Its goal is to find ways and means of facilitating positive health behaviour, such as a positive response to health interventions or a maximum utilization of the available health services. In other words, its goal is health action or practice.

Basically, health education utilizes the methods of systems analysis, holistic planning, and communicating health information in such a way as to render what is planned or communicated meaningful and agreeable to the target population. It also involves methods of bringing about the co-operation and active participation of the target population in defining their health needs and overcoming the problems, practicable ways of meeting the needs and overcoming the problems, participating in implementing and evaluating these plans, and constant feedback through effective communication between health workers and health consumers.

In its approach to the analysis of problems, health education is concerned with how far the success or failure of a health programme can be attributed to the programme initiators (or policy makers/planners), the health workers, the health consumers, and/or the environment in which the programme is introduced and administered. This approach is ultimately based on ecological thinking in terms of the interaction between *man and his environment.* The goals of such analysis is to evolve a comprehensive approach to planning and solving a health problem in the total setting of the consumer.

In short, health education is not just limited to 'health information,' as it has been narrowly conceived to be in the past by some people in Africa. Rather it is a combination of activities, which include health problem diagnosis with the consumers, educational planning and organizing with the consumers, establishing an effective process of communicating health information, environmental manipulation, human motivation, and evaluation and research with the consumers to ensure that any health intervention or programme may be acceptable, available, and accessible to the consumers.

Rationale for Studying Health Education as a Discipline

Health education as a professional discipline concerned with the forces which influence particular health behaviour is a complex discipline, because of its focus on human behaviour. Generally, it is difficult to predict human behaviour once and for all, because human beings respond to particular stimuli in their complex environment differently at different particular points in time, depending on the ecological variables or forces affecting them. In other words, the environment produces a significant influence on the consumers' health behaviours, and more often than not determines or conditions their behaviour toward health matters. *Whether health consumers are knowledgeable or not, the attitude which they bring to any health situation also determines what they will accept, do, or reject.* Thus, between health knowledge and health actions, the attitude of the health consumer is a major determining factor.

As remarked by Mico and Ross (1975), while *actions* are largely observable, *forces* are imperceptible – actions are the expressions of forces at work. These forces are attitudinal in their origin. Attitude has as its under current what are commonly referred to as needs, beliefs, values, interests, expectations, motives, perceptions, problems, biases, or prejudices. The force of each on action is both environmentally and personally conditioned at any particular point in time, and in terms of time and place, they each undergo a varying degree of change, being at times in constant flux and fluctuation, so as to make human behaviours almost totally unpredictable. All the same, attitudes, working through abstraction and predictions are nonetheless the vital force behind most, if not all, human actions. Since all health/medical programmes have behaviour correlates, these behaviours must be carefully investigated for their possible applications to protect and promote people's health.

The need for studying health education as a discipline concerned with people's health behaviour is also a result of the fact that *every human behaviour is caused.* Why health consumers accept and adapt certain health programmes, why they respond favourably towards certain health interventions, and why they utilize maximally certain health services must be carefully investigated. Educational process is utilized in the investigation and in facilitating positive health behaviours.

Foundations for the Practice of Health Education

For most of its principles, content, and methods, health education draws on the biological/health sciences, socio-cultural and behavioural sciences, and educational science. The contributions of each are briefly outlined below.

1. **Educational Contributions**

   Educational psychology, which is concerned with knowledge of how the individual learner learns, grows, and changes in his KAP, also include such activities as educational planning (for example, curriculum planning and instructional programmes), training, administration, supervision, and evaluation.

2. **Socio-Cultural and Behavioural Sciences Contributions**
   (a) Sociology - provides an understanding of the social structures and system which humans develop, and how these affect people's behaviours in groups, organizations, communities, or other large-scale systems.
   (b) Social psychology–contributes theories on the way people learn and change in social situations.
   (c) Anthropology–gives an understanding of the forces of culture, tradition, and custom in shaping people's behaviours.
   (d) Political science–contributes to an understanding of political phenomena, and how these shape the forces of power, policy, and governance.
   (e) Psychiatry–gives a basis for the diagnosis and treatment of behaviour affecting disease conditions.

3. **Health Science Contributions**

   From such subjects as human biology, anatomy, chemistry, environmental health, human nutrition, etc., health facts or information in relation to health and disease are derived.

Health education is, therefore, a discipline of disciplines and an application of applied sciences to health behaviours. Its distinctive philosophy, principles, and practices are embodied in its total mechanics and process (Ademuwagun 1977).

The Place of Information in Health Education

From the inception of its identification with health programmes (even though its distinctive role has been differently, but usually wrongly, interpreted) health education has been undergoing various role definitions.

At the beginning, health education was associated simply and primarily with 'health information.' Because of this interpretation, it is also associated with the production and distribution of health materials, such as audio-visual aids, in the forms of leaflets, posters, health films, and exhibits.

In many African countries today, the 'health educators' are usually remembered as members of the health team only during emergencies, such as epidemics of communicable diseases – for example, cholera epidemics. It is only on such occasions that many African goverments make some frantic efforts to see that the public is 'informed' by all means– by radio, television, rediffusion, pamphlets, and wealth of propaganda machinery – at all costs.

To the majority of health personnel, the 'health educators' are only good for 'telling the consumers' or 'informing' them of the causes of ill-health, of how to protect themselves against dangers of health or prevent ill-health, and of the available health services in their localities. The 'health educators are therefore usually expected to use all sorts of communication skills and 'teaching aids', such as mass-media information.

The underlying assumptions of this attitude are:

(1) That people's failure to take health precautions is a result of their ignorance of what to do. This assumption has been proved not necessarily true; because people may know what to do and yet refuse to do it (Ademuwagun, 1973).

(2) That lack of information of available health services is responsible for consumers' failure to make maximal use of orthodox health services. This has been proved as not necessarily true, in that many know and still opt for traditional medical care (Anon, 1975).

(3) That health propaganda conducted by radio, television, rediffusion, posters, leaflets, and the like will bring the required information within the reach of the 'hard to reach', and to many people at a time. This is not necessarily true, in that people usually see what they want to see (or are interested in seeing), and people read mostly what is of interest to them, and listen to (or hear) mostly only what is of interest to them.

At this juncture, we need to be reminded that all these behaviours are determined, caused, or conditioned by many factors in the total environmental setting of the consumers. Positive responses can only be expected from the consumers when the health information, intervention, or programme is consonant rather than dissonant with their felt needs, interests, values, beliefs, practices, and problems.

Take 'health talks' or 'health information' as an example. The mere fact that a health idea is accepted by a mother – for example, the idea that immunization of babies against tetanus is good for making them grow up healthy – is not necessarily sufficient for a mother to actually bring her baby to the clinic for immunization. It may be admitted that there may be initial acceptance of the ideas, owing to her interest in the survival of her child, and that the mother believes what is said and that she is interested in going to the clinic. None the less, to mention some intervening conditions which must be fulfilled to make her act accordingly: taking the baby to the clinic must be very high in the scale of her priorities at a particular point in time; the service at the clinic must not only be easily available, but accessible, to rule out problems of inconvenience; and the general perceptions and impressions of the mother about this particular clinic or any similar clinic must not motivate or militate against her positive response; and a host of other potential impediments could be added (Ademuwagun, 1972a, b; 1977).

The problem of what the consumers do or fail to do about health matters is fundamental to the practice of health education simply because all health/medical measures are useless unless they improve the health status of the consumers. Their health status will never be improved until they respond positively to health interventions, by taking measures such as:

(1) protecting themselves against common accidents, common diseases, and other hazards to health;

(2) promoting their health by doing those things that will make them healthier, such as eating a balanced diet (paying attention to quantity and quality), taking adequate rest and sleep and regular exercise, and having regular medical check-ups; and

(3) taking advantage of the available health care by doing such things as going to hospital (or health clinic) when sick, and making maximal use of the prescribed drugs and other medical prescriptions.

The goal of health education is positive health actions or response. And indeed, even the objective of those who saw (and still see) health information as the major function of health educators was also that through it the audience, consumers, or target populations would involve themselves in positive health behaviour. As already mentioned, this expectation has not always been met; in fact the approach has resulted more in failures than in successes in the health field. The reason largely lies embedded in the former neglect of the science of health behaviour, which is the sole scientific basis for the practice of health education.

It was later discovered by some field workers that 'health information', for a number of behavioural reasons, does not necessarily lead to health practice. Since then the traditional attitude of equating 'health information' with 'health education' has been changed; but not without tremendous efforts among professional health educators.

Information and Education

As a science of health behaviour, health education is also a science of *learning* and *change*, as has already been mentioned. Positive behaviours must be learnt or brought about through teaching-learning processes; negative behaviours must similarly be changed through teaching-learning processes. It is in this context that health education has traditionally been associated with *change* in health behaviours, as if to say that all consumers' health behaviours are negative.

In teaching people about health, information or fact is transmitted with the hope that the learner will eventually do something about the information or fact – that is, utilize it favourably as anticipated by the teacher. However, a professional teacher does not just give out information because he knows that mere acquisition of information by the learner does not necessarily produce the anticipated action or result, even though there are different intentions which may lie behind the giving of particular pieces of information. At times, a piece of information is just 'to be noted', or just 'to hear or know about'– to be informed. In this kind of information, no particular reaction is anticipated from the informed. But some educational information is expected to be acted upon by the informed person. Information is sometimes intended to produce a specific reaction. However, it has long been established that *knowing* is one thing and *doing* is another. Therefore, for information to be effectively educational – that is, to produce the anticipated total behaviours (KAP) – it must be organized, planned, and communicated with systematic educational methods and techniques.

The main behavioural objective of education is *growth* or *change* in the learners' knowledge, attitudes, and practices in whatever discipline they opt for. Therefore, in a pragmatic education programme, all facts or information which they are exposed to in various subjects or courses are systematically and sequentially organized and planned into integrated learning experiences, which are planned in the context of the functions which the learners are expected to perform when their schooldays are over. In this approach the growth and developmental needs of the learners – physical, social, emotional and intellectual, as well as the beliefs, values, and practices which stem from their peculiar needs, interests, and problems – are all taken into account.

Educationally, the discovery of relevance and meaning by the learner of what is taught to him by the teacher is fundamental to the objectives of the teaching-learning transaction process. The perceived relevance of meaning constitutes an internal motivation and dynamic force which facilitates relevant behaviours, particularly the application of the learned information, voluntarily and habitually by the learner, without necessarily referring to the source of his behaviour – the teacher. What is left in the learner, and particularly what motivates him to perform actions even after the teacher may have been forgotten, is called education. Educationally it is what the learner does that he has learned, not what the teacher does. Therefore, educational process is primarily concerned with helping the learners or targets of education to discover the relevance and meaning of what is taught them, so that they may take the necessary actions voluntarily through their own efforts, and act without waiting for external motivations. Once they do this, then they have internalized what is taught them, because the meaning has been discovered, and, therefore, acted upon.

The importance of the teacher helping the learner to discover the relevance and meaning of what he learns is the major focus of Comb in his article on 'Humanizing the Education.' On the relationship between 'knowing' and 'behaving' on the part of the learner, Comb said:

> There is a vast difference between knowing and behaving. Knowing comes from getting new information. Change in behaviour is a people's problem, the human side of the learning equation. It comes from discovery of meaning. The most important aspect of learning lies not in the giving of information but in the discovery of its meaning. Some of the most important learning we have has nothing to do with new information but everything to do with deeper and deeper discovery of the meaning we already know... The problem of changing meaning, however, is a slower, more difficult human task which cannot be done by an outsider. It has to be done by the learner himself. People need information of course. The danger comes when we lose our bearing. It is time we give attention to humanization and the discovery of meaning.

Information is one thing and education is another (Ademuwagun 1972; Miller 1966). While information may not always be intended to be acted upon by the informed person, the process of education is focused on bringing about growth and change in the learner through the acquisition of relevant information. To this end, information is merely a means in the education process. The information, however, must be organized and communicated by the teacher in such a way as to motivate the learner to action in a way consonant with the expectation of the communicator. In communication, according to Miller, (op. cit.) there is a conscious intent to affect the behaviour of the communicatee.

The difference between a merely *informed* person and an educated person, then, is that the latter applies what he knows for social/self-actualization and social/self-development. In other words, the latter grows or changes in his behaviour–KAP–while the former does not, or perhaps sometimes does in his knowledge and attitudes, but not in the real application or practice of what he knows.

What has been said of the relationships and the differences between 'information' and 'education' also applies to 'health information' and 'health education', even though health information is an integral part of health education, and not the same thing as health education. In the last analysis, health education has not taken place until positive health practice has taken place, that is, until there is measurable *growth* or *change* in the consumer's total health behaviour which is consummated in health practice.

After structural organization and planning of health information, effective communication of the information aids meaningful feedback, which helps in the discovery of the actual and potential impediments to the anticipated consumers' positive health behaviours. After discovery of impediments, strategies are evolved for removing or circumventing them. It is only in respect of the best way to communicate health information so that it may be relevant and meaningful – that is, produce an educational effect – that teaching-learning aids, often termed 'audio-visual aids', such as leaflets or mass media communication by radio or television, emerge in the practice of health education.

Relevance to the Practice of Health Education

When professional educators speak of the relevance of the educational process to the field of health, they have in mind the application of education methods and techniques to the science of health behaviour from the perspective which has been discussed above. The emphasis is how to bring about growth or change in the consumers' health behaviour (KAP) through assisting them to discover the relevance and meaning or value of what is discussed about health protection, promotion, and care.

Who 'Does' Health Education?

In 1958, an Expert Committee of the WHO on the Teaching of Health Personnel in Health Education of the Public declared:

> Every health worker who is in close contact with the people has a potential influence on the knowledge, attitude and health practices of the people with whom he works. In order that the best results accrue from these contacts, it is essential that doctors, nurses, midwives, environmental sanitation workers and others with specialized health knowledge become more conscious of their educational responsibilities and approach them with confidence, optimism and a variety of techniques. Many health workers already have to a greater or less extent the ability to educate or influence their patients, the family members and the general public. With a more systematic and specified training in health education this influence could be widened and increased in effectiveness (WHO 1958).

While all health workers agree with this position taken by the Expert Committee as to their health education responsibilities, the fact remains that most of them still have a problem of performing the roles effectively. One major handicap is that their pre-service preparation in the health education component of their functions has usually been very limited. Consequently, they have different and varying notions of what health education really involves. This is why the comment of the Expert Committee on the need for 'more systematic and specific training in health education' for these people is relevant.

According to the Expert Committee on Health Education of the Public (WHO 1954) the aim of health education:

> is to help people to achieve health by their own actions and efforts. Health Education begins therefore with the interest of people in improving their conditions of living, and aims at developing a sense of responsibility for their own health betterment as individuals, and as members of families, communities or government.

From this passage the fact that the goal of health education (whatever the educational method used) in health practice is made explicit. The same Expert Committee broke down the *aim* of health education into *general* purposes (WHO 1954) as follows (though the goal remains the same):

(1) to make health a valued community asset;

(2) to help individuals to become competent in and to carry on those activities they must undertake for themselves as individuals or in small groups, in order to realize fully the state of health defined in the constitution of the WHO;

(3) to promote the development and proper use of health services.

These purposes pre-suppose three mutually inclusive functions of health education:

(1) health protection – that is, the protection of oneself against accidents, the attack of diseases, etc,;

(2) health promotion – that is, doing those things which make a person healthier, happier, more productive, likeable, and better able to actualize his latent potentialities for social-self development; and

(3) health care – that is, planning realistic medical services which correspond to the exact health needs and problems of the people in their total environmental setting – and making medical services acceptable, available, and accessible, so that the consumers can make the best use of the services.

In essence, good, relevant medical care programmes require comprehensive planning. This might in fact be what the same Expert Committee had in mind when it declared:

> Health is but one of the elements, in general welfare of the people, and health education is only one of the factors in improving health and social conditions. It is, however, an indispensable factor, and should therefore be integrated with other social, economic, health, and educational efforts (WHO 1954).

Even though the 1958 WHO Expert Committee on Training Health Personnel declared that 'every health worker who is in close contact with the people has a potential influence on the knowledge, attitude and health practices of the people with whom he works'. This type of health education is only concerned with the professional functions of each of the health personnel mentioned.

Health education functions can be performed, if well prepared for as such, by such broad groups of people as:

(1) the non-professional, who only perform the health education components of their own professional functions; and

(2) the professional health educators, who specialize in health education (and even then these latter functions at different levels). As noted by the 1954 WHO Expert Committee:

There is a wide variety of health educators with specialized training for different responsibilities. For example, some may be working nationally, provincially, or locally in public health programmes administered by official health agencies, or by voluntary health organizations. Others may be employed in Colleges, Universities, or schools.

Professional Health Educators and other Levels of Health Educators

Every health worker is a health educator. Every health worker must of necessity, because of the objective of health education, be exposed to the health education component of his or her functions. The following question, however, must be asked:

1. How many physicians, nurses, midwives, public health inspectors, school teachers, etc., have really been exposed to organized and professional preparation in health education? What type of health education curriculum were they exposed to during their training?
2. What was the duration of their courses in health education – three months, six months, or nine months – during a period of three or five years of training as health personnel?
3. Who taught them – that is, what was the qualification of their teachers in health education? Were they professional health educators? What type of learning experiences were provided them while in training, so that they could build on these after occupying their different fields as professionals?

All other health and allied personnel, in addition to the professional health educators, must be equipped with knowledge, skills, and competencies in the health education components of their functions while in training. Thus the clinical medical doctors, the hospital nurse, the community nurse, midwife, the public health inspectors, teachers, adult educators, etc., must concentrate some attention on the health education aspects of their day-to-day functions. It will be unrealistic, if not absurd, to expect them to undergo in depth all that goes into health education as a specialized study and professional field – for that field is concerned with the whole science of health behaviour, with special emphasis on health consumers' behaviour towards common disease perceptions and health problems, and how to bring about positive health behaviour through the educational process. There are at least two broad groups of health educators:

1. those who perform the health education component of their own specialized functions and
2. those who are professional health educators with varied health education roles; and these, as shown below, are of different levels in their preparation and, of course, in their functions.

These role-differentials must be recognized and accepted as a fact before there can be a healthy practice of health education in the health team.

A line can thus be drawn between those 'doing' the health education aspect of their function,and those who actually specialize as health educators.

Principal Functions of Professional Health Educators

The 1954 WHO Expert Committee listed the following as the principal functions of specialists in health education: to strengthen and extend the educational functions of all members of the health team, and to supplement their health education activities on a sustained and organized basis. The health education specialists contribute to the health education team a fundamental understanding of the basic social sciences, just as other members of the team – the doctors, nurse, sanitary engineer, and others bring their particular skills to the solution of health problems.

More specifically, the functions of the health education specialist may include helping to create interest in, and definite opportunities for people to learn about health matters; taking part in studies of community problems or resources, and of means of reaching the people and in fostering co-operative relationships with health services and related agencies; assisting in the selection, development, and use of educational methods and media in accordance with local needs and possibilities; helping to plan and conduct training programmes in health education for health workers, school personnel, and staff members of other relevant agencies; explaining the health services which are available to the population; and helping to evaluate health education aspects of the whole health programme.

Areas of General Agreement on the Role of Health Education

Some areas of general agreement among professional health educators about the practice of health education are:

(1) it is concerned with the behaviours of the individual and the forces of needs, interests, beliefs, values, motivations, knowledge, and perceptions that influence those behaviours;

(2) it is a discipline of disciplines, and as such a discipline applied to health but drawing much of its content and methods from (a) the natural/health sciences; (b) the socio-cultural and behavioural sciences; and (c) the educational sciences;

(3) it is an educationally-oriented process;

(4) it is primarily consumer-oriented, in that its goal is the consumer's positive health practice or response to health interventions, its target ultimately the individual, even when conducted in a community setting; or through the mass media;

(5) it focuses on closing the gap between that which is known to be good for health and that which is actually being practised by the individual;

(6) it is concerned with comprehensive health planning using the education process; and

(7) its functions are increasingly becoming those of staff providing a planned array of facilitating services to the other personnel of the organizations concerned with health education and welfare. (These include: assisting others in the planning, implementa-

tion, and evaluation of their health-education services; in-service training of other personnel in the principles and methods of health education; and staff development training in general areas of professional skill development, team-building, intra-organizational problem-solving, inter-unit collaboration and conflict-resolution.)

It would appear from this list that research in health education is conspicuously missing as a distinct function fundamental to the practice of a pragmatic health education programme. Without knowledge of the consumers in their environmental setting (and particularly of their original traditional behaviours in terms of knowledge, attitudes and practices towards common local diseases and health problems) there will be no real basis for health educators to plan either for or with the people how to solve their problems, nor will they be able to plan how to investigate problems faced in the community. Behind the notion of change in the behaviour of people is the assumption that there is something already there which needs to be changed. But what can we change if we do not know what there is that should undergo change – is it negative knowledge, beliefs, values, perceptions, practice, and the like? Only research can reveal these, if jointly planned and carried out with the affected people. The resultant findings must be the basis of the practice of health education if we are interested in running a health education programme that works. Malinowski might well have been addressing himself to the question of the need to know the health consumers in their total setting when he said:

> We need to know about the social (and cultural) conditions which have educated original activities into definite and significant depositions, before we can discuss the psychological elements in society. This is the true meaning of social psychology...Native human nature supplies the raw materials; but custom furnishes the machinery and the designs. (Malinowski, 1977).

Today, the WHO has recognized the important position which research in health education occupies in the practice of health education. Now in Geneva there is a division of the WHO which is specially concerned with encouraging, sponsoring, and financing research in health education. But it was not until 1968 that a WHO Scientific Group on Research in Health Education met in Geneva to review the place of research in the practice of health education. Up till today, very little research in health education has been conducted in Africa. The time has come to initiate research in health education, and to document those projects already completed and those not yet completed – both for the purpose of general information and with a view to their possible replication.

Summary

1. *Health education* is not mere *health information* or *health instruction*. It is a whole complex of activities, including among them those which are intended to: facilitate the achievement of the objectives of any health programme or project; motivate the health consumers or the target population to make voluntary decisions and take necessary steps to improve their health through taking positive health precautions; facilitate the target population's involvement and active participation in identifying their health needs and problems and in planning for their solution; facilitate maximal utilization of the available health services in the locality; facilitate *change* or *growth* in the people's health *Knowledge, Attitudes, and Practices (KAP);* and help the health personnel to become more effective in the discharge of their health responsibilities towards the people.

2. The goal of health education is health practice or health action. To this end it probes all the actual and potential factors which are likely to be in operation before the consumer can actually practise health in his environmental setting. To do this effectively, the professional health educators are very much concerned with ecological thinking in health matters, and comprehensive community health planning in the context of the whole local environmental setting of man.

3. *Basic principles*

1. Every human behaviour is caused and, in effect, all health programmes have behaviour correlates.
2. Man's environment imposes a significant influence on his total behaviour: at times it even determines or conditions his behaviour.
3. The attitude which the individual brings to any situation, irrespective of what he knows, determines significantly what he will accept or reject, do or fail to do.
4. To participate in what affects his destiny is one of the fundamental cravings of man. Therefore, effective involvement and active participation of the consumers in community health programmes is fundamental to the realization of the objectives of such programmes.
5. What the learner does is what he learns, and not what the teacher does. To this end, we learn *to do* by actually doing.
6. Behind what a learner does is his discovery of the *relevance* and *meaning* of what he is taught – that is, how it fits into his total life patterning in terms of his beliefs, values, and practices, as well as his needs, interests, and problems at a particular point in time.
7. A *health informed* person is not necessarily a *health educated* person.
8. For any health behaviour to be voluntary and lasting, it must be self-motivated; it must be approached through an *educational* process.
9. Holistic or comprehensive health programme planning can only result from ecological thinking which takes into account man in his total environmental setting.

References

Ademuwagun, Z.A. (1970). Some Educational Principles in Public Health Programme. *J. Soci. Hlth*, Nigeria, V.

—(1972a). Major Impediments to Effective Use of Health Services. *J. Hlth Educ. 31.*

—(1972b). Information and Motivation in Health Education. *J.Hlth Educ. 31.*

—(1974). The challenge of Health Education Methods and Techniques in Developing Countries. *J.Hlth Educ. 33.*

—(1977a). Determinants of Pattern and Degree of Utilization of Health Services in Two Divisions of Western State, Nigeria. *Israel J. Med. Sc. 13.*

Ademuwagun, Z.A. (1977b). *Health Education:A Conceptual Approach.* Ibadan University Press.

Anon (1975). The Meeting-point of Orthodox Health Personnel and Traditional Healers/Midwives in Nigeria: Experience in the Pattern of Utilization of Obstetrics and Gynaecology Services in Ibarapa Division of Western State of Nigeria *Rural Africana, 26 (1974–75 Winter).*

Bennis, W.G. Benne, K.O., and Chin, R. (1961). *The Planning of Change.* Holt, Rinehart, and Winston, New York.

International Union for Health Education (1976). Health Education and Health Policy in The Dynamics of Development. *Summary Proceedings of the International Conference on Health Education, Ottawa.*

Knutson, A.L. (1965). *The Individual, Society, and Health Behaviour.* Russel Sage Foundation, New York.

Malinowski, Bronislaw (1977). *Sex and Repression in Savage Society* P. xv. Harcourt, Brace, and Coy, New York.

Mico, Paul and Ross, Helen (1975). *Health Education and Behavioural Science.* Third Party Associates, Inc., Oakland.

Miller, Gerald (1966). On Defining Communication: Another Stab. *J. Communication 16.*

Paul, B.D. (1955). *Health Culture and Community.* Russel Sage Foundation, New York.

Sommers, Anne R. (1976). *Promoting Health Consumer Education and National Policy* ASPEN, New York.

The Health Education Project Advisory Committee (1975). Making Health Education Work *Am. J. Publ. Hlth 65.*

WHO (1954). Expert Committee on Health Education of the Public.

—(1958). *Tech. Rep. Ser. Wld. Hlth Org. 89, 4* Expert Committee on Training of Health Personnel in Health Education of the Public. *Tech. Rep. Ser. Wld. Hlth Org. 156, 6*

—(1969). Research in Health Education. *Tech. Rep. Sr. Wld Hlth Org. 432.*

—(1975). *Health Education in Environmental Health Programmes.* WHO Regional Office for Africa, Brazzaville, AFR/HE/69.

Williams, Erol. (1975). Community Organization as a Health Education Process. Paper Presented at the Seminar on Environmental Sanitation, UCH, Ibadan, August 15-18, 1975.

Section B

Health Education

D.A. Ogunmekan

The Aims of Health Education

If a disease can be prevented by an alteration in behaviour, then the achievement of this altered behaviour enables its incidence in the community to be reduced. Some of the behaviour alterations that may be required in appropriate circumstances are the adoption of locally appropriate and correct feeding practices to prevent kwashiorkor, having one's children immunized and seeing that they take anti-malaria drugs. The achievement of these altered behaviour patterns on a really wide scale would reduce the incidence of many of the major diseases which now beset Nigerian children.

Lest it be thought that health education is merely the removal of ignorance, it is pointed out that it involves four things:

1. It supplies a person with enough new and correct knowledge about a disease to make the preventive measures required by scientific medicine seem reasonable.
2. It makes a person feel sufficiently keen about the importance of his own health to make him alter his behaviour and adopt these preventive measures.
3. It makes him concerned for the health of others.
4. It tries to make him feel so strongly about the first three that he supports and even initiates preventive action by the community.

Health education is a many sided endeavour of such importance that it must be furthered by every possible means. The newspapers, the radio, the television and schools all have their part, so also do hospitals and health centres.

The first point to realize is that *all* the staff, from doctor to sweeper have a part to play in health education both during the course of their work and in their other activities.

Many subtle intermediate stages of mind lie between the two extremes of ignorance or the wrong ideas on the one hand, and active conviction on the other. The successive stages it involves at various levels in the mind can be summarized in the following way by taking dysentery as an example. *A change in knowledge* – this is the first stage e.g. knowing that dysentery is an infectious disease. *A change in attitude* follows this. The patient now has a greater regard for the possible spread of disease. *A change in behaviour* is seen next. The patient begins to act on his belief and no longer disposes of his excreta in a latrine as an unthinking habit that requires no conscious decision. *A change in custom* is the last stage when care in disposal of excreta has become one of the cultural characteristics of the group to be handed on to children of the next generation.

Health education does not end with merely sticking up posters, distributing pamphlets, showing films or talking; it starts there. Instruction must be followed by demonstration and wherever possible a talk should be followed by what to do and why it is done. A Chinese proverb says, 'If I do it, I know'.

Because mothers are the most important target for health education, it is vital for them actually to practise what they have been taught.

In health education, one should endeavour to follow these seven points:

1. Decide how much of the available knowledge on a particular subject should be passed on to the community and to specific groups within it e.g. mothers.
2. See how these ideas can best be expressed in the vernacular.
3. Determine which beliefs, customs and attitudes are likely either to help or hinder the acceptance of this knowledge. See what can be done to circumvent any hindrances.
4. Try to discover which individuals or groups of people in the community are in a position to help or hinder the acceptance of this knowledge. See if it is possible to minimize the effect of the potential hinderers.
5. Make the most of the variety of teaching methods.
6. Make the most of teaching aids, having first determined that they are understood.
7. Endeavour to measure success or failure and make this evaluation an integral part of the educational programme.

Tuberculosis and kwashiorkor as examples of topics for health education.

N.B: It is possible for a person to believe in something which he does not practise or for him to practise something in which he does not belief. This divorce of practice from belief – this 'cognitive dissonance' as it is called, produces a certain psychological tension which is only relieved by the adjustment of practice to belief or vice versa. Thus having once instilled the belief that dysentery is infectious, it is important to strive to relieve the dissonance and complete the educational process by establishing the practice of careful excreta disposal. Dissonance may be relieved equally well by the loss of belief in which case, the educator is back where he began.

71

Tackling Major Disasters

G.O. Sofoluwe

The world has experienced major disasters from time immemorial; but they are now becoming more frequent. During the period of 1919 to 1951 there were 4.8 disasters per year, increasing to 10 disasters per year between 1951 and 1971, and increasing further to 13 disasters per year during the three years 1968 to 1971. Table 71.1 gives more details, together with the regional occurrence of the disasters during the three above-named periods.

Table 71.1
Disasters ranked according to region

Areas	**1919-1951**	**1951-1971**	**1968-1971**
Africa	33	29	9
Americas	42	35	6
Asia	89	77	24
Europe	49	35	3
Middle East	38	38	10
Total	**251**	**214**	**52**
Mean	4.8 disasters per year	10.0 disasters per year	13 disasters per year

Source of information: *UN Disaster Relief Organization (UNDRO), 1972*

Table 71.2 details the natural disaster which occasioned a major appeal on the part of the League of Red Cross Societies during the period of 1961 to 1970.

Table 71.2

Natural disasters occasioning a major appeal on the part of the League of Red Cross Society during 1961-1970

Area	Number
Asia	46
Africa	22
Middle East	20
Europe	13
Americas	11
Total	**112**

Source: *League of Red Cross Societies (1971)*

The natural disasters included floods, earthquakes, hurricanes, droughts, epidemics, famines, and volcanic eruptions. The numbers of each of these different types of disaster which occurred during the period 1968 to 1971 and 1961 to 1970 are detailed in Tables 71.3 and 71.4

Table 71.3

Number of Disasters by type 1968-1971

Type	Number
Floods	27
Earthquakes	8
Hurricanes	7
Droughts	5
Epidemics	2
Famines	2
Volcanic Eruptions	1
Total	**52**

Source: *UNDRO, 1972*

Table 71.4
Number of disasters by type 1961-1970

Type	Number
Floods	58
Earthquakes	19
Hurricanes	18
Droughts/Famines	8
Epidemics	6
Volcanic Eruptions	3
Total	**112**

Source: *UN Economic and Social Council, 1971*

In addition to the above-named types of natural disasters the following artificial causes have been responsible for further major disasters in Africa:

(1) aircraft crashes;
(2) railway accidents, especially derailments;
(3) serious road accidents;
(4) serious fires;
(5) wars and droughts causing large scale migrations of people across national borders and leading to the deaths of millions of people and livestock;
(6) serious explosions especially in chemical factories;
(7) the collapse of buildings and other structures involving injuries or dangers to persons and loss of lives.

To the above categories or lists of major disasters can be added the following factors:

1. In Africa, complex socio-economic and political forces have resulted in the expulsion of thousands of Africans from neighbouring countries to their countries of origin, even though some of them had been settled in those neighbouring countries for over forty or even fifty years. For example, Nigeria has within the past twenty years experienced the results of sudden expulsion *en masse* of thousands of Nigerians from Ghana, Zaire, and Fernando Po in Equatorial Guinea; whilst political problems have resulted in the disruption of the hitherto stable East African Community countries of Kenya, Uganda, and Tanzania.
2. Similarly, the decentralization of political power to regions, states, divisions, and local government areas has generated ethnic or tribal prejudices and conflicts, resulting in massive expulsions of persons from one area to another even within the same country.
3. Similarly Africa has within the last twenty years experienced a number of civil wars, military coups, civilian strikes and riots, and other such forms of civil strife, which have

resulted in the deaths of and injuries of many people; and sometimes in the mass enlistment of soldiers, who eventually have to be demobilized and rehabilitated.

All medical practitioners in Africa, especially community physicians, need therefore to have a working knowledge of how to tackle such major disasters; and perhaps some will be stimulated to team up with other professionals to prevent them.

Principles for Tackling Disasters

The following, in order, constitute a model list of the activities which should be undertaken to tackle such disasters:

A report should be made to the police.

The police officer nearest to the scene will proceed to the scene with a wireless equipped vehicle and alert the following officers:

the most senior police officer in the zone;

the principal or most senior medical officer (usually public/community health specialist);

the commissioner of police;

the chief or senior engineer, to deal with water supplies, etc.;

the chief military officer in command in the area, for the supply of military disaster relief facilities and equipment, such as for example army tents, kitchen, etc.;

the senior officer in charge of posts and telegraphs, to effect communication so that relief supplies and facilities can be summoned from more distant areas;

the police officer in charge of motor traffic; and

the provincial crime officer, to detect and prevent crime, looting, etc.

After assessment of the disaster judicious information needs to be relayed, so that a co-ordinated, comprehensive effort can be made to contain the disaster; to give prompt medical treatment to the injured; to identify the dead; and to contain the damage – for example, to contain or put out a fire, to redirect a flood, or to seal off the area so that an explosion does not set up a conflagration, etc.

An interministerial standing committee in the former Western Region of Nigeria in 1952 wrote a booklet detailing the following activities for the above listed officers:

The Police

The police should be the first at the scene to assess damage; they should set up an Incident Control Post and a Public Relations Bureau manned by both the Police and the Ministry of Information; they should contain and prevent crime; investigate crime; divert and control traffic, sealing off the area if necessary; maintain in chronological order a register of actions taken and make contacts; co-ordinate the activities of all the other governmental or voluntary agencies, such as the Red Cross, etc.; who will be involved in tackling the disaster; and should screen and examine all information to be disseminated about the disaster.

Fire Officer

Fire officers should contain and prevent the further spread of any fire; contain any flood, and rescue men in danger, etc.

Crime Officers

Crime officers should take into safe custody all valuables, freight, and mail; arrange for the identification of victims; take necessary photographs; and arrange for all necessary action to be planned under the Coroner's Act in respect of the dead. They should also liaise with the state, and national Criminal Investigation Department (CID) and Interpol if necessary.

Medical Officer

The medical officer should despatch ambulances, doctors, nurses and other members of the health team, and organize first aid, resuscitation, and transportation for treatment in hospital. The health officer should arrange for environmental health measures, including the provision of shelter, water supplies, sewage and refuse disposal facilities, the maintenance of food hygiene, and the control of communicable diseases, especially the prevention or containment of cholera, typhoid, typhus, plague, and other serious communicable diseases. He should also arrange for the immunization and feeding of children, and the pregnant, the old and feeble.

The welfare officer should render all necessary welfare services, alert voluntary organizations, such as the Red Cross, etc., and co-ordinate all medical and welfare activities.

Post and Telecommunication (P & T)

The P & T officials should ensure the serviceableness of all communication equipment; assist in the co-ordination of rescue operations; and undertake other activities in accordance with their available standing instructions on emergencies.

Engineers

The railways or airway engineers will take appropriate measures for the evacuation and rescue of victims. Many railway corporations now have a Manual of Accidents showing the activities necessary to tackle disasters.

Government engineers will need to arrange:

- for the availability of vehicles and other equipment, such as cranes, lifting gear, etc.;
- to provide a useable water supply setting up tests for potability and to exclude poisons in the water, and to prevent pollution; and
- to assist in salvage operations.

The Armed Forces – Army, Navy and Air Force

Members of the armed forces, who are always well trained and ready at short notice to effect disaster relief, will:

- organize manpower for rescue operations, for the clearing of forest, for path tracing, and for Bailey bridge construction;
- provide mobile health teams at short notice;
- provide special transport, equipped with four-wheel drive, etc.;
- provide field kitchens, ambulances, etc.;
- provide shelter, such as army tents; and
- provide mobile and static radio facilities.

Information and press releases need to be judicious and aimed at ensuring maximum rapid relief, and not run the risk of causing further panic or causing crime. Voluntary organizations, such as Red

Cross Societies, the St. John's Ambulance, and the Young Men's and Young Women's Christian Associations (YMCA and YWCA) are always ready and willing to assist in tackling disasters. Bilateral and international voluntary aid and prompt assistance from international agencies are always readily obtained.

As all the above are immediate and emergency measures which should be forthcoming within a matter of an hour or so it is necessary for all African countries to prepare themselves for tackling disaster by establishing a National Major Disaster Standing Committee, branches of which should exist at state, local government, and even political ward levels. Regular drills and meetings, even when no disaster occurs, should be held.

Lastly, there is a need for the committee to be supported by a university or a research institute, which should monitor on a local and on a world-wide basis the preventive measures employed against such disasters, and advise on modern and safer methods for tackling them.

Prevention of Natural Disaster by the United Nations Agencies

It is heartening to note that following a major disaster in the late 1960s the member states of the United Nations successfully established (from March 1972)a central office within the United Nations called the United Nations Disaster Relief Office (UNDRO) for the purposes of:
mobilizing relief more rapidly;
co-ordinating it more systematically to improve advance contingency planning and preparedness; and
harnessing modern scientific and technological knowledge for the prevention and mitigation of disaster.

Advanced countries such as the United States of America (USA) and the United Kingdom (UK) have now established research institutes to investigate the early-warning signs which are the first indications of the imminent occurrence of earth quakes, floods, hurricanes, and droughts.

Also among the UN agencies themselves UNESCO, WHO, the World Meteorological Organization (WMO), the UN Environmental Programme, and other UN institutions are now collaborating with UNDRO on preventive studies.

UNDRO was sited in Geneva, mainly in order to be near the League of Red Cross Societies, which had until that time borne the main brunt of disaster relief; and also to be near a convenient centre of communication, and especially of aerial transportation.

In the United Kingdom, the Institute of Development Studies of the University of Sussex and the Disaster Research Unit of Bradford University; and, in the United States of America, the Universities of Florida, Texas, New Mexico, Los Angeles, and San Fransicso are some of the numerous academic institutions now committed to the prevention of natural disaster and the mitigation of their effects.

Prevention of the Artificial Technological and Politico-socio Forms of Major Disaster

As the above are now almost peculiar to Africa and other emerging and developing countries, the key to their prevention lies in improved technological knowledge and practice, as well as in bolder attempts by governmental and private agencies to meet more quickly the basic human needs of over seventy per cent of the population of each of the African countries.

It is further necessary for African institutes of socio-economic research to establish a special Disaster Research Unit, which would not only actively prevent the wastage of resources arising from such disaster, but perhaps even turn the misfortune to economic fortune by inventing a number of economic and employment-yielding projects and appliances; for example, by designing emergency housing and forms of shelter, and so on.

Further Reading

1. Western State of Nigeria; '*Procedure for Detailed Information and Guidance on Tackling Major Disasters.*' Booklet Printed by Government Printers, Ibadan Secretariat.
2. Journal of Tackling Major Disasters, and
3. Publications from the United Nations Disaster Relief Organization (UNDRO).
League of Red Cross Societies 1971 UNDRO, 1972 UN Economic and Social Council, 1971.

72

The Effects of Social Change on the Health of Africans

P.C. Osuhor

Development and urbanization bring social changes. The influence of environmental factors on general development shows culture-lag in the utilization of the available health services. Stacey May (1968) is of the opinion that tropical medicine (community medicine) is the anchor for economic progress in the developing countries including Africa. But MacDonald (1968) on the other-hand, has also pointed out that too much of tropical medicine practice has consisted of a limited effort to reproduce the activities of developed societies, to the advantage of a few and to the great deprivation of the majority.

Medical programmes should develop at the same pace as and simultaneously with efforts to improve the education, economic, and social status of our populations. Each element must be in phase with each other for the maximum benefits to be derived.

We are a transitional and prismatic society, neither truly traditional nor really modern (Riggs, 1964). Perhaps out of this mixture of both the old and new systems, a culture and social norm acceptable to all will evolve; and we may be the better for it in terms of positive health (Osuhor, 1974).

In recent years, the role of human capital in the economic growth of a nation has been emphasized (Ebrahim, 1976). Since education and health are the means for human development, the health of the people has become a major concern of various national governments and international agencies (Akenzua, Ozigbo-Esere and Osuhor, 1984).

Gradually, various African nations are becoming increasingly aware of their health and medical problems. But as a result of their limited resources, including those of finance, rapid population growth rate and rural distribution of the population, the provision of facilities and personnel is not fast enough. There is again poor utilization of those that are available, for a variety of reasons such as culture-lag, distances involved, modes of transport, and the economics of hospital attendance.

There are also marked seasonal variations in attendance amongst the rural farming communities, depending on whether it is the planting or the harvest season (minimum attendance owing to farm work) or the dry post-harvest season (maximum attendance attributable to post-harvest leisure (Osuhor, 1977, 1982).

It is estimated that 60-80 per cent of all hospital admissions and cases in Africa are controllable and/or preventable. This means that if there were properly planned public and community health care systems, most of the diseases that reach the costly hospitals could be prevented or controlled before hospital attendance became necessary (Akenzua et al, 1984). Comprehensive medical care, which is the totality of all aspects of medical practice, both curative and preventive, should be the ultimate aim, in order to achieve maximum benefit for the majority of the population.

The concept of Health For All by the year 2000 (HFA/2000) has increasingly gained international acceptance (Bennett, 1979 and WHO, 1979). It has also become quite clear internationally but more so in developing countries that the strategy which holds the most promise for achieving HFA/2000 is Primary Health Care (PHC) – (Alma-Ata, 1978 and WHO, 1980), the seven principles of which were set out by the WHO (WHO, 9175) and re-emphasized later (Sidel and Sidel, 1977).

It is estimated that in many African countries, about 80% of the population are in the rural areas and engaged in subsistence agriculture. Most of them cannot read or write. These high levels of illiteracy are in turn intimately associated with adverse socio-economic and socio-cultural factors with their implications of poverty, anaemia, subnutrition, malnutrition, bad housing, infections and infestations. Some recent social and socio-economic changes have brought their own problems on the health of Africans.

Increased scopes in tourism have increased the infection rates of HIV/AIDS and other related sexually transmitted diseases(STDs). Environmental destruction in the form of excessive timber extraction, desertification due to excessive use of firewood and charcoal fires in arid and semi-desert zones is occuring at an alarming rate. The destruction of the ozone layer by such activities is said to contribute to less rainfall, excessive heat and therefore, less food. The viscious circle of poverty, undernutrition and disease is ever so present. Ecological imbalances also occur, as some animal and plant populations are almost wiped out for their economic values.

Toxic wastes dumped by the developed countries and also from badly planned industries in Africa are posing serious health and medical problems especially various cancers and skin diseases.

War, skirmishes, military coups and unstable governments have helped to seriously disrupt family lives and create homelessness, poverty, degradation and starvation with the resultant health and medical implications.

High inflation has brought depressed economy to most African states. Food is scarce and communicable diseases are rife.

Road traffic accidents (RTAs) have reached epidemic proportions as the economically active segments of the population are being killed daily on the roads with the attendant consequences of early widowhood, poverty and social disruptions. This subject is dealt with elsewhere in this book.

Due to negative sócio-economic changes, there is an alarming rate in brain drain from Africa to various developed countries in recent years. Medical doctors, engineers, agriculturists, economists and nurses are seeking better conditions in these countries. This trend is bound to reflect adversely on various health and developmental programmes unless the various governments halt the adverse conditons that prompt these professional groups to leave their countries, where they are greatly needed, for better standards of life elsewhere.

In order to improve the quality of life of the population, especially in the rural sectors, various governments have instituted social and economic reforms. In Tanzania and Nigeria the governments have launched Universal Primary Education (UPE) schemes, so as to eradicate illiteracy amongst the population in developmental processes. Post-primary and post secondary institutions have been expanded. All these measures will in turn help to improve the health of the people.

In Nigeria and Ghana there are massive programmes in nutrition (Operations Feed the Nation – OFN); with the accompanying water development, including dams, irrigation systems and bore holes.

The health problems of such ventures must be clearly defined so that preventive measures could be suitably applied. We should bear in mind the water impounding diseases and the diseases due to increased uses of fertilizers, pesticides and insecticides. Also accidents with agricultural and farm machinery are bound to increase in a highly illiterate society (Osuhor and Osuhor, 1978).

Nigeria has introduced various housing schemes and rural electrification. Manpower development, which includes the deployment of graduates of higher institutions through the National Youth Service Corps (NYSC) to both rural and urban areas, but especially to the benefit of the rural areas, has been intensified in Nigeria.

In order to combat the imbalance between the urban and rural areas in the provision of health facilities and personnel, Nigeria has instituted the Basic Health Services and the NYSC medical rural health programmes, whereby medical practice is brought nearer to the rural population. Through this scheme, Nigeria aimed to raise the medical coverage of the entire population from 20 to 40 per cent.

Target groups of the population have also been considered by various governments. The Maternal and Child Health (MCH) services have introduced Oral Rehydration Therapy (ORT) and Expanded Programme on Immunization (EPI). The use of the feeding bottle as a status symbol has increased amongst those sections of the communities who are ill-equipped educationally and economically to cope with this practice, with the attendant increase in the incidence and prevalence of the diarrhoeal diseases. ORT and EPI are helping to bring down the infant mortality rate (IMR) and the childhood mortality rate (CMR); so also the immunizations of pregnant women with tetanus toxoid. Female education has increased, thus delaying age at first marriage and therefore age at first pregnancy and delivery with the accruing benefits.

The role of dominant husbands in helping to reduce the high wastage of very young lives has now been well documented in African patrilineal societies; so also the influence of mothers-in-law (Osuhor and Osuhor, 1978).

Migrant workers have disrupted family lives; the incidence and prevalence of tuberculosis, STDs and violent deaths are high amongst them.

Traditional healers must be recognized as a part of our health care system. Therefore, adequate liaison channels must be opened between them and us if it is possible to work together as colleagues in the same setting. Perhaps, if we can incorporate the ingredients of modern and traditional medicine, we will have achieved a unique medical practice that suits the behavioural patterns of Africans (Osuhor and Osuhor, 1982).

While the environment is being modified, human behaviour in relation to the environment – for example, proper housekeeping and proper use of the available facilities and the available food – must be an important factor to be considered. At all levels of education – and that means primary, secondary, vocational, adult, informal and university – the basic elements of behavioural sciences and environmental health must form integral parts of health education programmes, so that ways of improving the health of the population with the minimal cultural disturbance can be evolved.

Given the high levels of illiteracy in Africa, adequate communication methods must be found which consider the cultural patterns in different communities. Painters, graphic designers, singers, cartoonists, composers and actors should be members of the health education team so that they would initiate, plan and produce meaningful and intelligible posters, plays and illustrations. The *Juju* musicians should be encouraged to compose songs about good health practices. Humour is recognized as a medium for conveying a serious message in African societies (Osuhor and Osuhor, 1978). A UNESCO survey has shown that 63.0% of all television programmes broadcast in Africa, are imported, mostly from the United Kingdom and America (Aborisade, 1976). Although the mass media now reaches a large audience, Kolade (1976) has stressed the need to develop and use local communication methods in the Third World societies. The bazzaars and the market places, being the foremost settings for meaningful communication in Africa, must be explored and used to the fullest advantage.

Since African societies are in various stages of transition – neither modern nor traditional in the real sense of the word – there may evolve the required ingredients for those changes in health behaviour that we need to effect in order to achieve positive health.

The effective organization and administration of the health services must be reconsidered, in order to provide the acceptable minimum of health services to the maximum number of people. Taking into account the available resources, two conditions must be fulfilled: firstly, environmental health activities must be co-ordinated; and secondly, they must be integrated in the public health services as a whole.

The establishment of effective machinery for co-ordination is also justified by the need for determining priorities among competing interests. For instance, the need for irrigation water may compete with the need for drinking water; the construction of impounding reservoirs for water supply may take up valuable agricultural land; use of pesticides or even fertilizers and improper disposal of agricultural wastes can lead to water-pollution problems. Effective co-ordination of environmental health activities, therefore, requires closer collaboration at the local, state, national and even international levels in the context of the broad field of environmental control.

The next step is the integration of environmental health services into the matrix of the general public health services. This implies that services that are at present composed of several units – for example, maternal and child health, environmental health, and communicable disease control – should be grouped together to constitute a more effective system. Each unit within this system should be broadly familiar with all aspects of health problems, and should be able to appreciate the role of the other units, in order to enable them to take part in concerted action. Integration of environmental health into the health services will make it possible, at lower cost, to eliminate gradually most of the diseases which weigh so heavily on national budgets; help to reduce the need for curative services; raise the general level of the public and communities' health, and hence the level of their productivity, which is so necessary to support economic growth. Finally, it will contribute to the overall improvement of living standards in the community, which is the ultimate aim of any development programme (Osuhor and Essien, 1978).

Africa is in a state of transition and therefore, conflicts do occur from time to time between the traditionalists and the modernists. The issues involved should be divided into those that are influenced by 'soft cultures'; that is, cultures and customs that we could change easily and influence immediately; and the 'hard cultures', which are those intimately associated with deep-rooted beliefs and religions and, therefore, may create antagonism in the community unless approached cautiously. It is almost certain that when these two parameters have been carefully identified, our health educational programmes in Africa will be more successful than they are at the moment (Osuhor and Osuhor, 1978).

Mortality and morbidity rates of various diseases are decreasing in Africa; in some countries, very slowly, yet in others, in a satisfactory and continuous downward trend. If the momentum of all the positive activities are maintained, then the health of Africans will be positively improved and not compromised by the various socio-economic changes that have occurred recently in Africa.

In situations of rapid economic and social change, the change in disease patterns can be observed as it happens. Thus, non-communicable diseases – for example, hypertension and diabetes – not widely reported among Africans only a generation ago, are now well recognized, side by side with the high rates of various communicable diseases.

References

Aborisade, B., (1976). 'Mass Media and Cultural Independence in Nigeria.' *New Nigeria*, March 2, 1976.

Akenzua, G.I., Ozigbo-Esere, I.J.M., and Osuhor, P.C., (1984). 'Community Response to Primary Health Care: Obadan Project in Bendel State of Nigeria', *Trop. Paed., 30,* 310-312.

Balachandran, V., (1976). Maternal Mortality in Kaduna, Nigeria. *Niger. Med. J., 5,* 366-70.

Bennet, F.J., (1979). 'Primary Health Care and Developing Countries'. *Soc. Sci. Med., 13A:* 505-14.

Davies, D.T., and Wilson, A.T.M., (1939). 'Personal and Clinical History in Haematemesis and Perforation'. *Lancet, ii,* 723-8.

Davies, D.T., and Wilson, A.T.M. (1973). Observation on the Life History of Chronic Peptic Ulcer. *Lancet, ii,* 1353-60

Ebrahim, G.J., (1976). 'A Model of Integrated Community Health Care. Community Health Care in a rural Area'. *Trop. Georgr. Med. 28:* 5-52.

Federal Office of Statistics, Nigeria (1972). *Housing Conditions in Selected Nigerian Towns and Cities, 1970-71.* Federal Office of Statistics, Lagos, Nigeria.

Finish Paediatric Team, (1976). *Report on Their Activities in Malumfashi District, Northern Nigeria, to the Institute of Health,* Ahmadu Bello University, Zaria (1976).

Gelfand, M., (1964). *Medicine and Custom in Africa.* Livingstone, Edinburgh.

Harrison, K.A., (1977). 'Maternal Mortality in Zaria'; *Faculty of Medicine Clinical Meeting, Ahmadu Bello University, Zaria, May 1977.*

Henshaw, N.E., (1974). 'A Survey of Dental Caries and Oral Hygiene in the Southern Zone of Nigeria'. *Niger Med. J. F,* 189-95.

Henshaw, N.E., and Adenubi, J.O., (1975). 'Periodonotal Disease in the Northern Zone of Nigeria'. *Niger Med. J. 5,* 152-9.

Hunponu-Wusu, O.O., (1976). 'Disorders which Shorten Life Among Nigerians; a Study of Mortality Patterns in the Age Group 15-44 years in Kaduna, Nigeria'. *Trop. Georgr. Med. 28,* 343-8.

Lambo, T.A., (1977). 'International Exchange and National Development.' *Pharm. Med. Sci. J. 1,* 193-202.

Lucas, A.O., and Gilles, H.M., (1973). *A Short Textbook of Preventive Medicine for the Tropics.* p.6. The English Universities Press, London.

MacDonald, J., (1968). 'Concepts; Medicus Mundi; International Organization for Medical Co-operation': On the *Promotion of Tropical Health* p. 7.

Obi, J., (1976). Analysis of Paeditric Medical Cases Admitted to Children's Clinic, Benin City', *Niger Med. J. 6,* 69-73.

Osuhor, Ann (1983). 'Dental Health of Primary School Children in Zaria City', Northern Nigeria. *Pub. Hlth. 97,* 17-23.

Osuhor, Ann (1983). 'Utilization of Health Personnel in Various Dental Health Activities in Nigeria'. *Niger Dent. J. 4,* 90-95.

Osuhor, P.C., (1974). 'The Family Systems in Nigeria'. *Report of Zonal Seminars, Nursing Division, Federal Ministry of Health, Lagos, Nigeria. August 1972, July 1973, and February, 974* pp. 7-17.

Osuhor, P.C., (1975). 'Transplantation Syndrome of Education in Nigeria'. Sunday Supplement, *Sunday Observer, Vol. VII, No. 428, 7 Sept.*

Osuhor, P.C., (1976). 'Stillbirths in Malumfashi: The Socio-Cultural and Socio-Economic Factors'. A Paper Presented at the Association of Physicians of Nigeria Scientific Meeting, Lagos 20-22 October.

Osuhor, P.C., (1977). 'Some Aspects of Community Medicine in Nigeria'. *Trop. Dr., 7.2.* 92-95.

Osuhor, P.C., (1978). 'Maternal Mortality in Malumfashi, Northern Nigeria'. *Pharm. Med. Sc. J. 2.* I, 35-39.

Osuhor, P.C. and Osuhor, Ann (1978). 'Factors in Culture and Change in Health Education for Adults in Nigeria'. *Convergence, XI, 2,* 63-68.

Osuhor, P.C., and Essien, E.S., (1978). 'Urbanization and its Effects on Environmental Sanitation'. *Pub. Health., 92,* 69-75.

Osuhor, P.C., and Hunponu-Wusu, O.O., (1978). *Family Planning Acceptors in Zaria, Northern Nigeria: the Socio-Economic Factors* (In Press).

Osuhor, P.C., and Etta, K.A., (1980). 'Morbidity Patterns in a Semi-Urban Population in Samaru, Zaria, Northern Nigeria'. *Trop. Paed., 26,3,* 99-103.

Osuhor, P.C., and Osuhor, Ann (1982). 'In Contact with Traditional Medicine', *Trop. Dr., 12,* 81-84.

Parish, W.E., et al; (1960). Hypersensitivity to Milk and Sudden Death in Infancy'. *Lancet, ii,* 1106-11.

Ponsioen, J.A., (1968). 'National Development: A Sociological Contribution'. *Publications of the Institute of Social Studies, Series Major, Volume XVIII.* Mouton, The Hague.

Riggs, F.W. (1964). 'Agrarian and Industrial: Toward a Typology of Comparative Administration': In *Toward the Comparative Study of Public Administration* (ed William J. Siffin) Department of Govern. Indiana University, USA., 1957 pp 23-116.

Sidel, V.W., Sidel, R., (1977). 'Primary Health Care in Relation to Socio-Political Structure'. *Soc. Sci. Med. 11:* 415-19.

Schram, R., (1971). *A History of the Nigerian Health Services.* Ibadan University Press.

Stacey, May, M. (1968)., 'Concepts; Medicus Mundi; International Organization for Medical Co-operation'; on the Promotion of Tropical Health. P. 7.

Susser, M.W., and Watson, W., (1962). *Sociology in Medicine,* Oxford University Press.

Teitelbaum, M.S. (1974). 'Population and Development: Is a Concensus Possible?' *A Ford Foundation Reprint Foreign Affairs.* pp 742-60.

Waboso, M.F. (1973). *Niger Med. J.* 3, 100.

World Health Organisation (WHO, 1975). *Promotion of National Health Service,* Geneva, (A 28/29).

WHO/UNICEF. (1978). *Report of International Conference on Primary Health Care.* Alma-Ata, (ICPHC/ALA/78.10).

WHO. (1979). *Science and Technology for Health Promotion in Developing Countries* 33, 399-406.

WHO. (1980). *Decisions of the Health Assembly.* Chron. 34: 258-63.

73

Social Security in African Countries

G.O. Sofoluwe

The aims and objectives of a social security system are:

(1) to guarantee every resident (which include both permanent citizens and temporary residents) a minimum standard of living in certain specific respect including income, housing, food, education, employment, health and pension;

(2) to provide aid and support in certain emergencies including the death of the breadwinner, sickness, unemployment, retirement, and financial distress;

(3) to provide relief during emergencies which affect large numbers of people, for example wars, earthquakes, floods, and tornadoes;

(4) to redistribute a person's income more evenly during his life cycle;

(5) to attempt to narrow gaps which cause social conflicts between different social classes;

(6) to attain national solidarity, so that one working age group cohort will support both those who are too old to work and those who are too young. The old people would have at one time supported the present working age group as well as having supported an older age group now dead. The young will in the future become the working age group and will support both their old parents and their own children.

All these requirements used to be met by the system of extended families who lived in small villages or parishes. In fact it is the provision of all the above that has cemented groups of people to form tribes, and in more recent times, nations. Urbanization and industrialization has tended to disrupt and fragment this simple system, with serious social consequences.

In summary, therefore a social security system is intended to provide for all citizens the basic human necessities of life, with the ultimate aim of ensuring peace and stability.

Social Security System in Africa

Historically, man in Africa has always lived on the soil, and in fact now almost 80 per cent of the population in all African countries are still peasant farmers.

Up till 1968, most still lived in small villages of about 500 people, who were mostly descendants from one family, and who therefore could not intermarry but had to marry people from nearby villages. Such small populations still constitute over 80 per cent of human settlements in African countries.

Such small communities are often self-sufficient and are able to provide housing, food, employment, traditional medicine, traditional education, and a pension – even though on a limited scale. They are still able to meet objectives 2, 3, and 5 listed overleaf. With regard to objective 4, a successful or wealthy relative takes the responsibility for his less successful and poorer relations.

For example, for those who live in remote villages in Africa, there is no unemployment, even among the handicapped, as they are still able to farm. If the head of the household dies, his eldest son or his next oldest brother assumes full responsibility for the household, including marrying all the wives of the deceased, except the son's mother. Thus aid and support during such emergencies as the death of the breadwinner, sickness, or physical or other incapacitation are provided by the village and also by the clan or tribe.

During natural disaster and during wars – as for example during the Sahelian drought in West Africa – families and villages moved *en masse* and even if they are scattered initially, the successful members of the village will immediately begin to gather the others together so that the village regroups again in another place.

In West and North Africa tribal markings, often on the face, help the members of a village, or an ethnic or tribal group to recognize each other, and this has made regrouping possible even after the people have been widely scattered by inter-tribal wars – or by the once notorious slave trade.

Gaps between the social classes do not exist in the rural areas. As professions run in families, the eldest son in each household attains a chieftaincy title; all villagers, including the ruler, still live in mud houses; all eat practically the same sort of food and wear the same kind of clothes. Many causes of conflict have thus been removed, and African villages therefore enjoy considerably more peace and tranquility than the towns.

Divorce, juvenile delinquency, rape, drug addiction, and other social problems are very rare (often non-existent) in African villages: but they are now more prevalent in African towns. In these towns it has been impossible to provide the sort of comprehensive 'social security' that still exists in African villages.

Nowadays, however, with the advent of Western education and industrialization programmes, and the massive rural-urban migration of the working-age group, the stable village social security systems are tending to be less complete, whilst both governmental and private agencies are unable to cope with the massive influx into the towns which have almost no social security system at all.

Thus many Africans retain their roots in their villages and enjoy cheap food, sincere love, land, and a peaceful and tranquil place to live even if they are ill or retired.

Most African countries have realized the great potential of rural areas for meeting social security needs, and hence the government resettles soldiers discharged from the army in their villages. In other African countries, people retiring from civil or commercial jobs are now voluntarily returning to retire in their villages. The villages are now being provided with electricity, basic health facilities, and schools and are being gradually industrialized, especially by their most successful offspring.

The Future Development of Social Security in Africa

The situation in rural Africa, described overleaf, is not ideal for newly emerging African nations. Since it is based on clans, tribes, and ethnic groups, it tends to discourage the fusion of such groups into nations. It has caused civil wars and military coups, as one group attempts to dominate the other.

Attempts are now being made to develop national social security systems in all African countries. Unfortunately the successful development systems in Europe and America depend on there being over 80 per cent of the population employed in the money sector, rather than in peasant farming.

In 1960 in Nigeria for example, only 1 per cent of the population were earning salaries from the government, industries, or trading companies. A beginning was however made with this group by the establishment of workers' compensation and National Provident Funds. All employers of labour, including the government, are now encouraged to give housing loans or build houses for their workers, to provide at least one subsidized meal a day, to assist the workers with the education of their children, to provide some health services, and to operate superannuation, if not a full pension scheme.

The main problem is to generate enough cash to provide comprehensive pensions available on an equal basis to all people in the community. A brief history of the scheme and some details of the provisions, sources of finance, and operation of the scheme will now be described to enable the reader to understand its principles. These will be based on their rich traditional heritage, their human and other resources, and a well tailored industrialization programme. It is hoped that the tremendous social problems encountered by the world's pioneers of industrialization can be avoided.

The History of Social Security Schemes

Originally, it was the responsibility of the family of a small society like a village to take care of the sick or disabled. It is still so in many countries in the world. In Europe in the Middle Ages it was the task of the church to care for the poor and the sick even if the community as a whole played its part in practice even at that time. It is still more or less so in some parts of southern Europe, like Spain, with a conservative political system.

In the north of Europe, in the sixteenth century, at the time of the reformation, when the state appropriated the property of the church, it took responsibility for the church institutions for the care of the poor and sick. The state, however, soon found this an excessive burden, and transferred responsibility to the local parishes. They had a duty to sustain the sick and support the poor, at a very basic level and this was financed by charity. In some countries, for example, Sweden, it was decreed around the middle of the eighteenth century that the parish's care of the poor and sick should be financed by local taxes. In this way, the principle of the responsibility of the society was established and at the same time the financial source was created, but it was still very primitive in a conservative community.

The first traces of an economic protection against illness may be found within the craft guilds of the Middle Ages. In these associations of craftsmen, a primitive insurance system on a voluntary basis was sometimes developed, as a precursor to the voluntary insurance cash which centuries later was given considerable attention by various national movements, to result eventually in the creation of National Insurance against illness.

The capitalist industrial society created a large labour class in the nineteenth and the beginning of the twentieth centuries. At the same time there was in many countries still a class of poor farmers in small farms.

Investigations into the extent and causes of poverty made between the close of the nineteenth century and the Second World War showed that it had two main causes (1) failure to relate income during earning to the size of the family and (2) interruption or loss of earning power.

Some measures were taken to support such families whose incomes had been interrupted or discontinued. They consisted of a nation-wide scheme of social insurance, covering the whole population and providing maternity, widowhood, sickness, unemployment and industrial injury benefits, retirement pensions and a death grant, supplemented by a state scheme of social assistance providing for those whose needs could not be met, or were inadequately met, by social insurance.

The underlying principle of social insurance is that all persons within its scope contribute at an agreed rate to an insurance fund, to which employers and the state also contribute. The understanding is that in certain situations they can claim benefits from the fund at standard rates, without any test of need. The benefits are claimed as a right provided that the requisite number of contributions have been paid.

This method of providing against contingencies to which all are liable was widely adopted by trade unions and friendly societies during the nineteenth century. The first health and unemployment insurance schemes in Europe in the beginning of this century were very limited in scope, but they were subsequently widened to include sickness and unemployment benefits for all manual workers and for non-manual workers with a limited income.

The Social Policy

To define the social policy a description may be quoted, which was prepared by the Swedish government for a memorandum to the United Nations: social policy is based on solidarity between and within the generations.

> Sweden has a system of general pensions for all citizens. Those of active age pay the pensions of those who have left gainful employment. We have general children's allowance for all children and study allowances to all young persons who are studying. These allowances are paid by the active generation. When the children reach active age, they, in turn, will pay the pensions of the next generation of pensioners. They will also be defraying the general children's allowances for the new cohorts of children, who in the future will have to pay their old age pensions, and so on.
>
> There is also a general sickness insurance covering all citizens. So long as we are healthy and able to work, we pay for the sick. And when we ourselves need support and care–for shorter or longer periods–then it is the others, those who are healthy and able to work, who have to pay for us. This can serve also as a description of the idea of solidarity within social policy as a whole.

In order to guarantee and maintain this solidarity, society must be provided with resources. One-sixth of the Swedish gross national income is set aside for social insurance, family benefits, medical care and social care. The costs are met from state and municipal taxes and social insurance fees, which can also be described as taxes. Prerequisites for this social policy are an active economic policy and full employment in the country.

A National Insurance System in Sweden

An insurance system is aimed to give the citizen support against the economic consequences of *illness* as well as of *disablement, childbirth, old age* and the *death of the family breadwinner.* In addition to this, there are *unemployment insurance* and *industrial injuries insurance* (workers' compensation).

Sweden was the first country to make basic (social security) pensions available on an equal basis to all people.

Organization

The insurance system may be organized and administered in different ways.

In Sweden the National Insurance is administered by the National Social Insurance Board and – under supervision of that Board – by Public Insurance Benefit Societies. There is one such society in each county and in the three biggest cities. These societies have smaller local branches. This decentralized organization has partly its base in the growth of health insurance and the Benefit Societies which were developed from the voluntary insurance societies when insurance became compulsory in 1955.

Participation

From the age of sixteen, it is necessary to be registered with a Benefit Society. Also foreigners who are residents of the country are insured under the National Insurance Acts of 1962. A foreigner taking up residence in Sweden has to report to a Benefit Society within two weeks for registration.

Pension Insurance

There are two kinds of pensions: (1) the basic, mainly, flat rate pensions and (2) the supplementary pensions. The main difference is that one receives the basic pensions irrespective of income (even a millionaire gets his basic pension), whereas supplementary pensions are dependent on earned income. There are four kinds of basic pensions: (1) old-age pension, (2) disability pension, (3) widows' pension, and (4) children's pension.

The Old-age Pension

This can be claimed from the age of sixty four years or with reduction from sixty three years of age or with a corresponding increase from the age of seventy years. The benefit for a single person amounts to 90 per cent of the so-called base amount valid for that month. This is a method of maintaining a realistic purchasing power of benefits, since the base amount continuously fluctuates at the general price level. There is now an increasing sum every year in a ten-year period for those who have none or a small supplementary pension. At the end of this period, in 1979, the basic pension would be 120 per cent of the base amount. It is now about 7,000 Swedish croner (more than ₦1,000).

The Disability Pension

Before becoming eligible for the old-age pension, an insured person may be entitled to a disability pension if for medical reasons his working capacity is considerably and permanently reduced. There are three grades of benefits, depending on the reduction in working capacity. Although it was stated earlier that a basic pension is granted without any rules or means test, income from work is taken into account in the assessment of the reduction of his working capacity.

The Widow's Pension

This is granted irrespective of the widow's age if she has in her care a child under sixteen years of age or if she was thirty six years old at the time of her husband's death, it is reduced if the widow was less than fifty, but after fifty she is entitled to full pension. The principle is that there is a difference in the want for a young able-bodied widow and an old woman who cannot be expected to be employed.

The Children's Pension

Payable to a child who has lost one or both parents before sixteen years of age. Different supplementary benefits may be added to the basic pension, such as a child supplement to a pensioner with children under sixteen years, or a disability supplement if he is severely handicapped and unable to take care of himself. Also a wife's supplement and municipal housing supplement, both according to special regulations is subject to a means test. Under certain conditions a disability allowance may be granted to someone who is not entitled to a pension according to the Act.

Only Swedish nationals, who are resident or have been census registered for a certain number of years, are eligible for a basic pension. A foreign national is excluded unless he can refer to an international agreement, convention, or treaty. Quite a number of such agreements have been signed with other countries.

Supplementary Pensions

The National Supplementary Pension system known as ATP, began in 1960. It is implemented in stages over a period of twenty years. When fully operative, the system will guarantee the average retired person with at least thirty income-earning years behind him a basic and supplementary pension whose total purchasing power is roughly equivalent of two-thirds of the working income he enjoyed during his fifteen best-paid years. The supplementary pension is entirely employer-financed. No working person runs the risk of forfeiting any of his future ATP benefits by changing jobs, since all employers pay their ATP contributions into a national fund.

Supplementary Social Services

Local government provides various free or low cost services to pensioners living on their own: 'home Samaritans', delivery of goods and library books, special transport arrangements, gymnastics, and loans or grants for converting individual flats to suit their physical limitations. The same authorities also operate old age homes and nursing homes for those unable to care for themselves.

Health Insurance

Health Insurance Benefits are of two main kinds: (1) compensation for medical, dental, and hospital care expenditure and (2) a cash benefit, called sickness allowance.

Compensation for Expenditure

The conditions are (a) treatment must be necessitated by illness (preventive measures, e.g. vaccination, is not included), (b) the illness must, in the doctors opinion, render medical care necessary.

The Local Insurance Benefit Society (IBS) pays the cost of hospitalization (usually direct to the hospital), ambulances, surgery and laboratory tests.

The fee for out-patient care at hospital clinics, district medical offices and other public facilities is low (at present, 12 Swedish Croner per appointment regardless of treatment) for the patient who pays cash, the main part will be paid by the IBS.

An earlier system, which was considered circumstantial and rather troublesome, both for the people and the authorities, is still working, if the patient chose to visit a private doctor. The choice of doctor is free. A private practitioners bill, as well as for physiotherapy and private convalescent care will be reimbursed by three quarters to the patient, according to a standard fee schedule, as well as half the price of dental care.

Some medicine and drugs are entirely free, such as for diabetes, epilepsy, TB, cancer etc. For others, no one has to pay more than 15 Swedish Croner (approximately ₦2) regardless of the real price and how many different drugs are bought on the same prescription. What the chemist does not get from the buyer will be refunded by the Social Insurance Board.

Sickness Allowance

In order to provide sufficient protection against the economic consequences of illness, a cash benefit is paid to working people above sixteen years of age. There are (a) a basic sickness allowance, and (b) supplementary allowance, which varies according to income. Until recently this was constructed so as to compensate about 90 per cent of the ordinary take-home pay (within normal income brackets). Now this is changed. The sickness allowance is now about 90 per cent of the earning income and ordinary tax is drawn (paid).

The principle is that when a citizen is sick, he shall not be dependent upon charity, it is his right to have the same economic standard of living as when he is working and has earnings.

The basic allowance is very low (about ₦1 per day). The upper limit for the supplementary and basic allowance together is about eight times that amount.

On the birth of a child, every mother is eligible for a six-month leave of absence from employment with a benefit corresponding to the regular sickness benefit. For part of the time, this benefit is payable to the father instead of the mother, if he is staying at home and she is going to work.

Either parent can receive a regular sickness benefit if forced to stay at home from work in order to care for a sick child.

A housewife without work outside her home cannot have supplementary sickness allowance. She will get only the basic allowance. There are however, the following voluntary allowances.

The voluntary sickness allowance can be added to the compulsory and this is directed mainly to housewives and students, i.e. a person who for six months or more is not or to a slight extent engaged in gainful activity. The insured person has to pay extra contributions to the IBS and the daily allowance is limited to about twice the basic allowance. There is also a waiting period of eighteen days.

When the health insurance was made compulsory in 1955 and the national supplementary pensions were introduced in 1960, it was held by many that it would mean the end of private health insurance. The opposite turned out to be true. For example, the average ratio of individual private life insurance – already higher than in any other European country – increased by about 10 per cent.

An important aspect of health insurance specifically for people who have been ill for a long time consists of treatment and/or rehabilitation which may help to restore working capacity or to shorten the sickness periods. The IBS are reminded of this, which one might consider an aspect of their important controlling activity, by ruling in the National Insurance Act which states that they have at least as soon as sickness allowance or compensation for hospital care has been paid for ninety consecutive days – to investigate whether any kind of treatment (rehabilitation) is possible or suitable. Vocational rehabilitation is administered by the National Market Board and its local organizations. When an IBS adjudges a case involving a long sickness period where rehabilitation might be useful, the matter is discussed by a special team set up by the IBS, to which representatives from the Labour Markets authorities also are summoned. The sooner rehabilitation can start, the better the results to be expected.

A child supplement may also be added to the sickness allowance depending on the number of children.

Maternity Insurance

There is one situation in which sickness allowance is paid even if the insured person is not technically ill. It is when a woman stops working because of pregnancy that she is paid a maternity allowance (at present about 1000 Swedish Croner, approximately ₦150), and as mentioned before a benefit corresponding to her sickness allowances.

Complaints

If an insured person is dissatisfied with a decision made by a IBS in a matter concerning his benefit, his complaint may be pursued by filing an appeal with the Social Insurance Board. If he is still not satisfied after the Board has reached a decision, he may appeal to the National Insurance Court, whose judgement is final.

Industrial Injuries Insurance (Workmen's Compensation)

There is still a special act for this insurance, but illness caused by industrial injury is dealt with as any other illness in accordance with the health insurance provisions, so long as it does not last more than ninety days. It is supposed to be even more closely fitted into the National Insurance legislation in the near future.

Unemployment Compensation

It is the only form of social insurance that is still voluntary. The trade unions operate unemployment insurance societies which union members are eligible to join. The government contributes two-thirds of the necessary funds and participating employees the rest. To qualify for daily benefits while unemployed, the insured person must register as a job seeker at the National Market Board

Office. Under certain conditions a person who is not a member of one of the societies can receive an unemployment benefit directly from the local National Market Board Office.

Families with children receive a number of benefits aimed at easing their economic situation. The government pays a tax-exempt child allowance of 1500 Swedish Croners a year to the parents of each child under sixteen, regardless of the family's income level. Infants, children under sixteen and pregnant mothers are included in a systematic programme of preventive health care. Children receive free school lunches. Families with below average incomes whose monthly rents or mortgage payments exceed a given level are eligible for partial housing allowances from both central and local governments, provided their homes meet minimum physical standards. Local governments provide free family advisory and child welfare services when needed, and operate a variety of recreational facilities for children and teenagers.

Finance of Social Insurance

Compulsory Health Insurance is financed by contributions from employers and employees and State grants. The latter cover about 15 per cent, the employers contribution about 45 per cent and the employees about 40 per cent.

Basic pensions are financed by the State, about 60 per cent, the insured persons about 25 per cent and the municipalities about 15 per cent.

Supplementary pensions are to some extent financed by contributions from employers, based on the remuneration of their employees, amounting to between 10 and 15 per cent. A self employed person has to pay his own contribution. A person's contributions are charged on his tax account and collected together with his income tax.

If Industrial Injury Insurance and Unemployment Insurance are added to the other items of Social Insurance the total financial sources are, the State about 30 per cent; municipalities about 5 per cent, employers about 35 per cent, insured persons about 20 per cent and 10 per cent from interests on funds.

The total expenditure in the social field amounts to close to 20 per cent of the Gross National Product.

A Summary of the Swedish National Social Security Scheme

A social security system is described which is comprehensive, covers the entire people, is founded on solidarity between generations, social classes and regions, is aimed to narrow the gap between rich and poor, distributes income more evenly over the life-cycle, and provides public services.

Many activities in this section were started on a voluntary basis and subsequently taken over by the public sector. They have grown in response to changing needs. Efforts were concentrated on finding generally applicable solutions. Two main approaches were adopted: (1) the preventive approach was aimed at abolishing unemployment, preventing occupational injuries, preventing diseases through better housing and health services, limiting working hours and providing for vacations; (2) the supportive approach operated in cases where a need had already arisen. New and more rational methods of assistance than the old poor relief were sought, they were found in a system of a compulsory national insurance, designed to offer security in situations known to involve grave financial risks or strain for a larger number of people, i.e. sickness, old-age, disability, etc. Now the national insurance, consisting basically of four different insurances – sickness insurance, maternity insurance, the basic pension, and the national supplementary pension is the backbone of the social security system. These insurances have emerged, one after another, and are continuously being improved. They are now co-ordinated in a uniform and essentially simple organization.

The state has assumed increasing responsibility for the individual's financial security in the event of illness, incapacity, old-age, death of the family provider, etc. Responsibility for personal care, for services, and for various types of preventive measures rests primarily with the communes, while responsibility for health and medical services rests with another type of authority, on regional level, the county councils.

In all sectors, however, the state retains ultimate control as the legislating and supervisory body. Research and higher education are other sectors in which the state directly assumes the main responsibility. In many cases the state also contributes towards the financing of social security.

Social benefits, which are identical for all, are financed mainly by taxation; while those adjusted to individual income are usually financed by charges paid by the insured person and/or his employer,

Health and medical services, care of the aged, support for families, and services for people at work, are financed by taxation.

The general view of social security has been altered in the last decades. Previously such measures were regarded purely as a burden on the economy of central and local government. Today social policy is regarded as an important positive factor in that it offers the individual not only greater security but also a greater chance of making an active contribution to production and the life of the community. In other words, it is accepted that social policy is also a good investment, one that pays off in the national economy.

74

Undergraduate Training in Public Health in Africa

D.A. Ogunmekan

Many African Anglophone medical schools have been developing their own curricula and have allowed adequate time for learning about community health and most have spaced the subject through several years of study, some through all the years of the course.

Objectives for Undergraduates

Faculty Objectives

The goals of the undergraduate programmes in Faculties of Medicine are to produce doctors of high quality and in such numbers as are required to meet the health care delivery needs of the nation at community and hospital levels.

These objectives can be achieved by:

1. Designing teaching and evaluating courses which portray man as an integral part of his total environment – biological, physical and social.
2. Demonstrating to the students through their involvement in community health practice that manipulation of the environment including health services administration can be carried out to benefit the health of the individual and the community.

The student should be able to demonstrate that he has knowledge of the appropriate measures (promotive, preventive and curative) that can be used to identify and solve the health problems of individuals, families and communities.

He should have the skills to assess the health of a community and describe how social, cultural, demographic, ecological and economic factors can affect the health of a community.

He should also be able to apply health management techniques for delivering health care services with the assistance of other members of the health team for the prevention and control of prevalent communicable and non-communicable diseases.

To achieve these objectives, the following courses are taken:

1. Medical sociology, including demography.
2. Statistics, including vital and health statistics.
3. Epidemiology and the control of communicable and non-communicable diseases.
4. Environmental and occupational health.
5. Disease survey skills (projects).
6. Maternal and child health/family health.
7. School health.
8. Health promotion, including health education.
9. Health planning and management.
10. Experience in primary health care delivery in a rural or urban area by students who have completed some clinical postings.

Many Faculties of Medicine have developed programmes of field work carried out in health centres or mobile clinics.

Objectives for field work relate to gaining understanding of and ability in carrying out 'community diagnosis,' the planning of services and also managing and evaluating these services. The teachers in field work should be viewed as facilitators. Students have an opportunity during a field rotation to do projects along guidelines laid down for them. Another teaching method that is increasingly being used is the 'self-instructional' unit which can be used to reinforce the teaching in the evenings.

Other undergraduates who require courses in Community Health:
Both nursing and health education are tending to extend from the Ministry of Health auxiliary training schools and have some levels of courses now given in the universities. Sometimes, such courses start as diplomas given by the university with the goal of providing teachers and administrators in these fields. However, often, the initially small university department expands, gains more staff and financial support and is able to offer a full degree course.

Whether at diploma or degree levels, nurses and health educators who will be in high administrative posts should have some concept of the importance of community health. They should learn to assess community needs, plan and organize a programme, administer primary health services, evaluate them and work with people and their leaders.

Dentistry faculties or schools also find that community health is an essential part of their curriculum. Preventive dentistry, health education, community survey techniques and epidemiology are all subjects that the dentist needs.

75

Medical Education in Rural Public Health: the Ibarapa Model

William R. Brieger

The advent of primary health care (PHC) has encouraged many medical schools to rethink about their approach to training. Some, like the College of Medicine, University of Ibadan, are leaders in the field, having established a rural public and community health rotation fifteen years before the Alma Ata Declaration. In this chapter, The Ibarapa posting will be examined as a model student training programme in public and community health.

First it is necessary to define what is a training programme. Training is a series of planned learning activities that emphasize acquisition of specified skills and competencies along with knowledge, attitudes and values needed to ensure appropriate application of these skills. Training is particularly associated with professional and practical education. It goes beyond imparting information toward providing opportunities to practice in a real life situation. Training presupposes some level of general education or experience upon which to build.

Training also implies service and can therefore be either pre-service or in-service, with the former usually being the longer, preparatory phase. Professional training is therefore a continuous process that does not stop once service begins. It is in the area of basic, pre-service professional training, where the Ibarapa programme generally fits. Ibarapa is a component within the design of a larger professional training curriculum for medical and other health sciences students. Consequently it is necessary to examine how this rotation integrates with the larger course of study as well as to consider its internal structure and organization.

Curriculum Models

At least, four broad models for curriculum development in medical education exist, (1) subject centred, (2) integrated, (3) competency based and (4) problem solving (Barrows and Tamblyn, 1980; McGahie et al 1978). Subject centred curricula are probably the most common as well as the most traditional. The approach is a natural extension of the general education system. Subjects like mathematics, physics and government are covered in the secondary school curriculum, while anatomy, physiology and pharmacology make up the medical course of studies. Each subject is taught in a discrete manner with an emphasis on memorization, but little room for student involvement or initiative. The subject centred approach is probably the least responsive to the current challenge of PHC which demand looking across traditional subject boundaries toward fostering intersectoral collaboration and community involvement.

The integrated approach is interdisciplinary and often focuses on major organ systems as a point of departure. Theory and experience are brought together, for example, the knowledge and activities of the biochemist, internist, physiologist, surgeon, psychiatrist and social worker can be brought to bear on the study of the gastrointestinal system and the management of problems emanating from there. Questions have been raised about students' ability to remember the variety of issues presented during an integrated period of study, which has led to a compromise variation of this approach that utilizes a core curriculum of essential foundation courses to precede the interdisciplinary experience.

A competency based curriculum is built around the real functions which a medical doctor or health worker is actually expected to perform. Once the competencies or performance objectives have been determined, they can be arranged in a systematic manner, such that the knowledge and skills can be built upon and learning can be sequenced from simple to complex. This approach encouraged student initiative in mastering competences at the student's own pace.

Problem solving is a natural human learning process. When applied to medical education, it facilitates learning about an individual patient's need, a difficulty in health service delivery or resolution of a health research question. Problem based learning fosters development of diagnostic and reasoning skills and encourages the student to become an active seeker of knowledge, not a passive receiver. This approach shares with the integrative model the need to draw on the resources of various disciplines simultaneously.

Underlying Philosophy

Underlying these four approaches to medical training is a broader philosophical issue about education, whether it is teacher centred or student centred. The subject centred approach is generally focused on teacher determined needs otherwise known as a directive approach. On a continuum of ever increasing levels of student involvement in learning, one would find next, the integrated approach followed by competency based education with problem solving providing the most involving challenge to students. It should be noted that the more student or learner centred an approach,the more resources, especially personnel, are needed to facilitate learning.

In reality most medical schools are an amalgamation of approaches. Preclinical education is often more subject and teacher centred. As students advance in their studies, they are given more room to solve problems and take initiatives. At Ibadan today, medical education is still very much departmentalized and therefore subject centred. The Ibarapa posting is the exception.

The Ibarapa posting (or rotation) was established in 1963 for the primary purpose of distinguishing the Ibadan M.B.B.S. curriculum from its London parent. Ibarapa was meant to be the heart of the new curriculum that would make medical education truly relevant to the needs and environment of Africa generally and Nigeria specifically. The rural Ibarapa District in southwest Nigeria was to serve as a living community health laboratory for student faculty services, research and teaching (Ogunlesi, 1965; Gilles, 1965). A collaborative state, local government, community and university approach to delivering health services was established.

As presently organized, the Ibarapa posting is an eight-week rotation in the fourth year of medical training. At this point, incoming students have had introductory rotations in medicine, surgery and paediatrics. They have also had the lecture format courses with some field trips in public health. Ibarapa provides the first hands as an exposure to the latter discipline.

Ibarapa Adaptation

Ibarapa began and has continued as an interdisciplinary programme. There has been continuous staff input (consultants, lecturers, registrars, technicians) from the University of Ibadan and the teaching hospital, the University College Hospital (UCH). The Departments of Medicine, Surgery, Preventive and Social Medicine, Paediatrics and Obstetrics and Gynaecology are involved at both the decision making and teaching levels. Timely input from the laboratory sciences, radiology, psychiatry, ophthalmology and other departments has enhanced both student learning and community service.

The Department of Preventive and Social Medicine (PSM), which is administratively responsible for the rotation, is itself interdisciplinary. Faculty and staff with the following areas of postgraduate public health specialization are represented: maternal and child health, epidemiology, biostatistics, health education, environmental health, health management, social medicine and occupational health.

Ibarapa has always followed the integrated model of medical education by drawing on these various resource disciplines. Experience with patient education (including the social and behavioural aspects of health care) is integrated with clinical teaching. Family health activities pay attention to the environmental conditions where pregnant women live and young children play. The school health visits incorporate child health, clinical screening, health education, environmental sanitation and nutrition as well as management of health resources such as the first aid box and the training of teachers to use it.

Practical field experiences are also brought into the seminar room where staff from various backgrounds interact with students. Students present their observations on health management issues in Ibarapa and can expect reactions from a health educator, medical officer, community nurse or public health inspector. During a seminar on essential drug supply, a physician may challenge students' views on which drugs are appropriate for locally endemic conditions. The health educator may introduce the issue of compliance with medical regimens. The public health nurse may raise concerns about the need to provide drugs in a form appropriate for small children.

One concern with the integrated model is that in the attempt to incorporate all relevant issues, staff may loose sight of the specific task students should master. In recent years therefore, Ibarapa staff have given serious thought to the competency based model (Brieger, 1978). This has been done in the context of the length of the rotation and its timing within the overall medical curriculum.

The posting at present is divided into six major week long rotational activities: Environmental Health, Health Education, Maternal and Child Health, Occupational Health, Primary Medical Care and General Practice. A list of competencies has been developed for each. These take the form of skills which the student is expected to practise at least once during the rotation. Due to the integrated nature of the training, the practice of a specific skill is not limited to any one specific week's activity. Students are given a full list of the competencies during the orientation week and are expected to avail themselves of any opportunity to practise throughout the posting. For example, the health education competency of providing individual counselling can take place during environmental inspection of a market stall, while on a home visit or in the ward during clinical activities. An abbreviated sampling of these competencies follows:

1. Primary Medical Care:
   - diagnose and treat a child with malaria
   - set up an intravenous drip and regulate it
2. Laboratory Practice:
   - perform packed cell volume test and interpret results
   - make total white cell count
3. Maternal and Child Health:
   - book a pregnant woman in antenatal clinic
   - palpate to determine gestational age, position and presentation
4. Health Education:
   - deliver a group health presentation
   - provide individual patient counselling
5. Environmental Health:
   - assess the sanitary condition of a dug well
   - inspect an eating establishment to identify factors that promote or threaten health
6. Occupational Health:
   - identify occupational related diseases in local work sites
   - determine health problems in a local farm village

Ibarapa is not without a problem solving component. In the early days when there were few students per posting, students in pairs or individually were assigned to specific villages or neighbourhoods. Therein they would study the problems and resources of that community and develop recommendations to solve the identified problems. Today this process has been formally integrated with the regular supervision of volunteer village health workers. A visiting student team discusses with villagers the nature of their problems. Then they plan with the village health worker possible ways to implement solutions to the identified problems.

Student research projects provide another avenue for problem based learning. Teams of approximately six to eight students choose a research topic which they will pursue throughout the eight weeks of the posting. They are required to set their own objectives, choose an appropriate research design, select their study population, develop methods and instruments (ensuring reliability and validity), carry out the study, analyse the data and present the findings. A major portion of the posting's final week is taken up with preparation and presentation of project reports. Although these student have had biostastics and epidemiology as subjects during their earlier years in medical school, it is often only after they reach Ibarapa that they begin to understand how to apply these skills.

Organization and Logistics

After looking at the content and approaches to learning in Ibarapa, it is necessary to look at some organizational and logistical aspects of the training. One cannot talk about gaining competencies and solving problems unless the training itself is situated in actual ongoing health services. To that end, the Ibarapa Programme is intimately involved in the provision of preventive and curative services for all seven towns and the hundreds of small hamlets in the district.

The Ibarapa Programme manages a health centre in collaboration with the state government, maintains links with the district hospital and a private clinic, supervises local government maternal and child health clinics in several towns, provides family visiting outreach services, maintains a self-sufficient volunteer primary health care programme, provides a model school health service and assists the local government health office in environmental surveillance. Medical students are brought directly into this milieu as health team members.

The staff who teach and guide the students are practitioners who provide the services just mentioned. They are employed by the University, the Oyo State Ministry of Health, the Ibarapa Local Government or are community volunteers. They are dedicated to their work and to the communities they serve. Even though they are not paid to teach per se, they devote much of their professional and personal time to the learning needs and welfare of the students. They demonstrate how it is possible for professionals to find job satisfaction in a rural community.

Direct input by academic university staff helps students integrate their learning experiences in the community with the content of lectures and practicals held at the main campus. Visiting academic staff from Ibadan also provide supervision and encouragement to the Ibarapa based personnel.

Time is a major logistical consideration for the Ibapara training programme, both the amount allocated and the point in the medical student's career when the posting occurs. Concern is always raised that students should not be exposed too late after a clinical bias may have taken hold, nor too early before they have the requisite knowledge, skills and maturity to appreciate the complexities of community health.

To solve this training problem, many schools phase students into the community gradually. Even in the preclinical years special field trips can be arranged or students can be assigned to follow up specific families to learn about the social and environmental dimensions of health. Practical service postings occur later after students have crossed over to the clinical side. The Department of Preventive and Social Medicine at Ibadan has attempted this approach. Its courses 'Man and His Environment' in the preclinical years and the 'Introductory Course' when students first enter their clinical studies do take the students out into the community for field trips and offer theoretical input which can later be applied in Ibarapa.

Two problems confront this approach. If the duration and intensity of exposure to the community is not long enough, these courses will amount to only a fleeting memory and have little impact on student attitudes. A second and worse fate is that the students may see such courses as being in competition with their 'real' priorities, that is passing the preclinical exams. The University needs to consider ways to increase the time available for and the legitimacy of these community oriented courses. Otherwise the time (eight weeks) allocated to public and community health in the Ibarapa posting may be inadequate to achieve its founders' goals – that of developing physicians who not only appreciate, but can also function in the rural African environment.

Other Students

So far, this chapter has described the Ibarapa Programme as it affects medical students. In the context of primary health care, Ibarapa is open to all health science and related students. During much of the 1970s, student nurses from the teaching hospital were posted regularly to Ibarapa. The Ibarapa experience stimulated their tutors to open their own community practice site in a small village just north of Ibadan. At present, student midwives from the teaching hospital have just completed their third annual posting in Ibarapa. Public and Community Health Officers (a type of public health nurse clinician central to Nigeria's basic health services scheme) who are being trained in Ibadan have been coming on six week rotations to Ibarapa for ten consecutive years as part of their one year professional training.

Students in Ibarapa therefore come from different curricula, different levels of competence, different amounts of experience and different priority learning needs. Since Ibarapa posting has developed a competency based approach to training, it is easier to accommodate a variety of students. Student midwives would share the basic skills which are expected of medical students in the area of maternal and child health. However, their needs concerning environmental health would focus more exclusively around the home setting, while future physicians as potential medical officers of health would require more detailed experience in public health laws and community-wide sanitation.

Community Health Officers would have all primary medical and preventive competencies in common with medical students, but would require additional skills in service management at the local level. This sensitivity to similarities and differences among the various cadres of health workers, balanced against community needs, makes curriculum planning more logical and easier.

Apprenticeships

Finally there is a third group of trainees that come to Ibarapa who might best be called apprentices. They are the postgraduates and diploma students in various public health courses at the University. For them a posting in Ibarapa is more like a period of apprenticeship than one of instruction. They are expected to undertake self-directed learning utilizing resident staff as resource people. They work together with local staff on existing programmes and services in the clinic and field, but also design their own projects. Their model of learning is definitely problem based as they cope with the daily realities of service delivery.

A major group of these mature students are the medical registrars from the teaching hospital in Ibadan. The Departments of Medicine, Paediatrics and Obstetrics and Gynaecology send all their registrars for a period of service in Ibarapa. The Department of PSM and the UCH General Outpatient Department (which participates in the national postgraduate general practice training programme) send their own registrars to Ibarapa on advanced rotations with specific learning objectives in hand.

Since its inception in 1975 the African Regional Health Education Centre at the University has been posting some of its master and diploma students to Ibarapa for their three-month internship. Many of the master students stay on to undertake their dissertation research. They understudy the resident health educators and take increasing responsibility for existing health education services such as primary health worker training and patient education and develop new services.

Present Assessment

Recommendations from the recent World Conference of Medical Education in Edinburgh (August 1988) provide a timely standard by which to measure the contributions of the Ibarapa posting (WHO 1988). These include the following:

- enlarge training settings to include all health resources of the community.
- shift emphasis to self-directed learning.
- build a curriculum based on professional competence and social values.
- ensure the curriculum reflects national priorities.
- train medical teachers as educators, not just content experts.
- complement instruction on patient management with health promotion and prevention
- use a problem solving approach.
- select medical students based on personal qualities, not just academic ability.
- facilitate co-operation among sectors.
- ensure admissions policy reflect national needs.
- increase opportunities for interdisciplinary teaching, research and service.

Clearly, the Ibarapa Programme measures up quite well, having been established and maintained with many of the above goals in mind. The only issues that Ibarapa cannot address, e.g. admissions policy, are ones beyond the responsibility of one posting or department.

Future Directions

The above recommendations also point directions toward where the Ibarapa posting needs to move. While professional competencies have been spelled out, they should constantly be reviewed. The issues of professional values needs more attention. More in-service training on competency based and problem oriented learning would be of benefit to Ibarapa staff.

At the service level, more attention to intersectoral collaboration is needed. Formal links need to be forged among the various local government agencies in Ibarapa: health, agriculture, education, social development, information and culture and others. More community involvement such as the volunteer primary health workers' programme needs to be fostered, and the medical student needs to be involved in all these efforts.

In February 1989, at the 25th Anniversary ceremony of the Ibarapa Programme, Nigeria's Federal Minister for Health Prof. O. Ransome-Kuti, suggested that the bulk of medical training should take place in settings like Ibarapa. The Ibarapa Programme staff and the community are ready for such a challenge.

References

Barrows, H.S and Tamblyn R.M. ***Problem Based Learning: An Approach to Medical Education.*** New York: Springer Publishing Company, 1980.

Brieger, W.R, 'Developing Service-based Teaching in Health Education for Medical Students'. *Health Education Monographs* 1978; 6:354-358.

Gilles, H.M. 'Teaching Preventive Medicine in the Tropics'. *Lancet* 1965; 2: 280.

McGaghie, W.C., Miller, G.E., Sajid, A.W., Telder T.V. 'Competency Based Curriculum Development in Medical Education: An Introduction'. Geneva: ***World Health Organization, Public Health Papers No. 68, 1978.***

Ogunlesi, T.O. 'The Ibarapa Project, a New Look at Ibadan'. ***Journal of the Nigerian Medical Association 1965; 2:*** 168-172.

World Health Organization. 'World Conference on Medical Education'. In ***WHO News and Notes. World Health Forum 1988; 9:*** 623-625.

76

Postgraduate Education and Training in Public Health in Africa

O.O. Hunponu-Wusu

Introduction

The keywords in this chapter, which are postgraduate, education, training, and public health, are defined and explained in their ordinary and special usages. Their significance is illustrated with examples which are largely drawn from the West African countries.

Medical Education

Education may be described as the learning and the development which results from the process of training, or the process of teaching and training, or the academic discipline which deals with teaching and learning methods in schools. Medical education can be described as education carried out or acquired in Medical Schools or Faculties of Medicine, Colleges of Medicine or Health Sciences of Universities and tertiary institutions of learning. Postgraduate medical education or training is education which is carried out at the postgraduate level either for a higher degree, a certificate or a diploma.

Until comparatively recently, the attention of the authorities of many medical schools in Africa had been to concentrate on the establishment of undergraduate programmes and courses with the main objective primarily as an instrument for training and also for the development of health manpower. For instance in a statement from the Medical Council of Nigeria in 1984, the national objectives in medical education to guide new medical schools in the country were as follows:

1. to produce medical doctors with internationally acceptable knowledge of the scientific foundations of medicine but with a clear orientation towards the health and medical problems in Nigeria.
2. to train these doctors so that they have in addition to practical skill for handling common health problems and medical emergencies, a strong inclination to broad Community Health, Preventive Medicine, as well as the ability to lead a health team and manage a small health service.
3. to train as well, other cadres of health manpower in such a way as to constitute a health team.

One can observe from the foregoing the value placed on training in the local setting, and the importance of public health in the national objectives of medical education. Again the emphasis on public health and the community was illustrated in another example by the Faculty of Health Sciences of the University of Ilorin which has a Community-Based Experience and Services (COBES) programme, a medical education philosophy which prepares doctors for community service by exposing them to the health needs of the populace which reside largely in the rural and peri-urban areas, in addition to their recognized role as hospital-based physicians.

Thus in many medical schools in Africa, public health is taught as an undergraduate subject throughout the whole course of training for five years while in a few others, the subject is taught for about four years. This illustrates the emphasis given to and the orientation for public health.

Postgraduate Medical Training

Many of the new medical schools in Africa had been pre-occupied with the training of undergraduates and the setting up of academic standards. The issue of formal national or local postgraduate training had not however been given enough attention. Moreover, only in a handful of centres are there sufficient numbers of teachers with adequate academic and professional experience to make local or national postgraduate training comprehensive and meaningful. For example in the whole of the Anglophone West African region there is only a total of six approved centres for the training of residents for the Part I Fellowship Examination in the Faculty of Public Health. The six comprise of the four accredited centres in Nigeria, namely the University Teaching Hospital and University Departments of Community Health situated in Lagos, Ibadan, Zaria and Ilorin and one each located in Accra and Kumasi, both in Ghana.

In the West Africa Region, the two main bodies/agencies for accrediting and assessing centres for postgraduate professional training in public health are:

1. the West African College of Physicians, which is a constituent part of the West African Postgraduate Medical College and
2. the National Postgraduate Medical College of Nigeria.

These two bodies accredit centres for the training of residents and postgraduate medical students in public health, assess the qualifications of individuals for the different parts of the examinations, and also assess those individuals who present themselves for the Fellowship examinations of these Colleges in Public Health as far as the consultant level.

Public Health

Public Health is the science and art of preventing diseases, prolonging life and promoting health through organized efforts of the society. It is the study of health and diseases in groups of people or populations. The specialist in public health seeks to identify the etiology of diseases, the prevention of illnesses and the provision of medical care. This discipline has been called various synonyms such as Community Health, Community Medicine, Preventive Medicine, Social Medicine, Epidemiology et cetera and these terms have been used interchangeably in this context. The basic tools of this specialist are in behavioural sciences, epidemiology, health statistics, information systems and management science.

Postgraduate training in public health should therefore cover all these relevant areas.

The Need for Local Postgraduate Training in Public Health

The marked progress which has been achieved during the last three decades in the establishment of medical schools for the training of doctors in Africa had not been paralleled with similar substantive improvements in the total health care services to the populace of our countries. The need, importance and urgency for postgraduate training in public health has not been fully recognized for quite some time while the training of public health personnel, which is essential for the effective delivery of health services and the adequate coverage of the population still lags very much behind. Paramount on the list of reasons for an inadequate delivery of health care to the populace are the lack of these public health personnel to carry out community health care, and the inability to fully apply the basic principles of public health to the implementation of the health programmes.

It is increasingly realized however that in order to improve the health of our nations, it is mandatory to train more public health medical personnel *pari passu* with those of the allied health workers in community health, to elevate the status of public health personnel and to apply the scientific and public health principles in the protection of the health of these communities.

Most countries in Africa have established the system of Local Government Administrative Areas (LGAA) or Local Government District Areas (LGDA) or their equivalents for the entire country. In addition to other professional personnel in the municipal services of these LGAA, each LGAA, rural or urban, should have at least a Medical Officer of Health with the appropriate qualification and experience to carry out the health functions in the area. Unfortunately, however, many LGAA or LGDA have no Medical Officers of Health, many LGAA have no health services component while these services are poorly developed in others. This realization of the acute shortage of public health personnel made Sofoluwe in 1979 to work out estimated manpower requirements for community health specialists in Nigeria. Taking into consideration the attrition rate, and that 75% of specialists in any branch of medicine will offer full time services in their area of consultancy and based on the then existing 308 LGAA in Nigeria, he stated that within the decade 1980 and 1990 there was a need to train 308 x 4 = 1232 community health specialists for the Local Government Administrative Areas for the entire country. That would mean that the existing ten University Departments of Community Health should produce about 10-12 community health specialists per year for the next ten years!

A similar plea for the training of public health specialists had also been made by Hunponu-Wusu in 1979, and in 1980 in the occasional publications of the Department of Community Health of the College of Medicine of the University of Lagos.

Because of the needs of African countries, the specialty of public health should therefore be the pivot of all specialist training schemes. Government policies should be accordingly directed towards producing public health specialists or community physicians in sufficient number (quantity and quality) to man the primary health care services of the community in order to attain the desired goal of Health For All Africans by the year 2,000.

The Postgraduate Programmes

Postgraduate training in public health in Africa is mandatory for the successful practice of public health. An adequate postgraduate training has as its basis, a sound and thorough undergraduate training in public health. Experience has shown that those whose undergraduate training are weak or deficient, or those with inadequate exposure in tropical public health find postgraduate training in public health in Africa considerably much more difficult. However through review or refresher courses, and up date seminars and workshops, one can correct one's weaknesses even before embarking on postgraduate training.

The Fellowships of the West African College of Physicians (FWCP) and the National Postgraduate Medical College of Nigeria (FMCPH)

These two fellowships are open to medical practitioners with basic medical degrees or other registrable medical qualifications. In addition the candidate must have completed one year internship and should have worked for at least another year as a medical practitioner i.e. the candidate should have completed or be exempted from the National Youth Corps Service in Nigeria.

The doctors in training are offered residency positions in accredited centres in hospitals. The centres are accredited by the West African College of Physicians or by the National Postgraduate Medical College of Nigeria on the recommendation of the Faculty of Public Health. The list of such accredited training centres is published by the respective colleges from time to time. Each training institution is expected to issue a certificate of training to each resident who has satisfactorily completed the prescribed training. The resident undergoing the Fellowship of the Medical College in Public Health (F.M.C.P.H) residency training in Nigeria must be registered simultaneously with his training centre and with the National Postgraduate Medical College whose secretariat is in Lagos. The registration of each resident with the college must be processed through and supported by the training centre. This registration with the college confers on the resident the status of an Associate Fellow of the College.

The Fellowship Training

The professional training in approved institutions is for a period of not less than four years while the training and the examinations for the Fellowship are in three parts namely:

1. Primary Examination.
2. Part I Examination, and
3. Part II Examination.

Primary Training, Basic Sciences as Applied to Public Health for the Primary Examination

While in the West African College of Physicians, the training for the Primary examination is to run *pari passu* with the Part I training in order to emphasize the relevance of the applied basic sciences to the practice of public health, in the National Postgraduate Medical College of Nigeria, there is no formal period earmarked for training in basic sciences. One is expected to update one's knowledge by tutorials, workshops and seminars privately in order to pass the examination. Indeed some accredited centres only take as residents the Primary examination privately so that they can thereafter officially start their training earnestly for the Part I examination.

The basic subjects in the Nigerian syllabus for this part of the examination are human ecology, microbiology and parasitology, therapeutics, biostatistics and epidemiology whereas immunology, psychology and medical Sociology are also included. Therapeutics is excluded in the West African syllabus for this examination.

Junior Residency Training for the Part I Examination

This training is designed to equip the resident with the relevant knowledge and practical exposure in the practice of public health for a period of not less than two years after the commencement of the training. To be eligible to sit the Part I examination, the candidate must have passed the Primary examination of the National Postgraduate Medical College of Nigeria or that of the West African College of Physicians and must produce proof of at least two years work in approved post/posts in the field of public health or produce evidence of having passed the Master of Public Health (M.P.H) degree or its equivalent in addition to a minimum of one year field experience. By the end of the junior residency programme, the resident should be able to:

1. demonstrate sufficient theoretical and practical knowledge in certain key sub-specialities of public health namely: epidemiology, medical statistics, environmental and occupational health, public health administration/health management, primary health care and health research and planning.
2. head or lead a primary health clinic and perform some of the essential duties of a Senior Assistant Medical Officer of Health at the Local Government level or a Senior Registrar in the Ministry of Health.

Senior Residency Training for the Part II (Final Examination)

The Part II examination shall be taken after at least two years of further training in any of the sub-specialities of public health underlisted:

1. Medical Sociology.
2. Medical Statistics.
3. Environmental Health.
4. Occupational Health.
5. Epidemiology.
6. Health Education
7. Public Health Nutrition
8. Family Health.
9. Community Mental Health.
10. Health Service Planning/Management
11. International Health.
12. Primary Health Care.

The candidate must during the period of training spend at least six to nine months working on a relevant community health project or a dissertation subject, and he must be under the supervision of one of the recognized consultants who must be a Fellow in the Faculty of Public Health. The candidate shall at the end of two years period, present his project or dissertation for the Part II examination, and also present himself for a *viva voce* on the practice of public health. Such a subject of study must have been previously approved by the Faculty Board of Public Health. The dissertation or project is intended to test the candidate's ability to apply the knowledge and skills already acquired in the training programme to solve public health problems.

Poor Intake and Small Production

The Department of Community Health of the College of Medicine of the University of Lagos/The Lagos University Teaching Hospital first started the four year residency training programme of the National Postgraduate Medical College of Nigeria in public health in 1975. This was followed by the Department of Preventive and Social Medicine of the College of Medicine, University of Ibadan in 1976 and the Department of Community Medicine of the Ahmadu Bello University , Zaria in 1978. The Department of Community Health of the University of Ghana Medical School, Accra, Ghana, and the Department of Epidemiology and Community Health, University of Ilorin have also been training residents in public health.

For the West African Fellowship examination, the Nigerian Fellowship examination and from all the accredited centres, the intake of students is grossly small and inadequate to meet the urgently needed manpower development in public health for the West African subregion. Consequently, as of February 1991, only four Fellows, F.W.A.C.P., have been produced and admitted by examination in the Faculty of Public Health since its inception of the community health examination in 1979 of the West African College of Physicians. As of February 1991, only twenty Fellows, F.M.C.P.H., had been produced and admitted by examination in the Faculty of Public Health since its inception in 1975 of the public health examinations of the National Postgraduate Medical College of Nigeria.

The Master of Public Health (M.P.H.) Degree

The Intermediate Stage

In order to achieve the objective of producing more community physicians urgently for the local manpower needs, both academic and non-academic, it became obvious that medical schools should provide an intermediate training programme – The Master of Public Health (M.P.H) or its equivalent which can be offered as a one- or two- year training programme.

The Department of Preventive and Social Medicine of the College of Medicine of the University of Ibadan with the assistance of the World Health Organisation started a two-year Master of Public Health degree in Health Education at the beginning of the 1975/76 academic year. This course which is largely for non-medically qualified personnel to produce health education specialists is a very important contribution in Africa to the training of public health personnel. It is the first African Regional Health Education Centre (ARHEC) for the Anglophone member countries of the World Health Organisation in Africa. Candidates have been admitted from the following countries, namely; The Cameroons, Ethiopia, The Gambia, Ghana, Kenya, Liberia, Malawi, Nigeria, Sierra Leone, Swaziland, Tanzania, Uganda, Zambia, and Zimbabwe (arranged alphabetically). ARHEC has produced about 98% of all the professional health educators in Nigeria and about 95% of all health educators in Africa (Ademuwagun 1991). By 1987, the College of Medicine of the University of Ibadan has produced 86 of these graduates of Master of Public Health (Health Education) and by 1990, a total of 103 graduates had been produced.

The Department of Community Health of the College of Medicine of the University of Lagos established a one-year Master of Public Health degree for medically qualified personnel in 1980. By 1988, the College of Medicine of the University of Lagos had produced 66 of these graduates of Master of Public Health and by 1990, a total of 105 had graduated. These Lagos M.P.H. graduates constitute the largest single contribution to the development and training of public health doctors in West Africa and it is a remarkable achievement in the course of a decade.

Although the Department of Community Health of the University of Ghana Medical School, Accra, Ghana started an M.P.H. programme in October 1979, only three persons qualified as M.P.H. graduates in 1981 and another three in 1983. The course has since been stopped. Furthermore, the Department of Community Medicine of the College of Medicine of the University of Calabar also started a two- year Master of Community Health programme in 1984 with four candidates, but the institutions had only produced a few qualified personnel.

M.P.H. Degree and Part I Fellowship Examination

Holders of the Master of Public Health degree from Universities are now exempted from the Primary examination and the course work of the Part I examination of both the West African College of Physicians and the National Postgraduate Medical College of Nigeria. Holders of the Master of Public Health degree are now eligible to sit the Part I examination irrespective of whether they have been residents in public health or not.

In this way, the faculty is able to attract M.P.H. degree holders for the Part I examination. This policy has thus made it possible to attract graduates with the M.P.H. degrees but who are working in the Local Authority or State Ministries of Health to start and continue their professional fellowship training. After passing the Part I examination, the candidate needs to continue in approved posts and work under a Public Health Consultant for the supervision of his training for a period of two years before he can present himself for the Part II Final examination. Thus the M.P.H. degree must certainly be regarded as a way of improving the recruitment of medical doctors into the field of public health.

The Identified Problems

The factors which have been identified for the production of the small number of public health specialists may be broadly categorized as follows:

1. University Teaching Hospitals which have the responsibility for the training of public health residents have few training posts or positions for these residents. Furthermore these teaching hospitals have drastically limited the residency admission into the discipline of public health as only a few vacancies exist in accredited centres in each year. Consequently, only a few people can be taken for the Fellowship admission. This is a major contributory factor for the paucity of public health specialists.
2. There are no incentives to attract young doctors into the discipline.
3. Some consider that the four-year residency training programme is too long although the four-year residency period is common to all the Faculties in the two Colleges.

Opinion and Attitudes to the Practice of Public Health:
A Study of the Responses of 53 Fellows of the Colleges in the Faculty of Public Health

In order to assess and find solutions to some of the problems in the practice of public health, a survey of 53 Consultants, Fellows in the Faculty of Public Health of the National Postgraduate Medical College of Nigeria who possess the F.M.C.P.H., and who are also Fellows of the West African College of Physicians, F.W.A.C.P. in the Faculty of Community Health was carried out on their opinion and attitudes to the practice of public health. As an indication of the direction of the expert opinions and suggestions of those already practising in this field, a profile study of community health and community physicians in Nigeria was undertaken on 53 Fellows who comprised the study population. Osibogun (1989) working in my department in Lagos found that all Local Government Areas in Nigeria should have a Medical Officer of Health who has been trained as a specialist in public health, and that 57% of them considered that the period of residency training of four years was adequate. While 85% of the 53 specialists considered that they obtained job satisfaction from their practice, 53% considered that the practice of public health in Nigeria should involve more clinical work than it at present does for the specialist; 47% considered that it should involve more clinical work for the trainee than it does at present 57% of the 53 specialist respondents considered that housemanship programmes for internship doctors should include a rotation through the Department of Community Health.

Of these 53 specialists,

(a) 68% of them considered that doctors who specialize in public health should be given extra incentives above their colleagues in other disciplines.

(b) 77% stated that doctors who work in the discipline of public health should receive call duty allowance and

(c) 83% of them affirmed that community physicians should receive clinical supplementation.

The reasons why many people are not attracted to the discipline are:

1. the lack of prospects of private practice,
2. the inability to practise public health as an individual physician after retiring,
3. lack of attractive career structure,
4. inadequate facilities – human, material and especially financial resources for the effective practice of public health; and
5. ignorance about the speciality.

The Challenges in Africa

The problems must be seen as challenges and opportunities to rise to the occasion and not as a means of giving excuses, reasons or explanations. The modern public health specialist or community physician is a well trained medical practitioner whose interest touches on almost every specialty of medicine, and on almost every human endeavour. He is mostly needed in the effective delivery of health care for the populace, particularly is he needed in the struggle of Health for All Africans by the year 2,000. He is a force to be reckoned with, a tower of strength up to and beyond the year 2,000 and into the next century. Many doctors and specialists who have spent several years in curative services and who finally find themselves in administration or in the practice of public health have often found it challenging. But a career in public health should not be relegated to the declining professional years when intellectual ability may be substantially diminished. Working as members or even leaders of the health team in primary health care settings should be a rewarding experience for young physicians or doctors. These opportunities abound in our African countries and young community physicians should seize the bull by the horns of these opportunities in order to foster public health manpower development for the African region.

Even though postgraduate education and training is slowly increasing the manpower strength in the field of public health in Africa, yet there are several posts still to be filled by zealous and enterprising community health specialists, or community physicians who are interested in working in academic settings at the University Departments of Community Health in the Teaching Hospitals or in the Colleges of Medicine; or by serving as consultants in the Federal, State or Local Government health departments; or by serving as specialists in industries, factories, corporations and in the private sector in commercial enterprises in solving the health problems including the control of communicable and non-communicable diseases. The demand for public health specialists is aggravated by the population explosion, the rapid industrialization, the rural-urban migration, the poor environmental conditions, the unavailable and meagre medical resources and the abject poverty of the populace so rampant in many countries in Africa.

Recommendations

In order to attract more doctors into the specialty of community health, to improve the quality of training, and to increase the production of public health specialists and community physicians, the following recommendations are now proffered:

1. There should be an unambiguous clearly stated government policy to encourage the production of public health specialists or community physicians.
2. Appropriate policies should be evolved to obtain a more equitable production of public health specialists vis-a-vis those of other specialists.
3. Appropriate steps should be taken to include incentives for the training and career of public health doctors.
4. A large quota of admissions of all residents should be devoted each year to the intake of public health residents until the shortage of public health specialists is corrected.
5. Establishing the Master of Public Health (M.P.H) Degree Programmes in several university centres will greatly increase the public health manpower production. The Master of Public Health (M.P.H) Degree should also be a registrable post-graduate qualification with the individual country's medical council which is charged with the responsibility of the registration of qualifications of all practising doctors.
6. The Department of Community Health in the University Teaching Hospitals should be allocated hospital beds for the admission of in-patients. As community health is a clinical subject, the allocation of hospital beds to this department will definitely serve to emphasize more the clinical aspects of the subject and to attract those that are interested in the clinical practice of community health. The practice has been in existence for several years for example in the Department of Preventive and Social Medicine, University College Hospital, Ibadan, Nigeria which has hospital beds for the admission of in-patients.
7. Postgraduate training in public health should not be limited to the accredited centres in the University Teaching Hospitals, but some aspects of the training can be carried out with

advantage of 'designated or approved centres' in the Local Government Health Authority Departments, in the State or Federal Ministries of Health, industries, in corporations and in commercial enterprises.

8. Introduction of residency rotation in public health through 'designated or approved centres' in the Local Government Health Authority Departments, in the State or Federal Ministries of Health, in industries, in corporations and in commercial enterprises will produce trainees who will be willing to make a career in any of these fields and areas where they have been successfully trained.
9. In order to improve the postgraduate training, a sound undergraduate training in public health should be well established by making the curriculum community based and orientated, and to span throughout the whole of the five years or at least four years of the undergraduate period in the medical school.

Summary

The keywords of this chapter are explained with respect to their special usage and connotations. The reasons for postgraduate training in public health are outlined, and the patterns of the Fellowship training in public health for the West African College of Physicians and the National Postgraduate Medical College of Nigeria are described. The Fellowship examinations indicate a low rate of registration for the examinations and a poor residency admission rate for public health which are not commensurate to the requirements of these countries. However the Master of Public Health Degree and similar one year courses provide a quicker alternative way of training more public health personnel who will render public health and primary health care services at various grades and posts. In order to elucidate the solution to the identified problems the results of a cross-sectional knowledge, attitudes and practice study of 53 public health specialists, community physicians who are Fellows of the College in the Faculty of Public Health are given to indicate the direction of their expert opinion. Recommendations on the ways of solving these problems which should be considered as challenges in the practice of public health in Africa have also been proffered.

References

Ademuwagun, Z.A. (1991) Personal Communication

Faculty of Public Health. National Postgraduate Medical College of Nigeria. Residency Training Programme in Public Health. *A Handbook for Residents and their Teachers.* Revised 1990. Page 21.

Hunponu-Wusu, O.O. 1979. Proposal for the Establishment of a Master of Public Health Degree at the College of Medicine, University of Lagos, Lagos. In the *Occasional Publications of the Department of Community Health No. 3* CMUL, Lagos.

Humponu-Wusu, O. O. 1980. Proposal for the Establishment of a School of Public Health at the College of Medicine University of Lagos, Lagos. In the *Occasional Publications of the Department of Community Health No. 6* CMUL, Lagos.

Medical Council of Nigeria. *Guidelines on Minimum Standards of Medical Education in Nigeria.* 1984 Page 6.

Osibogun, A.O. 1989, 'Community Health and Community Physicians in Nigeria – A Profile Study.' F.M.C.P.H. *Project Submitted to the National Postgraduate Medical College of Nigeria, Lagos.*

Sofoluwe, G.O. 1979. 'Manpower Requirements for Community Health Specialists in Nigeria *Mimeograph.*

West African College of Physicians. 'Constituent College of the West African Postgraduate Medical College.' *Training Programme and Syllabus for the Fellowship Examination and Diploma. 1976.* Page 4.

PART TEN

Health and Wealth in Africa – Ventures for Generating Wealth and Employment Opportunities through Active and Better Health Promotion

77

Seychelles and Mauritius – Examples of a Healthy Paradise in Africa

G.O. Sofoluwe

This chapter highlights brief details about how malaria, yellow fever, typhoid, cholera and other diseases which at one time, decimated all human existence including white, yellow and black races, was by the judicious efforts of mostly the United Nations agencies especially the World Health Organisation; World Bank and United Nations Development Programmes within ten to fifteen years, turned the two islands into a healthy paradise for all human races.

Yellow fever was eradicated before the 1950's and malaria was eradicated before 1961. The efforts of Bruce Chwatt on malaria eradication requires urgent attention of all human kind interested in turning misery to a healthy paradise.

The writer was directly involved in 1970/72 when he was the World Health Organisation (WHO) Regional Adviser who directed a WHO/UNDP project on Port Health Project which included building an international class kitchen for the preparation and serving of healthy food on aeroplanes to convey tourists to the Seychelles as well as develop an innovative environmental sanitation project including innovative training of local staff to build and maintain a healthy chlorinated water supply to all the villages and human settlements; devise and maintain affordable sewage systems including sewage ponds which also grew fresh water fish; and to make the remote villages not only healthy for rich tourists but also for the poor villagers who were made rich by the tourists.

In September 1986 a unanimous resolution was made at the WHO/African Regional Assembly to assist as soon as possible:

1. the provision of pipe borne chlorinated water supply to the inhabitants, however humble, in all the forty three countries served by WHO in the African region;
2. to provide sewage systems, specifically water closets; septic tanks leading to sewage stabilization ponds or eventually sewage systems;
3. to liaise with the World Bank and United Nations Industrial Development Organisation UNIDO; to develop industries to provide electricity for lighting; refrigerating and other purposes for all the peasants in all human settlements as was exhibited at the venue which was the WHO/AFRO Headquarters in Congo Brazzaville by such a successful and existing Solar Energy Industry in Zaire by a Belgian company.

4. to ensure that peasant farmers have a special community food farm in every village through the assistance and supervision of WHO, UNICEF and FAO (Food and Agriculture Organisation), and
5. to ensure that all families have self contained affordable housing units. A special United Nations Agency Habitat – now exists in Kenya for this purpose.

The examples of Seychelles and Mauritius deserve this chapter because of the excellent speed of the realization of first class health which generated wealth and a first class peaceful coexistence of all human beings – of all races, white, yellow and black in these two islands – a very truly successful achievement of United Nations and Commonwealth ideals.

By 1990, the Australian Government had assisted Mauritius to pipe chlorinated water supply to all village huts which the U.K. County Council of Staffordshire and some UK Authorities, acting as Executive Agencies for the World Bank have transformed Mauritius to a tourist paradise.

Seychelles in addition is now a paradise to which all human beings can travel without the *fear of contracting malaria*, a no mean achievement for a previous white man's grave: all can and do survive without any vaccinations or immunizations for yellow fever, and cholera. The previous poor peasants are now clean and healthy tourist companions. They are now wealthier and have been rescued from their previous abject poverty.

All African countries need to emulate the small countries of Mauritius and Seychelles.

Peaceful sharing of all created resources especially the abundant sunshine are the main essentials for transforming other African countries, especially the other numerous island countries to paradise.

It must also be mentioned that travellers to the small island country of Saint Helena also like Seychelles Isles did not require to take antimalarials, or require immunizations against yellow fever and cholera as at December 1990.

This chapter is to convince all African countries that there is so much goodwill in the world now flowing out from the richer countries to make them stop hiding under their easy let out of imagining poverty.

UNIDO has lists of industries, industrialists, retired professors, scientists, business men and women who would gladly invest in Africa to turn it into a paradise like Seychelles, Mauritius, Saint Helena, Lesotho, and Kenya.

Bibliography

The Travellers Guide to Health Prepared by the Department of Health and the Central Office of Information, printed in the U.K. for Her Majesty's Stationery Office, London. 22.02. 1990.

78

Health and Wealth in Africa – The Lessons of Nairobi, Kenya

G.O. Sofoluwe

This short chapter, details, truthfully, a full and lengthy discussion by the writer and the Town Clerk of Nairobi City Council in Kenya about 1978. Nairobi City Council is now Nairobi Metropolitan Agency.

The writer was in 1970 a World Health Organisation (WHO) short term consultant to the Government of Kenya to assist them to prepare and develop the country's health manpower for the decade 1970-1980. He was luckily also the WHO Regional Adviser from 1970-1972 to implement not only his proposal but to supervise the implementation of WHO and all other United Nations Agencies Health Projects in that country.

Fortunately for Kenya, no oil was discovered and one of Africa's statesmen who worked till his death for peaceful co-existence, co-operation and fair trading with all countries of the world and who defined an African as stated in the preface – as any human being of any race or colour or creed – the late Jomo Kenyatta, ruled Kenya during the transition to and the first decades of independence.

Tourism was the main foreign exchange earner and as such many people visited, traded and lived in peace in Kenya. All those who have visited Nairobi from 1970 onwards will agree that the city could pass for any city in the developed countries of United Kingdom, United States of America, other European countries and modern cities in Japan and Singapore.

Jomo Kenyatta's 'Harambee' (that is self help) was actively augmented by huge investments from well wishers from any part of the world; his humility to invite experts and give them trusting and loving free hands led to the following health and wealth generating achievements. This will concentrate only on Nairobi as detailed by the then Town Clerk of Nairobi to the writer.

Investors were invited to develop Nairobi as one of the best cities of the world – no double standards. The investors would state their conditions – including how much interests and the period of time they wished the capital interests to be repaid and they were given free hands to collect their capital and interests.

Another important question was as to whether the investor who would be given an automatic Kenyan citizenship if he liked, would continue his citizenship or would leave Kenya after the unification of his project. The objective was that the project should not die with the investor leaving Kenya but that if he wanted to leave he had to train Kenyans or his own relatives, or others of his choice to assume and continue the donated citizenship to actively continue the existence, maintenance and further development of the project.

Such was the success attained as now described below. The area of Nairobi City near Jomo Kenyatta's Airport was developed by a consortium of British investors who constructed everything even including streets, concrete seats; drive in cinemas with kisosk restaurants and so on.

The investors who left trained Kenyans or their nominated successors and in most cases the housing, commercial and other projects were absorbed by the Nairobi City Council which has now grown to be the Nairobi Metropolitan Authority or Agency.

The United States of America, Israel, Holland, Belgium, Germany, Denmark, Sweden, South Korea, Japan and many other developed countries have such successful investments in Nairobi and other parts of Kenya. The Annual Reports of Nairobi City Council till 1980 showed more revenue than expenditure. In addition, healthy chlorinated and piped borne water supply uninterruptedly flows to all houses; water closets exist with healthy sewage schemes: electricity flows uninterruptedly; food is in abundance which unfortunately occasionally attracts plague. There are clean and beautiful parks; together with the world acclaimed National Park loaded with exotic lions, etc. just within easy reach of Nairobi City. All the above made Nairobi not only healthy but wealthy and were mainly achieved by opening Kenya to all human beings of all races, colours and creeds.

The writer was also fortunate to assist in the development of Thika, the industrial special city, near to Nairobi. No industry was opened for work until all the prospective workers had been living comfortably in healthy houses with piped chlorinated water supply; water closets, wash hand basins, healthy sewage and drains, community food farms, electricity, health centres with the children in clean schools and facilities of clean markets, shops etc., Thika has been the only industrial estate in Africa that the writer has seen which put its workers and their families into a state of healthy living before the industries were allowed to open for work.

Poverty and lack of money were transformed by love and humanity to an open door policy which opened the main doors to health and wealth for all human beings in Nairobi, a worthy example waiting to be copied by all who still say they are poor, and to all African countries.

Bibliography

Nairobi City Council Annual Reports 1970–1982
Oral Communication by Mr B.O. Getonga, Town Clerk, Nairobi City Council, 1978.

79

The Twinning of Institutions:Accra City Council – Colombo Municipal Council with Staffordshire County Council

M. J. Simpson

Introduction

Many international agencies including the World Bank and the United Nations are concerned about the need to ensure an effective transfer of professional skills, technical know-how, and strengthening of institutions to deal with the problems of Africa.

During the 1980's the concept of technical twinning as a method of delivering technical assistance was developed. The early Twinning Agreements were between single function entities such as water supply and electricity supply utilities, and bodies such as a port authority all of which had only single or limited functions. However, there have been some interesting developments relating to technical twinning by linking a British Local Authority with a comparable African and Sri Lankan Local Authority. This experimental multi-function twinning may be relevant as a way of helping African communities to improve their performance and to strengthen their institutions in the area of community health.

The Staffordshire Experience

In 1985, a 'twinning' arrangement was agreed between Staffordshire County Council, a Local Authority in the United Kingdom and Accra City Council, the capital city of Ghana as a small part of the Accra District Rehabilitating Project which was supported by the World Bank. The objectives of the project were road construction, road rehabilitation, road maintenance, area improvement, municipal revenue mobilization and the associated institutional development, including training.

The components of the Accra project with which Staffordshire County Council were involved were road maintenance and revenue mobilization and the associated institutional development. The duration of the Accra project was for five years, terminating on the 31 December, 1989.

In 1988, a 'twinning' agreement was reached between Staffordshire County Council and Colombo Municipal Council, the capital city of Sri Lanka, which was also supported by the World Bank. The twinning arrangement is a small part of a larger municipal management project.

The areas of responsibility with which Staffordshire County Council are involved are waste collection and disposal, financial management, administration, computing and the associated institutional development including training.

The Colombo project is ongoing.

The Twinning of Institutions – Its Use as a Technical Assistance Delivery System – World Bank Technical Paper No. 23

The Twinning Concept

'Twinning can be defined as a professional relationship between an operating entity in a developing country and a similar but more mature organization in another part of the world. The services provided by the latter differ from those of a consulting firm in the following respects:'

(a) 'The supplier of technical assistance has *operating experience* in similar functions.'

(b) 'Twinning provides opportunities to integrate technical assistance *and training*.'

(c) 'There is *flexibility to alter the work programme* over time and the possibility of very *long term co-operation*.'

(d) 'The technical assistance supplier *may lack world-wide experience*.'

(e) 'The supplier may lack experience in the consulting profession.'

Operating Experience

'The major advantage of a twinning arrangement to provide technical assistance is having an operating entity stand behind the technical assistance supplier's work. Thus, the entity that provides the assistance can draw upon its own in-house resources in the relevant functional areas, offering services as needed in the client's complementary functional areas. For example, a supplier entity in a twinning arrangement can train client staff as it trains its own in operating or maintaining equipment. Also, the experts in the field have had practical experience in jobs similar to those which the client's staff are performing. For a client, a twinning arrangement means that the technical assistance comes from a very credible source – another entity actively and successfully engaged in the same type of operations.'

Description of Local Authority Involved

Accra City Council and Colombo Municipal Council are in many respects similar to Staffordshire County Council. Each of the authorities has similar though not identical statutory responsibilities, and their organizational structures are based on a common legal and administrative tradition. Officers and members from either authority visiting the other are to a considerable extent familiar with the powers, duties and systems operating in the other authority.

Although Accra and Colombo are largely urban authorities whilst Staffordshire includes urban and rural areas, in many respects, they are comparable. All Authorities have similar problems although very different in scale.

Accra, 1984-1990

The secondments to Accra by Staffordshire staff spilt into short term and long term. There have been short term visits amounting to approximately 30 man weeks, long term secondments of 60 man months, (2 Officers) relating to Highways, and 36 man months (1 Officer) relating to financial matters. The short term visits to England by Accra Members and Officers have been similar at approximately 30 man weeks.

During the work in Accra the important interrelationship between health and other functions have become apparent. There is a very obvious health benefit from improved systems for waste collection and disposal but what is less apparent is the considerable health benefit achieved by the proper design and maintenance of highway schemes and the associated drainage works. A well designed highway drainage scheme not only drains the highway adequately but also ensures that there are no water traps providing a breeding ground for mosquitos. Because the provision of technical assistance under the twinning arrangement also has public health responsibilities the range of matters to be taken into consideration are more readily apparent.

The Municipal Management Project – Colombo, Sri Lanka

In October 1988, Staffordshire and Colombo Municipal Council extended a twinning agreement involving short term exchange and secondments in the waste management field.

As a result of the experience of working with the County Treasurer upon the financial system relating to waste management, the twinning agreement was extended into the areas of general financial management, computing and administration and the associated institutional strengthening and training.

As British Local Authorities are both housing and market authorities, they are able to expose their partners to current practices in those fields and that partner is able to draw from that operating experience that which is relevant. The contribution that good housing and clean and carefully controlled markets can make to health cannot be overstated. Some of the Colombo self help housing projects are good examples of what can be achieved with very little resources by using the skills of the authority to design, the enthusiasm of the occupier to construct and the resources of the authority to get the project established.

Twinning Arrangements – Advantages

As the arrangements are essentially long term, institutional links have been built between Staffordshire and Accra and Staffordshire and Colombo and between individuals within the organization which go beyond the specific boundaries of the projects.

The long term nature of a twinning arrangement means that there can be a reduced risk of an inappropriate transfer of technical assistance or technology. A deeper understanding of the problems, possible solutions and consequences can be achieved when a longer timescale is deliberately chosen.

By exposing an operating entity such as Staffordshire to the critical scrutiny of colleagues from Accra over a period of time, they have been able to draw conclusions which have not been anticipated by those in Staffordshire, but which are of significant benefit to Accra. Equally, the scrutiny and questioning of systems is beneficial to Staffordshire.

The long term nature of the links and the wide spread of those individuals exchanging visits have greatly increased the mutual understanding and mutual respect of those participating.

Once a trust has been built up between individuals within the institutions, it is possible to examine not only successful schemes and systems to see to what extent appropriate lessons can be drawn, but also practices to be avoided and systems that are no longer applicable. Given the scale of Staffordshire's operation, and the length of time for which it has operated, the experience to be drawn upon is considerable.

The institutional links between like institutions enable the inter-relationship between the political, managerial, administrative, and technical problems to be fully evaluated. The specific links between direct service delivery and revenue collection can be an invaluable aid to performance. The political and institutional implications of an apparently simple technical decision are often apparent to an institution facing like problems and previous similar experience helps to make the process of institutional development more effective.

The timescale of the twinning arrangements has permitted the planning of successive visits to Staffordshire to secure an overview of processes which would not be possible over shorter timescales. A succession of short term visits spread over several years at specific points in the Staffordshire financial planning process gives a better insight into the institution and its operation than a view from a single point in time with a description of the parts of the process not current.

By explaining the Staffordshire institutions to Accra and Colombo staff across a range of functions and over an extended period including more than one visit, Accra and Colombo staff are able to draw conclusions that may be relevant to Accra and Colombo which are not apparent to Staffordshire staff.

Twinning Arrangements – The Future

There are lessons to be learned from Staffordshire's experience with their colleagues in Ghana and Sri Lanka which may well be relevant for other areas of responsibility and in particular in the community health fields. The benefits of long term links can be secured in the health and community health areas of responsibility as well as within the more technical and management areas.

Staffordshire is only one, albeit one of the largest local authorities in England. If the project is considered successful, there is scope for other projects in other parts of the world with similar administrations and legal backgrounds. The principles of twinning can be extended to health authorities and other community organizations.

Those participating in the twinning arrangements in Accra, Colombo and Staffordshire, have found them to be a rewarding and stimulating experience. Links of friendship, respect and understanding have been forged that will long outlast any formal arrangements.

80

Transmigration Village in Sumatra

Roselyn M. Taylor

'Transmigrasi' (transmigration) is defined as:

> '... the removal and/or transfer of population from one area to settle in another area determined upon within the territory of the Republic of Indonesia or for other reasons considered necessary by the Indonesian government.'

(Basic Transmigration Act, 1972: Clause 1)

This shifting of large amounts of people from one island to another has had a long history in Indonesia, dating from 1905 and Dutch colonial rule. The reasons for this policy are clear. Although smaller in area than Sumatra, Kalimantan, Sulawesi and Irian Jaya, Java has long been the most densely populated of all the islands. Population census figures of 1971 (see Statistical Pocketbook of Indonesia 1970 and 1971) show that the islands of Java and Maduria, with 6.64% of total land area, had 63.83% of the total population. This was coupled with an overall annual population increase of 2.37%. In 1972 the average per capita annual income was 97 US dollars. (The Strategy of Transmigration and Co-operatives in the context of National Strategy). It became increasingly obvious that Java was, and is, simply not capable of supporting its vast and rapidly increasing population. The census figures also show that the aforementioned Outer islands, with a total land area of 1,892,384 square kilometres, had a mere 29.7% of the total population.

However, transmigration is not simply a means of reducing population pressure on Java or of redistributing a maladjusted population. It is an attempt to provide labour and opportunity for the agricultural utilization of huge tracts of underdeveloped land in the Outer islands.

It is also, as the phrase '... for any other reasons considered necessary by the Indonesian government' shows, a deliberate political policy on the part of the government; a policy which gives them '*carte blanche*' to effect the removal of any person or groups of persons they should desire.

My objective is to set the particular transmigration site on which I carried out fieldwork, Rimbo Bujang, in the Jambi district of Sumatra, within the context of Indonesia's nationwide policies of transmigration and regional development.

Methods and Ethics

As the methods and forms of research is relevant to the possible interpretations of ethnographic data, I feel that it is important that one should explain the way in which field work was undertaken.

I spent five months in Indonesia from April to September 1986. The duration of my fieldwork was three months which were spent living in the mess. This is a building with twelve bedrooms, four bathrooms, a kitchen, and a living area. It is generally used by P.T.P. VI – P.T. *'Perkabunan'* (Plantation) the government owned estate company which runs transmigration projects and the employees who were either on short term contracts or had not yet found accommodation. The mess is situated a quarter of a mile from a small village clustered around a sawmill.

Fig. 80.1

The Mess

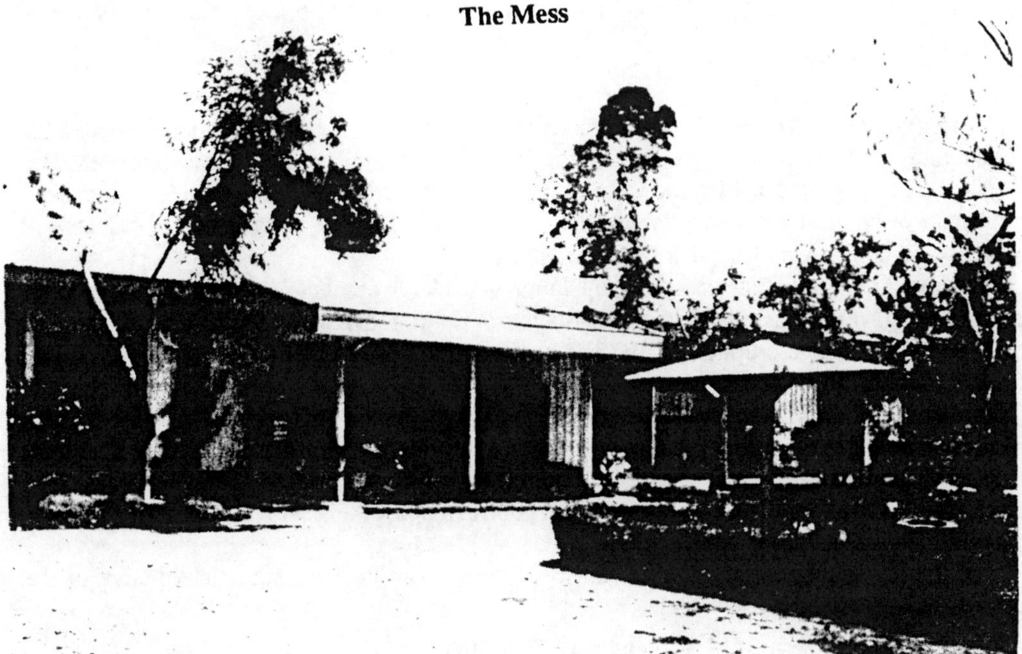

One hundred and ten heads of households (approximately a third of the total households in the village) were interviewed. In thirty cases a second follow up interview was undertaken. I attended the meetings of various *'Kolompok Tani'* (farmers work groups) and *'Penguluhans'* (information sessions) carried out either by P.P.T staff, who were concerned with rubber crops, or P.P.I extension workers, who were concerned with the food crops.

The third survey was conducted with the Javanese settlement, and concentrated on those members of the indigeneous population – the '*margaland*' – who had entered the rubber project, under the same stipulations as the migrants. The aim was to contrast the two situations.

The Situation of the Javenese

Rimbo Bujang (literally meaning 'virgin forest') is a transmigration project in the Jambi province of Sumatra, financed by the World Bank. The project area of approximately 35,000 hectares was virgin forest before land clearing began. The first transmigrants arrived in 1975 and the last in 1985.

There are currently over 6,000 families mainly from Central and East Java, living and working within the project.

Each transmigrant village has approximately 500 families. Each family has received five hectares of land, three hectares for their own use and two hectares reserved to grow rubber trees under the direction of P.T.P VI. Rp. 10,000 is given to each family per month as credit for maintenance of the rubber crop (Rp. 10,000 is approximately £7.00).

Most of the villages have a mosque, P.T.P office, market place, and a school, to SMP level. Those of the local population who wished to participate – approximately 2,000 families – received two hectares for rubber cultivation (all were landowners already) with the usual provisos for credit repayment.

Unit 4

This *'desa'* (village) was chosen as it was neither among the most or least economically successful villages, and would hopefully give an accurate reflection of the 'average' transmigrants. The village has a population of 501 families. The first migrants arrived in 1977 449 families came under the category of 'general transmigrants' and the remaining two families came under the category of *'spontan'* and did not participate in rubber cultivation.

An important feature of the village's population is the large number of people originally from the same area. Over 300 families come from Maglan in Central Java where a large area of land was destroyed by a volcanic eruption in 1976. Other common places of origin were Solo, Tegal, Boyolali, Sarakin, Biora and Klaten.

The majority of *'jalons'* (streets) in the village have a predominance of former Maglan inhabitants which, considering their general predominance, is not surprising. There was no instance of a street occupied by families solely from one place of origin. However, people from the same area do tend to stick together to a certain extent. *'Jalon'* 8 is a good example of this, with a mixture of a number of families from Tegal, Solo and Boyolali.

I feel that by setting out my data in statistical form, I can give an immediate picture of the situation, as I perceived it.

Family Structure

Average number of family members	6.8
Maximum per family	13
Minimum per family	1
Number nuclear family	104
Number extended family	3
Family with one parent	3
Average age male HH head	42.9
Average age female HH head	33.9

The Importance of Transmigration within the Context of Regional and National Development

In the mid 1960's, Indonesia began a *'Bimbingan Massal'* BISMAS (mass guidance) campaign in the agricultural sector. This entailed rice intensification programmes, infrastructural rehabilitation, agricultural extension, distribution of credit, fertilizer, pesticide and the new high yielding varieties (h.i.v) seeds. 1970 saw the inception of the *'kabupaten'* (district) programme. This entailed the allocation of funds from central government to each *'kabupaten'*. This sum was based on a set sum multiplied by the number of inhabitants. The funds were used to either construct, or repair existing, infrastructures such as roads, bridges, and irrigation canals.

Both campaigns have encountered serious difficulties. Between 1969 and 1974 there was a 4.6% increase in the annual average rice production growth. The average per hectare yield increased from 1.26 tons in 1968 to 1.80 tons in 1974. The new high yielding varieties were not the sole cause of this increase as many farmers did not use them. The increase in the availability of, and use of fertilizer was a very important factor in the growth.

Unfortunately, this initial success did not continue, despite the attempts of *'Repelita'* II. From 1974/5 there was a perceptible decline in the consumption of fertilizer, production of rice, and the numbers of farmers participating in the BISMAS scheme. One reason was the continuing poor irrigation facilities. It also became apparent that the high yielding varieties were not the solution to all the problems but, in effect the cause of some. The varieties were subject to increased pest infestation which led to harvest losses, as it was too early for the pesticide programme to have caught on.

It has been suggested that a major reason for the tailing off of interest, combined with a levelling of economic growth, was credit repayment. A substantial number of farmers either fell behind or failed to meet their credit repayments. This has not discouraged the government and other agencies from continuing a credit policy. However, much of the blame for credit defaulting must be placed on unrealistic expectations.

On transmigration and other development projects, the participants are expected to repay credit facilities given to them as soon as it is economically viable for them to do so. One of the reasons for credit repayment becoming such a major difficulty is the fact that the cost of living and other village infrastructures such as roads, bridges and irrigation is included in its evaluation. Basically, in the long term, the government and other funding agencies expect the total cost of building and running a project to be repaid by its participants. At the present time this expectation is ridiculously optimistic and there is no evidence to lend credence to it. For example, it was estimated that the cost of building one transmigrant house in East Kalimantan in 1981 would be Rp. 575,000 (approximately £400) (Transmigrant Feasibility Study, 1982:107). The average income of farmers in Unit 4 was Rp. 30,000 (£21) per month. The average expenditure on food, education, transport and kerosene totalled over Rp. 25,000. A further Rp. 2,000 was set aside for '*arisan*' or '*simpan pinjam*'. This leaves a total of Rp. 3,000 per month, or Rp. 36,000 per year but does not include the cost of clothes, schoolbooks or '*Hari Raya*'. On this evidence, it can be assumed that including infrastructures in credit repayment is not a feasible notion.

There has been an increasing recognition that a failure of the transmigration policy would have a disastrous effect on regional and national development. It would result in discouraging smallholder agriculture and funding from donor agencies. This has resulted in an increasing amount of research within Indonesia itself into the reasons for project failure and the necessary prerequisites that can encourage project success.

A recent comprehensive study in Bunga Nas Lahat, South Sumatra (Mustari, 1985:49) concludes that although internal accessibility within the project (between home and land education facilities, health clinics and education) is important, it did not influence the willingness of the transmigration to stay. Factors such as land ownership, new hopes and a good harvest had much more influence.

There is an illuminating study into the psychological aspects of a new environmental setting

(Unjod, 1979:55). A comparison was made between transmigrants of Bojonegoro who stayed in Rimbo Bujang and transmigrants of Wonogiri who stayed in Sitiung. The reason for this was different transmigration patterns.

The entire village migrated from Wonogiri to Sitiung which entailed the continuation of the previous social and political system, with its obligatory ties and existing stratification. Also there was no available land in Wonogiri so there was no choice but to move in order to survive. The move from Bojonegoro to Rimbo Bujang would fall into the category of '*transmigrasi umum*' (general transmigration). It was not a shift of entire villages but of individual families from mixed origins. So the people saw the project as not only an opportunity for increasing wealth, but also social and political status. It is important to note that in this case, transmigration was voluntary and there was some land available in the farmers place of origin.

With the information it is not surprising to find that transmigrants from Bojonegoro to Rimbo Bujang shared a greater ability to adjust than transmigrants from Wonogiri. It makes a very relevant point that the importance of self-motivation should not be underestimated. Although a policy of voluntary migration is paid lip service, the reality is quite different.

Despite claims to the contrary, there is a large element of forced participation. Rural farmers who have lost their land because of natural disaster are offered help in the form of joining a transmigration project. This was the case for those farmers in Unit 4 from Maglan.

To a certain extent, the notion of quantity of numbers rather than quality of development is still adhered to. When the first transmigrants arrived in Rimbo Bujang they had been promised that all the land would be cleared, a house with a latrine would be ready and electricity would be available. They arrived to find that the land had not been properly cleared and was still infested with lalang. The houses were built, but with inferior materials and no latrines. The promise of electricity has still not been fulfilled after eight years. Given that situation, it is not surprising that approximately 40% of the original migrants abandoned the project within a year.

Indonesian anthropologists have shown a great deal of interest in transmigration policies and their effects. This research and ensuing information does not appear to have had any detrimental effect on transmigrants in general. On the contrary, it has proved to be in their best interest, as the two examples given show. It must be remembered that a great many Indonesians are willing to migrate. Such is their abject poverty.

Bibliography

Ayres, R.L. 1983. *Banking On the Poor*. London: MIT Press.
Barnes, J.A. 1979. *Who Should Know What?* Middlesex: Penguin.
Chambers, R. 1983. *Rural Development*. USA: Longman Inc.

Darmawan, A. 1976. *Konsep Lingkungan Tempat Kediaman Transmigran Di Daerah Pasang Surut Banguasin Berdasarakan Pertumbangan Aspek Sosial Budaya.* Bandung: Institut Teknologi.
Foster-Carter, A. 1985. *The Sociology of Development.* Lancashire: Causeway Press Ltd.
Geertz, C. 1960. *The Religion of Java.* USA: University of Chicago Press
Geertz, C. 1963. *Agricultural Involution.* USA: University of Califonia Press.
Geertz, C. 1967. *Peddlers and Princes.* USA: University of Chicago Press
Geertz, C. 1968. *Islam Observed.* USA: University of Chicago Press
Gjessing, G. 1968. The Social Responsibility of the Social Scientist. *Current Anthropology* Vol. 9. 373-377.
Gough, K. 1968. New Proposals for Anthropologists. *Current Anthropology,* vol. 9.378-381.
Hansen, G.E. (ed) 1981. *Agricultural and Rural Development in Indonesia.* USA: Westview Press Inc.
Hardjono, J.M. 1977. *Transmigration in Indonesia.* Kaula Lumper: Oxford University Press.
Hardjono, J.M. 1980. Assisted and Unassisted Transmigration in the context of Repilita III Target. *Prisma,* LPES Vol. 18.
Harriss, J. (ed) 1982. *Rural Development.* London: Hutchinson & Co.
Holt, C. (ed) 1972. *Culture and Politics in Indonesia.* USA: Cornell University Press.
Hymes, D (ed) 1974. *Reinventing Anthropology.* USA: Random House.
Jay, R.R. 1969. *Javanese Villages.* USA: Massachusettes Institute of Technology.
Keivelitz, U. 1985. *The Socio-Cultural Impact of a Development Project in its Evaluation from the Perspective of the Local Population – The Case of Abai Siat, West Sumatra.* Padang: Unpublished Research Paper.
Kievelitz, U. 1985. *The Pre-requisites for a Smallholder Organization: Socio-Cultural Situation , Social Structure and Peasant Attitude in Nucleus Estate Smallholder Project OPHIR, Pasaman, West Sumatra.* Padang: Unpublished Research Paper.
Koentjaraningrat, (ed) 1967. *Villages in Indonesia.* New York: Cornell University Press.
Kurim, M.M. 1985. *The Effect of Internal Accessibility on the Willingness to Stay of Transmigrants. Case Study of Bung Mas Lahat Development Area, South Sumatra.* Bandung: Institute of Technology.
Loeb, E.M. 1972. *Sumatra, Its History and People.* Kuala Lumpur: Oxford University Press.
Mair, L. 1984. *Anthropology and Development.* London: Croom Helm.
McNeill, D. 1986. *Making Aid Projects More Suited To Local Needs.* Edinburgh: Centre of African Studies.
Naim, M./Agus, H. 1981. *Tree Crop Farming System in Koto Padang, Sawahlunto/Sijunjung District, West Sumatra.* Padang: Unpublished Research Paper.
Peattie, L. 1981. *Thinking About Development.* New York: Plenum Press.
Robertson, A.F. 1984. *People and the State.* Cambridge: Cambridge University Press.
Rustan, U. 1986. *The Rise of Small Towns in Rural Marketing. Development Case – The Rural Market in Transmigration Area.* Bandung: Draft researeh proposal.
Srisioewarni, 1974. *Studi Pola Migrasi di Pulau Java.* Bandung: Institut Teknologi.
Wrigley, G. 1961. *Tropical Agriculture and the Development of Production.* London: B.T. Batsford.
Transmigration Area, Development Group 1882. *Transmigration Feasibility Study, Muara Wahau and Sangkulirang, East Kalimantan.* East Kalimantan: TAD.

81

A Model Health Service for Cocoa Plantation Workers in Santa Isabel, Equatorial Guinea in West Africa, in the Late 1960s

G.O. Sofoluwe

Health generates abundant wealth not only for employers but also for employees as well.

The fact that in 1966 the infant mortality rate of the poor and generally low income cocoa plantation workers in the whole island of Fernando PO, Santa Isabel in Equatorial Guinea was 20 per 1000 below the 24/1000 in the United Kingdom in that year clearly illustrates that the most important determinant to drastically improve health in Africa as well as the whole world is the provision of

1. pipe borne chlorinated water even into huts made of barks of trees;
2. water closets;
3. wash hand basins;
4. showers, and
5. electricity.

Hence all African countries need to improve their friendly relationship with investors and make the right use of the World Bank, UNIDO, ILO, WHO, UNICEF, UN Habitat and other United Nations and bilateral national agencies to provide the above listed facilities for all human settlements and inhabitants of Africa.

The details described below were research investigations made by the writer when as the Chef de Mission and Honorary doctor to the Nigeria Sports Contingent comprising of footballers and basketball and volley ball players to the first Independence Celebration of the neighbouring country of Equatorial Guinea. In 1966 he had by very good accident to visit the huts of Nigerians who were cocoa plantation workers on the island. The writer saw, confirmed data and was able, fortunately, 4 to 6 years later to have the opportunity to be the WHO Regional Adviser to directly assist the health services of Equatorial Guinea and to practically confirm that the data mentioned below were very accurate.

As by accident of nature again, cocoa requires very special soil chemistry before it can grow. There must therefore be a comprehensive soil analysis survey of every inch of any proposed cocoa plantation for maximum success and profitability. In addition Santa Isabel as opposed to the Rio

Muni, the mainland part of the country of Equatorial Guinea, was an island completely surrounded by water. The Spanish cocoa plantation workers therefore provided piped chlorinated water which could be tapped from every inch of the island thus making it easy to shift the huts of the workers to anywhere on the island and provide them with water taps, water closets, wash hand basins, showers, and electricity in every hut!

As the huts must be easily moved, they were built not with cement or mud blocks or even grass but with barks of trees which could last several moves to different sites.

The writer visted the 1000 bed hospital and in 1966 it had less than 200 patients mostly consisting of the newly recruited Nigerian plantation workers who were more or less shedding their intestinal parasites etc., before the effect of chlorinated water, water closets and electricity were to have drastic effects on improving their health.

Equatorial Guinea, especially Santa Isabel, was definitely the only country in Africa with a remarkably low infant mortality rate. The evaluation of health and health services for plantation workers in the four countries of Malaysia, South India, Sri Lanka and Zimbabwe by Laing (1986) showed that the lack of attention of the provision of chlorinated piped water, water closets, showers and electricity were responsible for the lack of a drastic rise in the level of health despite the small rise due to improved earnings.

This chapter has described a most successful venture when the health of plantation workers in Africa was improved to the comparatively high level of their European plantation owners and supervisors.

It is definitely a venture to be intensively studied, and vigorously and actively copied to every detail throughout all African countries.

Bibliography

Laing, Richard – Health and Health Services for Plantation Workers – Four Case Studies – Evaluation and Planning Centre for Health care 1986 EPC Publication November 10. ISSN 0267-5994 Series Editor Gill Walt.

Sofoluwe, G.O. 1973 'Occupational Health and Economic Development in African Countries' *Arch. Environ Health, Vol. 26,* April 1973.

Evaluation and Planning Centre for Health Care, London School of Hygiene and Tropical Medicine, Keppel Street, (Gower Street), London WC1E 7HT.

82

Health and Wealth in Africa

G.O. Sofoluwe

Godlee (1991) on *Cholera Pandemic* in the BMJ Vol 302 of 4th May 1991 wrote:

> *World Health Organisation* (WHO) estimated that providing safe water and sanitation for Latin America 'i.e. pipe borne water, water closets and sewers' could cost US$5 billion (£2.9 billion)a year for the next 10 years. Capital investment on this scale is, said Professor Drassar, beyond the financial capability of most governments, let alone those in the Third world. 'If our sewers collapsed in this country (i.e. United Kingdom) we would not have the money to replace them', he said. The installation of sanitation and sewerage in Victorian Britain was 'in real terms probably one of the largest capital investments ever made'.

WHO also estimated that cholera epidemic could cost Peru above US$ 100 million in *lost* revenue from exports and tourism and in damage to the social infrastructure.

Thus, Godlee emphasized the importance of safe pipe borne water, water closets and sewerage on the health and wealth of any nation. The only two previously developing countries which have crossed the rubicon to development were Japan and Singapore. They were successful because they made the provision of the pipe borne and chlorinated water, water closets as well as other environmental sanitation facilities such as healthy houses and electricity available and affordable to all their citizens within a specified space of time. All inhabitants, whether poor or rich whether they resided in urban or isolated rural areas were completely covered within a period of thirty (Japan) and ten years respectively.

Four thousand died in London, U.K in the three days between 5 and 8 December, 1952 due to the London Smog Disaster. This stimulated the setting up of the Beaver Committee on Air Pollution in 1953, the acceptance of the report in 1954, the declaration of the whole city of London as a smokeless zone in 1955 and the enactment of a Clean Air Act for the whole country of the United Kingdom in 1956.

Thus in four years, the 4000 deaths due to smoke pollution in London resulted in multi-disciplinary identification of the root causes of the death; manufacture of new appliances to eradicate the scourge and phenomenal improvement in the health and wealth of all inhabitants in the U.K.

Thus an estimated loss of £295.5 million per annum was due to only the non clinical effects of new industrial and other techniques and procedures; manufacture of affordable central heating; well insulated affordable houses and generation of such new employment opportunities as are listed in chapter 17.

The eradication of yaws throughout Africa was possible only by the manufacture and injection of penicillin to all Africans in their respective villages. This also led to the generation of employment opportunities for those employed by the medical field units or grands endemics in Anglo and Franco phone African countries.

Similarly the more recent eradication of smallpox throughout Africa was accelerated by the setting up by WHO of three centres in Nigeria, Senegal and Zaire for the manufacture of smallpox vaccines.

Research to boost productivity in the hot and humid West Africa and to stop the practice of taking siestas (sleeping during the hours of twelve noon to fourteen hours) by the medical research council of Great Britain in Lagos led by Dr W.L. Laddell and their co-operation with Professor S. Hatch of the Institute of Occupational Health in Pittsburgh USA lead to the manufacture of the Air Conditioner (the opposite to central heating in colder climates) which still awaits further development to affordable costs to the majority of the African populations by the future governments, industrial and business concerns in Africa.

The drastic improvement in health, the massive wealth and new employment generated by improved sanitation of all the peoples in Japan, Singapore and other countries in Europe are worthy examples to be copied by African countries immediately.

The very successful attempts by Kenya, Seychelles, St Helena, Mauritius and Santa Isabel up to the late 1960s' clearly indicate that such a bold scheme will meet with phenomenal success and is feasible and achievable.

Africa cannot escape making huge capital investments on sanitation similar to that ever made in Victorian Britain which was stimulated by Chadwick; we must also be ready to make colossal investments similar to that made in San Francisco, Los Angeles and all the states of the USA stimulated by Shattuck, and the more recently reported in Singapore by Wai On Phoon in this book if all African countries were serious on erasing the titles of 'Poor and Unhealthy' and wish them to be replaced by 'Healthy, Wealthy and Developed'.

Sofoluwe, Ogunbi and O. Ransome Kuti in 1968 clearly identified indoor smoke pollution as being mainly responsible for the huge carnage due to broncho pneumonia among the under five year old children in Nigeria as accurately documented since 1900 yet the advocated provision of affordable houses to effectively prevent and eradicate such has not been made possible even though bold attempts and some success in that direction have been made and achieved.

Sofoluwe identified serious lead intoxication among the several 100,000 lead accumulation battery chargers and repairers in Lagos, Nigeria in 1971. By 1990, however, a drastically reduced number of such battery chargers and repairers are now to be found in Lagos or other parts of Nigeria mainly because Nigeria now locally manufactures, and sells enough lead accumulator batteries at affordable prices to those who utilize them.

There is thus a need for the creation of a multi-disciplinary Ministry in Health and Wealth in all African countries. These should be concerned mainly with active health promotion as well as wealth and employment creation. It is however necessary that the first priority attention on this should be devoted to improving sanitation, i.e. provision of affordable pipe borne safe water, water closets, sewers, electricity, affordable healthy houses, community food farms, refrigeration, leisure, keep fit and health screening centres.

All state and regional authorities should have such Ministries of Health and Wealth and all local Government Authorities should have Directorate of Health Utilities ensuring that all appliances for sanitation and electricity are always in good working order and generating employment for the same in all villages or human settlements of whatever size in population or area.

Health and wealth are achievable ventures in Africa.

Index

I

K

L

M

N

O

P

T

U

V

W

X

Y

CPSIA information can be obtained at www.ICGtesting.com
Printed in the USA
BVOW07s1412140314

347684BV00010B/250/A

9 789780 304904